Color Atlas of
Tissue Response *to* Biomaterials

Color Atlas of Tissue Response *to* Biomaterials

Mira Mohanty MD FIC Path
Head, Division of Implant Biology
Scientist In-Charge, Histopathology Laboratory

A Sabareeswaran MVSc Path
Scientist
Histopathology Laboratory

Sulekha Baby BSc MLT
Scientific Officer
Histopathology Laboratory

Joseph Sebastian BSc MLT
Technical Assistant
Histopathology Laboratory

Caroline S Diana MSc
Research Fellow

Biomedical Technology Wing
Sree Chitra Tirunal Institute for Medical Sciences and Technology
Thiruvananthapuram, Kerala, India

Foreword

MS Valiathan

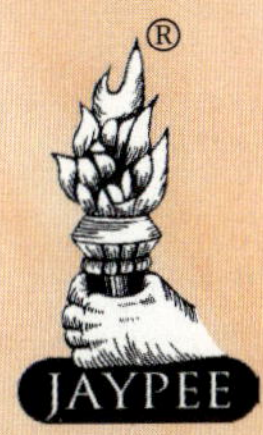

JAYPEE BROTHERS MEDICAL PUBLISHERS (P) LTD

New Delhi • London • Philadelphia • Panama

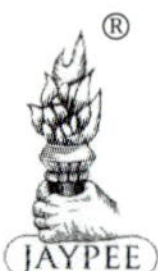

Jaypee Brothers Medical Publishers (P) Ltd

Headquarters

Jaypee Brothers Medical Publishers (P) Ltd
4838/24, Ansari Road, Daryaganj
New Delhi 110 002, India
Phone: +91-11-43574357
Fax: +91-11-43574314
Email: jaypee@jaypeebrothers.com

Overseas Offices

J.P. Medical Ltd
83 Victoria Street, London
SW1H 0HW (UK)
Phone: +44-2031708910
Fax: +02-03-0086180
Email: info@jpmedpub.com

Jaypee Medical Inc.
The Bourse
111 South Independence Mall East
Suite 835, Philadelphia, PA 19106, USA
Phone: + 267-519-9789
Email: joe.rusko@jaypeebrothers.com

Jaypee Brothers Medical Publishers (P) Ltd
Shorakhute, Kathmandu
Nepal
Phone: +00977-9841528578
Email: jaypee.nepal@gmail.com

Jaypee-Highlights Medical Publishers Inc.
City of Knowledge, Bld. 237, Clayton
Panama City, Panama
Phone: + 507-301-0496
Fax: + 507-301-0499
Email: cservice@jphmedical.com

Jaypee Brothers Medical Publishers (P) Ltd
17/1-B Babar Road, Block-B, Shaymali
Mohammadpur, Dhaka-1207
Bangladesh
Mobile: +08801912003485
Email: jaypeedhaka@gmail.com

Website: www.jaypeebrothers.com
Website: www.jaypeedigital.com

Inquiries for bulk sales may be solicited at: jaypee@jaypeebrothers.com

Color Atlas of Tissue Response to Biomaterials

First Edition: **2014**

ISBN: 978-93-5090-738-2

Printed at: Ajanta Offset & Packagings Limited, New Delhi

FOREWORD

Implants, such as lens, heart valve, pacemaker, vascular graft, joints, hydrocephalus shunts and many others, occupy a central place in medical technology which has grown by leaps and bounds in recent decades. Development of implants after World War II was delayed until a series of physiologically inert materials such as teflon, silicones, dacron, and metals such as 316 series stainless steels and Haynes 25 became available. While inertness has been the prime requirement for implant materials, recent advances in cell biology have raised the prospect of tissue-engineered materials, which may become the new and unstoppable wave in the construction of implants during the forthcoming decades.

It has long been known that the body provides a hostile environment to implants made of supposedly inert plastics, metals and alloys. The tissue response to implanted materials covers a wide range of inflammation, hyperplasia and occasionally, even neoplasia. The response would depend on the physico-chemical characteristics of the implant and host factors, such as the kind of tissue, site of implantation and the animal species receiving the implant. Even when an implant is linked firmly to the host and remains functional like a prosthetic joint or heart valve, it should be noted that the connection at the tissue-material interface is no more than a smooth mechanical linkage by collagen and not a union at the molecular level. This is precisely what makes the tissue material interface in all tissues—soft and hard, vulnerable to implant failure.

However, the success story of implants is undeniable; their use has exploded and impinged on practically every speciality in surgery; they account for a multi-billion dollar global industry, which continues to grow; their research and development has become a major discipline in science and technology with societies, journals and an extensive literature. In spite of these striking developments, the absence of an atlas on the manifold tissue responses to prosthetic materials, highlighting wide-ranging histopathological changes has been a glaring deficiency. There is little doubt that such a publication will be highly useful not only to the pathologist who studies the slides from tests of newer materials but also to the medical and veterinary scientists, toxicologists, engineers and others who are involved in the making of the implants story. It is the gap, which Dr Mira has sought to fill by preparing the present atlas based on her vast experience at the Sree Chitra Tirunal Institute, Thiruvananthapuram, Kerala, India. A highly competent pathologist, Dr Mira set up her Division of Implant Biology at the Chitra Institute three decades ago when few such Divisions existed in the world. It received plenty of tissue samples and case histories from the Devices Laboratories as well as the Hospital of the Institute, which provided a rich source of varied material for Dr Mira and her group. Their painstaking study over several years has culminated in this splendid atlas, which begins by a lucid description of the preparation of tissues for microscopy and goes on to deal with implants in soft tissue, implants in bone, preclinical evaluation of biomaterials and devices during research and development (R&D), study of retrieved implants and finally, experimental artifacts, which can complicate the interpretation of slides. Each chapter is profusely illustrated with excellent photographs and graphic descriptions, which will benefit investigators and students of this new branch of pathology, which will grow in proportion to the steady expansion in the range and variety of new implants.

Dr Mira and her colleagues deserve our thanks for their admirable effort in preparing this valuable and much-needed atlas.

MS Valiathan MBBS MS FRCS (England) FRCS (EDIN)
FRCPS (C) FRCP (London) DSc

National Research Professor, Government of India
Founder Director, Sree Chitra Tirunal Institute for Medical Sciences and Technology
Thiruvananthapuram, Kerala, India
Former President, Indian National Science Academy
Former First Vice-Chancellor, Manipal Academy of Higher Education
Manipal, Karnataka, India

PREFACE

Biomaterial science encompasses both material and biological sciences. Residence of a material in biological tissue depends both on material characteristics and on the adjacent tissue. This is what makes this science interdisciplinary. Research into material-tissue interface requires a comprehensive understanding of events in the tissues adjacent to material. This is best understood by microscopic examination of the interface.

Books on biomaterial science abound with details regarding different materials, their physical and chemical characteristics and their interactions with tissue. However, visual detail is what is most informative for the material scientist. This is brought forth in this atlas, which is a collection of gross features and photomicrographs of events taking place at the material-tissue interface. The book brings to the reader first hand details regarding the sequence of events that occur in different tissues following implantation of different types of material. It informs the young researcher briefly of the common procedures used in the laboratory for preparation of tissues for microscopy, how to identify different cells in tissues, and how to assess responses elicited in tissues, essentially how to evaluate whether a material is compatible with tissues or not.

Our laboratory is a nodal laboratory for receiving different types of tissues for assessment of suitability of different types of materials for medical devices. We feel that it is appropriate that this laboratory provides a means to educate students and researchers in material science about the morphological features and changes identified over a time period post-implantation.

Mira Mohanty
A Sabareeswaran
Sulekha Baby
Joseph Sebastian
Caroline S Diana

ACKNOWLEDGMENTS

All the photographs in this atlas are of tissues received in the histopathology laboratory for testing of biocompatibility of materials and for preclinical evaluation of devices. They belong to a collection over three decades. We specifically thank Professor MS Valiathan, for giving us this idea of putting together these pictures in the form of an atlas. We thank all the technical staff who have been in this laboratory during this time, for their contribution in providing these sections. We are very grateful to the Department of Science and Technology, Government of India, without whose financial help, this atlas would not have been possible. We also express our gratitude to the Director and Head, Biomedical Technology Wing of Sree Chitra Tirunal Institute for Medical Sciences and Technology, for their encouragement and permission to use the photographs for this atlas.

CONTENTS

1

Preparation of Tissues with Implants for Microscopy

A piece of tissue ⟹ stained section.

A section of tissue around/adjacent to an implant must provide clarity, and good contrast to give maximum information. All tissues on removal from the living body, either human or an experimental animal must be fixed, dehydrated, cleared, impregnated with an embedding medium, embedded, cut into sections and stained prior to examination under the microscope. These steps are described in the following pages.

FIXATION

Study of the cellular events in tissues around materials, requires perfect preservation of cell and tissue architecture. It also requires the preservation of the interface between material and tissue. It is this interface which gives information of how cells respond and behave in relation to various chemical and physical properties of materials. The clarity of what is seen under microscopy depends to a large extent on proper fixation of tissues.

Tissues undergo cell death, otherwise known as autolysis, when removed from the body. Visualization of changes in cells and tissues is difficult in autolytic tissue. Termination of the different biochemical reactions in tissues prevents this autolysis and can be done by fixation of tissues in certain chemicals. These fixatives terminate any ongoing biochemical reactions in the tissue and protect it from decay. The most common fixative used for all types of tissues (Muscle, skin, bone, brain, etc.) is formalin. This is available commercially as a 40% w/v solution of formaldehyde. Tissues are fixed in a 10% solution of this commercially available formalin. Formalin preserves cellular architecture and this is further enhanced when the fixative is buffered by addition of disodium hydrogen phosphate and monosodium dihydrogen phosphate, this solution being called a 10% solution of neutral buffered formalin with a pH of 7.0. An important point in obtaining properly fixed tissue is the need for proper penetration of the fixative into the tissues. When tissues containing small implants are to be examined, the implant when removed should have a minimum of 1 cm thick tissue all around to enable the fixative to seep into the tissue. Hence, when a large tissue, e.g. a limb with a prosthesis in situ needs fixation, it should be completely submerged in formalin and tissue pieces from the areas required for study should be taken as early as possible. These tissue pieces should have a minimum of 1 cm thickness all around to enable proper fixation. If a delay is anticipated before selection of tissues, deep cuts in the tissue can be given. Fixation must be for a minimum of 24 hours.

The amount of fixative should be at least nine times the volume of tissue. Most biomaterial studies require viewing the interface at the ultrastructural level. In such cases, the tissue should be fixed in glutaraldehyde. When an investigation into the surface morphology of a material and tissue is required, after removal in an in vivo experiment, glutaraldehyde is used as a fixative.

It is preferable to hold the tissue in running water for a few seconds before placing in fixative, to remove traces of

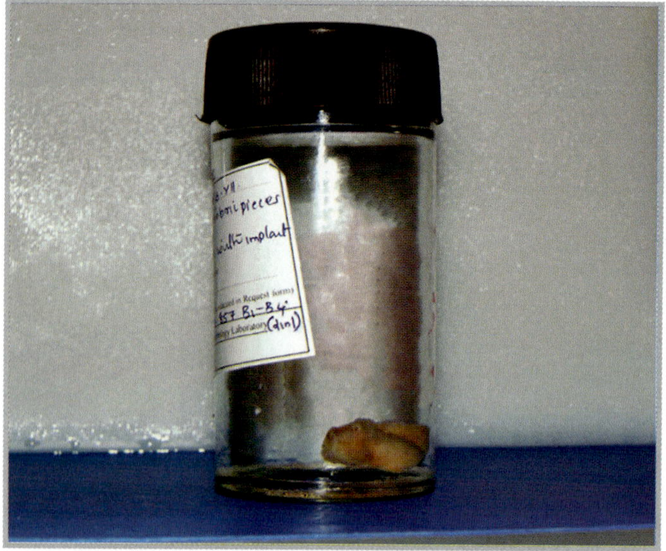

Figure 1 Block of tissue fixed in formalin

blood. Blood combines with formalin to form a deep brown pigment in tissues which when viewed microscopically may be mistaken for evidence of old hemorrhage. However, in some cases, the delicate nature of the tissue may not permit this as the tissue may be physically destroyed, e.g. the newly formed endothelial cell layer in a vascular graft or on a stent. In such cases, perfusion fixation is carried out, where the fixative is infused into the circulation of the animal prior to necropsy. When whole small bones containing implants are fixed in formalin, it is always desirable to cut both ends of the bone to permit formalin to enter the marrow from both ends for proper fixation.

GROSSING

Grossing is the terminology used by pathologists for the procedure carried out to describe what is seen in the tissue by the naked eye or grossly and to cut out pieces of tissues

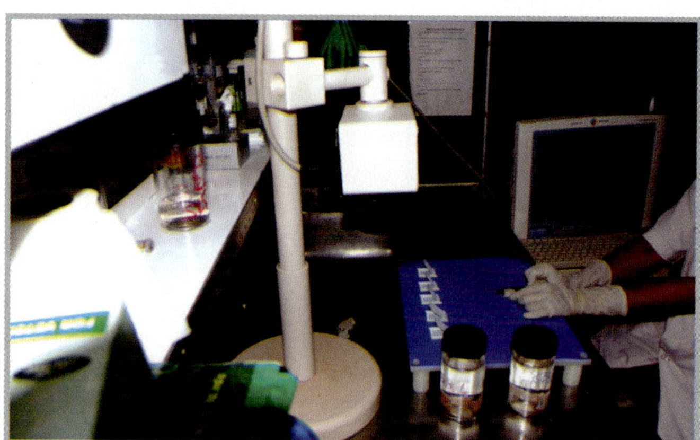

Figure 2 Grossing of tissue with adjacent macrophotography system

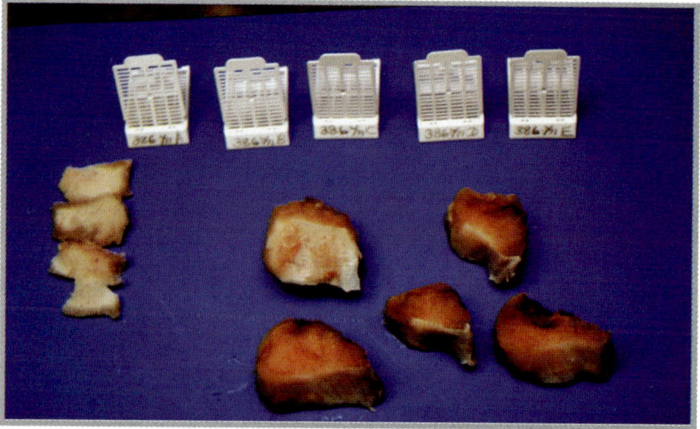

Figure 3 Pieces of skeletal muscle with implants ready for grossing

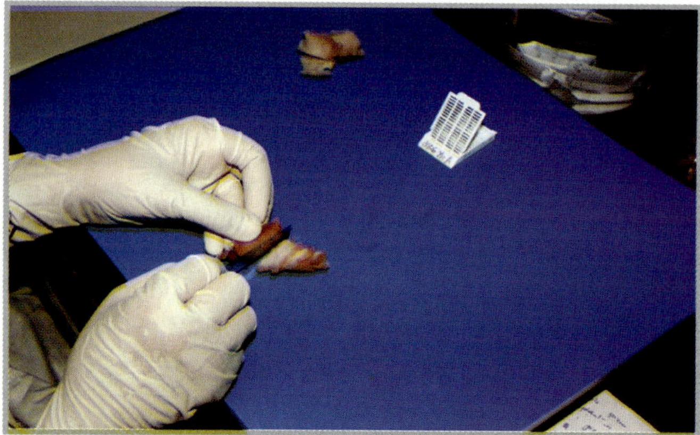

Figure 4 Cutting of parallel sections perpendicular to implant site

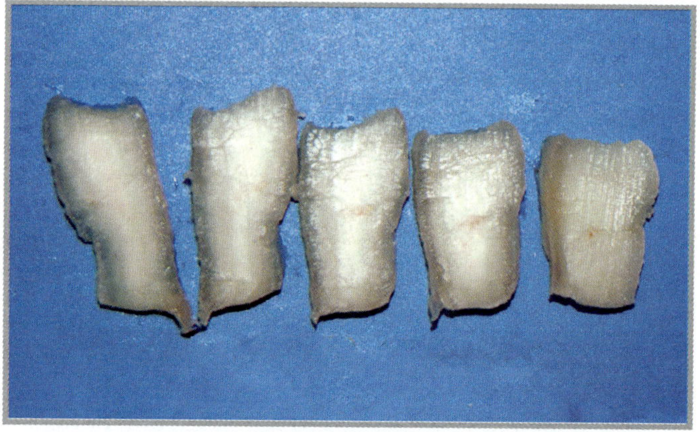

Figure 5 Gross sections of skeletal muscle with implant site in the center

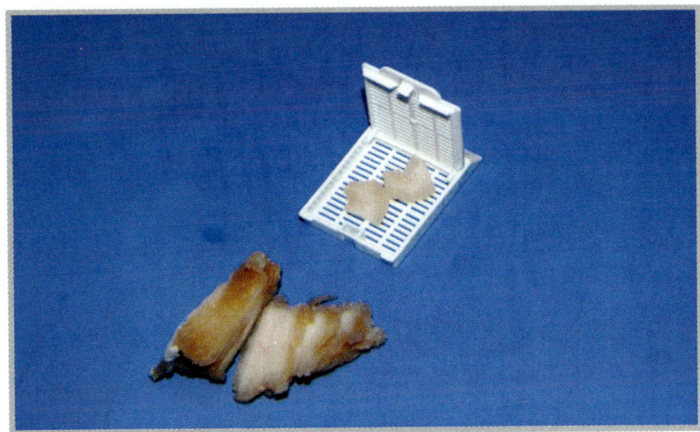

Figure 6 Gross sections of skeletal muscle with implant site in capsule for processing

from the areas to be investigated. This procedure also involves taking photographs of the implant/prosthesis in the tissue. After noting a complete description of the prosthesis/implant and tissue, photographs should be taken from all angles to give maximum information to anyone who wants to know how it looked prior to being cut up for investigation.

Seeing the entire specimen which may be only a small implanted material in tissue or a complete prosthesis, the decision should be made as to which areas need investigation. These areas are cut out carefully or trimmed in thin slices of at least 1 mm thickness and further kept in formalin. The material tissue interface, being important, the piece of tissue taken must include the material. This is possible only if the material can be cut through by metal knives at this stage and at the stage of cutting thin sections. If, it is a polymer, this is possible. If not possible, as in case of metals, the implant can be removed gently from the tissue without causing much damage to the implant-tissue interface. All tissue pieces taken should be properly labeled to denote the specimen and area from which it has been taken. The tissue is placed in a tissue cassette and the relevant laboratory identification code is written on the cassette with a graphite pencil to avoid being erased in due course in the processing solutions. Simultaneously, record must be made of description of the tissue and all observations made. The record must contain details of labels given for each piece of tissue (e.g. A-proximal implant, B-distal implant). Record must also be made by photography, preferably using digital techniques. The digital photograph is saved for record with a file name describing the feature in the image.

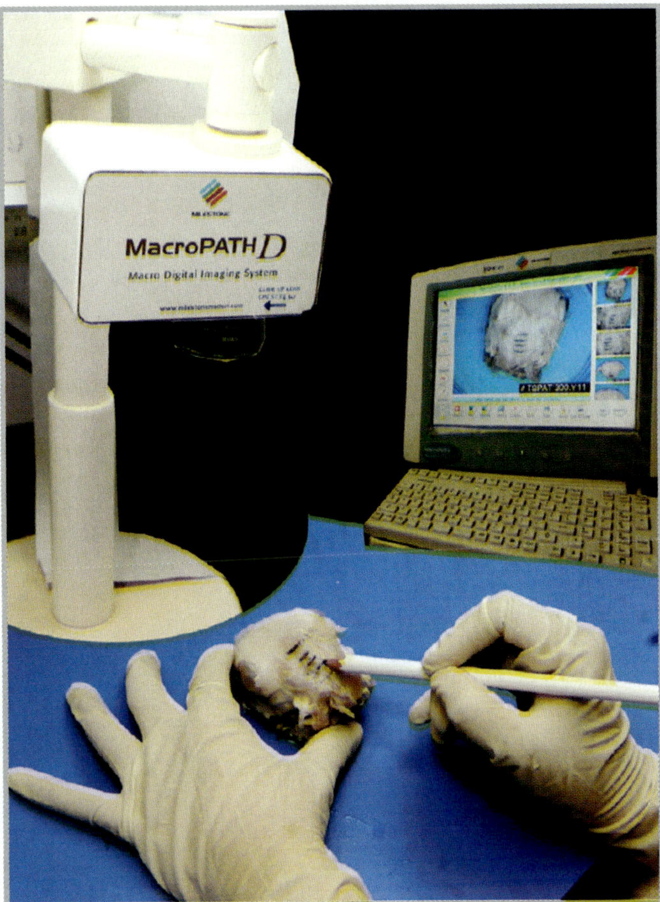

Figure 7 Macrophotography for record

PROCESSING

Sections of tissues cannot be viewed directly by transmitted light microscopy. Most tissues are soft and require a rigid support for sectioning. This support is usually provided by paraffin wax. Direct embedding of the tissue in wax is not possible, as the main constituent of the tissues-water is immiscible with the embedding medium. Hence, the tissues are usually processed prior to embedding in wax. The purpose of tissue processing is to replace the water in the tissues with a solution which is miscible with the embedding medium and this is achieved by the diffusion of processing reagents in and out of the tissues.

This processing is done stepwise through dehydration, clearing and infiltration. In an automatic tissue processor, the tissue cassettes arranged in a specimen basket are placed in the retort of the processor. Tissues are perfused with the solutions accroding to a pre-programmed schedule. Processing can also be done manually using beakers with different solutions and manually changing the cassette holder into every solution.

DEHYDRATION

Alcohol is a good dehydrating agent and alcohols of various types like ethanol, methanol, isopropyl alcohol, denatured

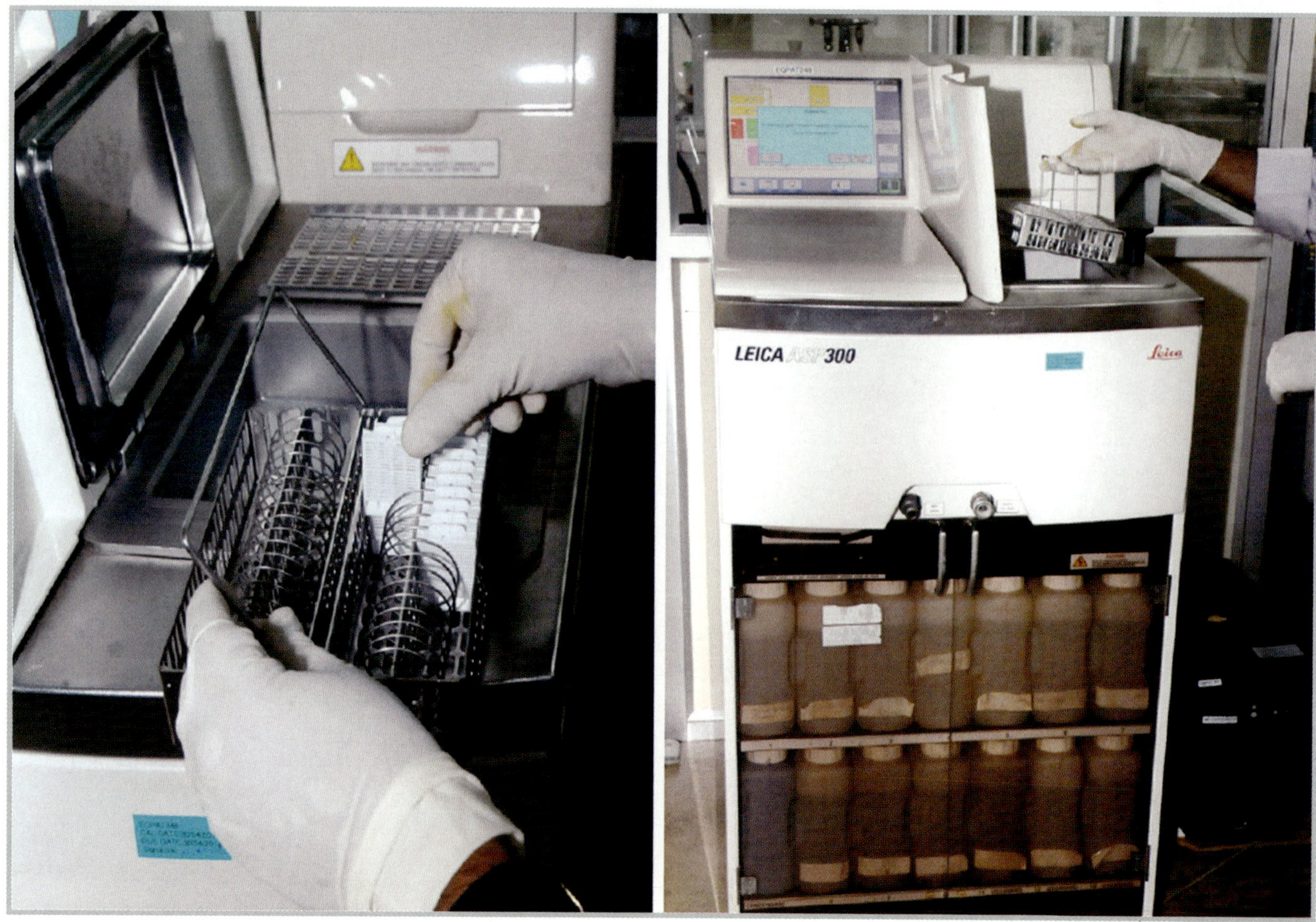

Figure 8 Basket with tissue cassettes loaded onto tissue processor

alcohol are used. Water is completely removed from the tissues using alcohol of increasing concentration. The slow passage of the dehydrating agent through the tissue prevents sudden shrinkage of the cellular membrane which will result in disruption of tissue architecture. Tissues are passed through ascending grades of alcohol. The duration is usually decided by the size of tissues, larger tissues requiring longer duration. The volume of alcohol used should be 50–100 times greater than that of the tissues to permit adequate dehydration and to prevent incomplete dehydration which does not permit infiltration of clearing agents and embedding medium. In addition to the water, some of the cellular constituents like lipids are also dissolved in the dehydrant. (Hence, these areas would appear as clear spaces in sections when observed by microscopy).

CLEARING

The next step involves replacing the dehydrating agent with a solution which is miscible with the embedding medium, the process being called clearing. For this, a solvent which is miscible both in the dehydrant and in the embedding medium is needed. Hydrocarbons, usually xylene is used. Cleared tissues are translucent, the refractive index of the clearing agent being similar to that of cellular proteins enabling the light entering the tissues to pass through it without much refraction giving the tissues a clear appearance. Hence, the translucency of the tissue is used as an indicator of proper clearing of tissue, opaque areas indicating incomplete dehydration. Chloroform/toluene can also be used as clearing agents but are flammable, cause skin degreasing and have varying degrees of toxicity.

Impregnation of tissues with embedding medium

The cleared tissues are next impregnated with molten wax. The melting point of the wax should be approximately 58° to 60°C. Higher temperature would damage tissues whereas lower temperature would prevent adequate impregnation. Applying vacuum to the container of wax

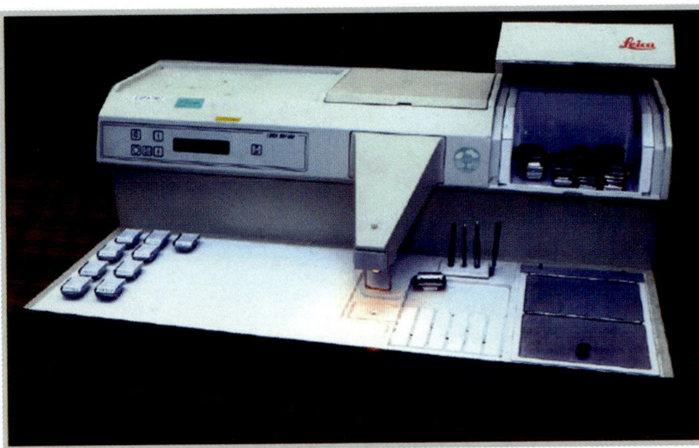

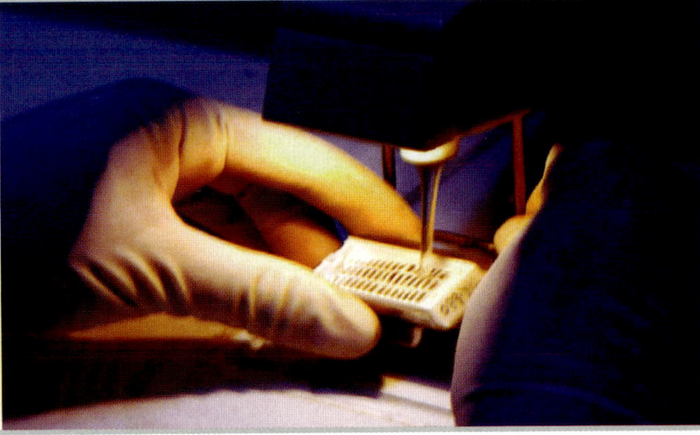

Figure 9 Embedding of tissue in paraffin wax in mould

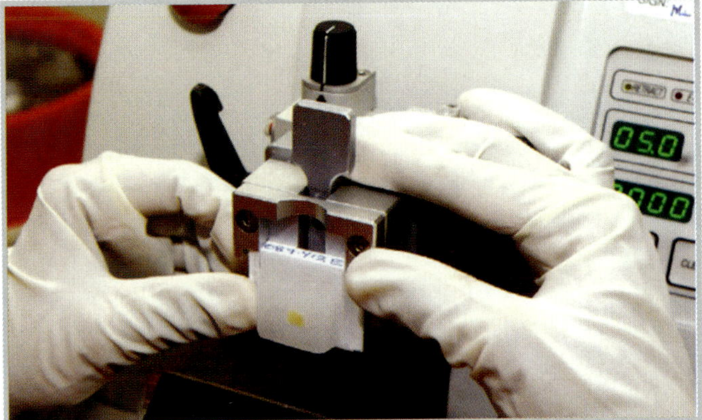

Figure 10 Fixation of paraffin block on a rotary microtome

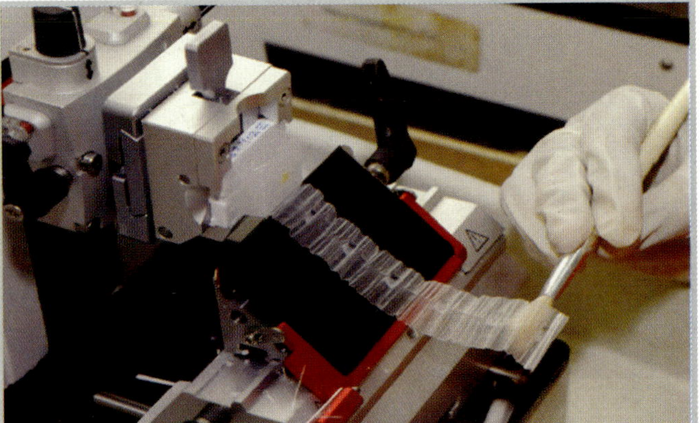

Figure 11 Ribbon of 5 μm thick sections

ensures better impregnation. The tissues are impregnated in three changes.

EMBEDDING

Each tissue is next embedded in a block of wax. Molten wax is poured into the mould and the tissue is placed flat into the wax. It is important to ensure that the side of the tissue which you want to examine by microscopy is placed face down into the wax, so that when the block is cut the desired section is obtained. Blocks are cooled and can be stored at room temperature in polythene bags prior to cutting.

SECTION CUTTING

Sections of the block of wax with tissue are cut using a steel/tungsten blade. The blade is fixed on a rotary microtome in which the block moves vertically with microprecise movement. The block is held tight in a holder to ensure stability during cutting. After initial trimming of the block thickness of the section is adjusted on the microtome. Usually, 5 micron thick sections are cut. The face of the block being cut is cooled using ice to avoid curling of sections. Sections are cut automatically and a ribbon of sections are picked up and floated onto water in a water bath which is maintained at a temperature of 45°C to 50°C. The process of floating the sections onto water, flattens out any folds in the section. A single section is picked up onto a glass slide and air dried on a slide stand. To enhance adhesion of section onto the glass, the slide can be smeared with egg albumin. Alternatively, charged or Poly-L-lysine coated slides can be used.

STAINING

Sections of tissues are stained with hematoxylin and eosin. Hematoxylin colors the nucleus of cells a deep purple and Eosin stains the cytoplasm of cells pink. This contrast

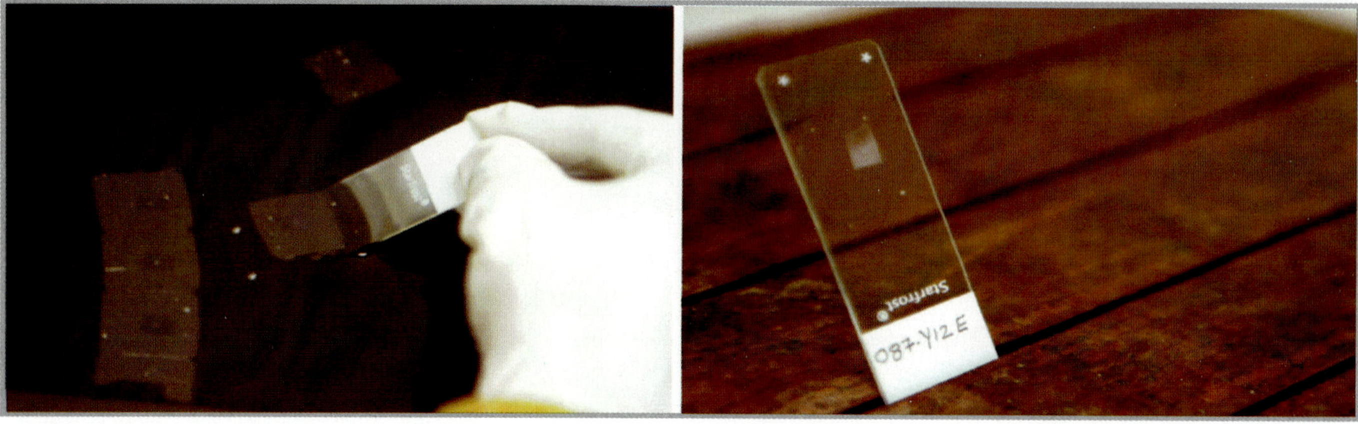

Figure 12 Paraffin sections for drying

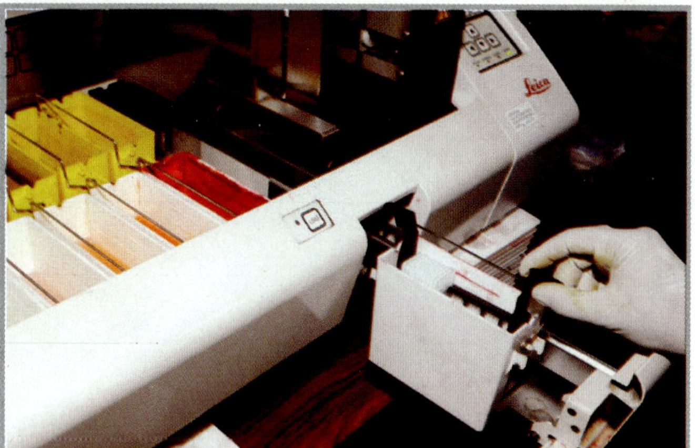

Figure 13 Loading of slides in a slide holder into an autostainer

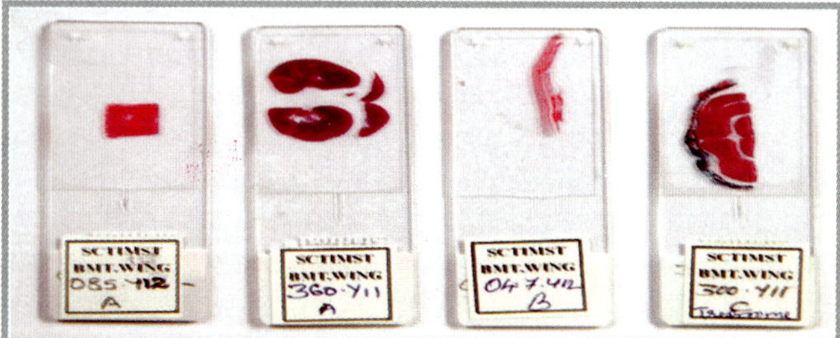

Figure 14 Slides with stained sections

is very essential for identifying different cells by their nuclear and cytoplasmic morphological characteristics. Slides with sections are warmed at a temperature of 50°C. The staining is carried out in different steps beginning with deparaffinization. This is to remove the paraffin wax which has impregnated the tissues. Deparaffinization is done by placing the slide with adhered section in xylene. As the tissues were dehydrated during processing, the sections are then hydrated in descending grades of alcohol and stained first with hematoxylin. Section is placed in lightly acidified alcohol for differentiation to remove excessive hematoxylin and then carefully dipped in lightly alkaline tap water for bluing.

The differentiation step is critically timed to prevent over or understaining. Following this, sections are stained with Eosin and dehydrated in alcohol of ascending concentration. Dry sections as such cannot be viewed under the microscope. So, they are covered with a fluid called mounting medium over which a coverslip of thin glass is gently placed. The refractive index of this mounting medium is the same as that of the coverslip. Xylene being miscible with this medium, sections after having passed in xylene are mounted in the medium and coverslipped. It is very essential to ensure that no air bubble enters the medium during coverslipping. It would prevent good observation.

Fixation and gross cutting of hard tissue with implant

Bone with implants are fixed in the same fixative as for soft tissue. Ten percent neutral buffered formalin with a pH of 7.0 is the fixative commonly used. It is very necessary that fixative diffuses through the marrow as soon as possible after removal of the bone. It is desirable to cut cross-sectional blocks of the bone with implant to permit fixative to seep through.

PROCESSING AND EMBEDDING

Bone with implants can be either decalcified to make bone soft, prior to processing or be processed as such

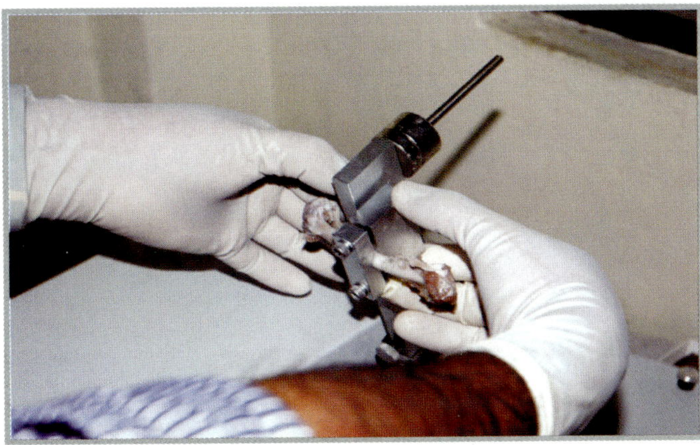

Figure 15 Fixing of long bone with implant on a low-speed saw before processing

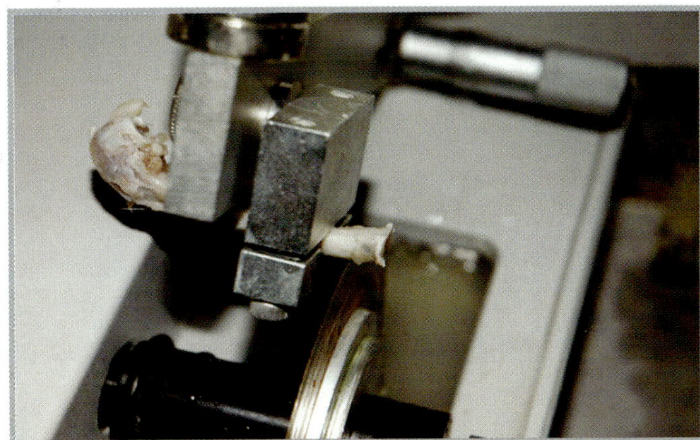

Figure 16 Cutting of block of bone with implant using a diamond wafer coated blade in a low speed saw

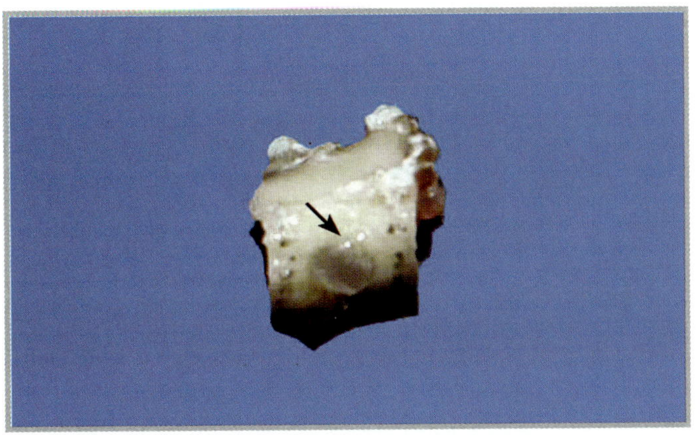

Figure 17 Block of bone with implant

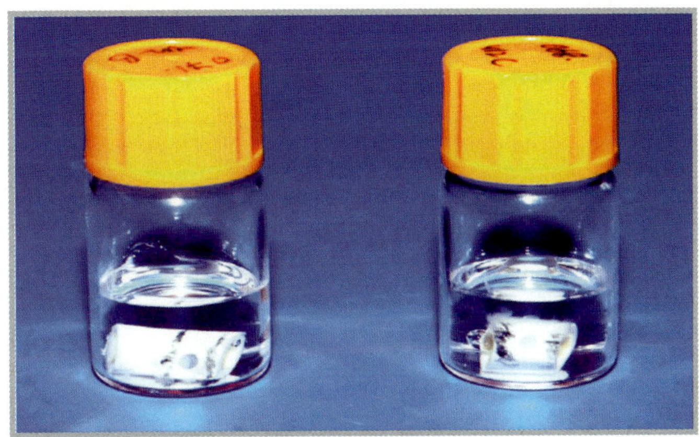

Figure 18 Blocks of bone with implant in resin

as undecalcified bone. As the decalcification process is carried out in chemical solutions, ceramic implants with calcium are also removed during the process. Undecalcified sections are preferred for assessment of biocompatibility as the implant bone interface is preserved very well. Following fixation of about two to four days depending on size of the block, the sample is dehydrated in ascending concentration of alcohol, defatted in acetone and then perfused with resin.

Paraffin wax which is used for embedding of soft tissue does not give adequate support to hard tissue. Hence, resins are used as embedding media. Most common resin used in our laboratory is methyl methacrylate which polymerises to polymethyl methacrylate, thus, providing a block which is easy to section in a saw microtome. The blocks of processed bone with implant are embedded in resin.

Vacuum is applied to enhance better impregnation with resin. It is very important that the embedding solution is free from air bubbles which will appear microscopically as black discolored areas in stained sections. It is also important that as the resin polymerises, the tissue with the implant should be aligned in the correct position. This will ensure that sections when cut, give a clear picture of the implant bone interface.

SECTION CUTTING

Thin 50 to 100 microns thick sections of the resin block are cut using special blades. Diamond wafering blades provide good thin sections. It is very important that the block blade interface is bathed in a coolant to prevent warping of the section by heat generated while sectioning.

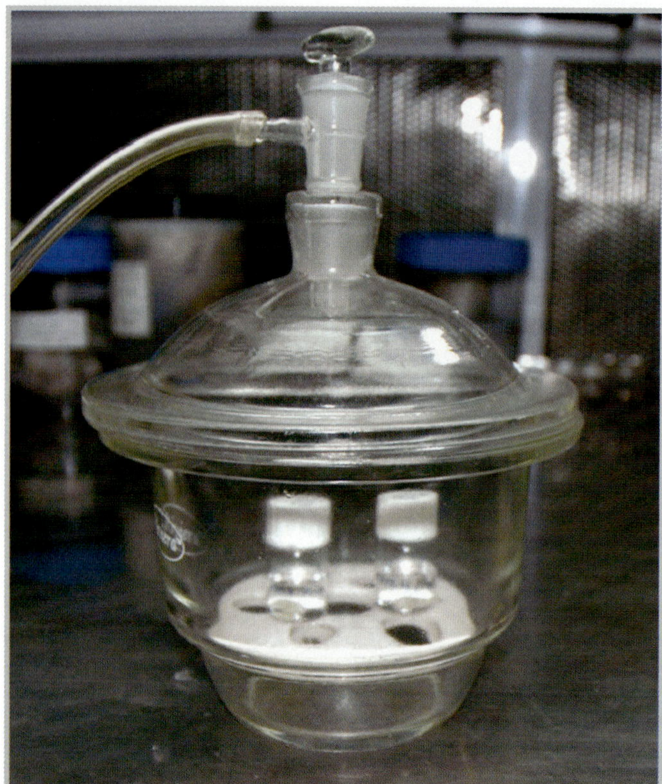

Figure 19 Application of vacuum for resin impregnation

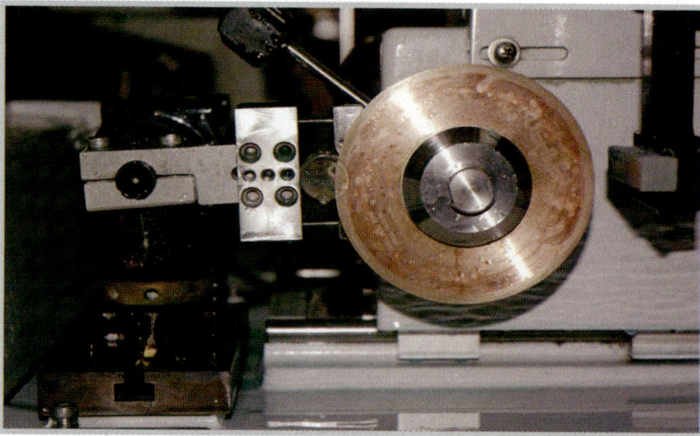

Figure 20 Thin resin section cut on a high speed precision saw

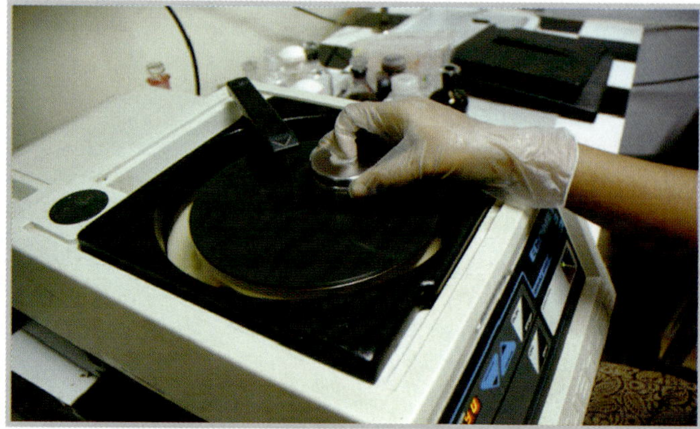

Figure 21 Polishing of section held in holder

GRINDING AND POLISHING

Thin cut resin sections are further ground gradually to a thickness of 20 to 50 microns using abrasive discs with different grit size for clear visualization of cellular details. Polishing is accomplished with muslin cloth to make the section diffraction free.

STAINING

Sections of bone are stained with hematoxylin and Eosin or with Stevenel's blue, the latter being preferred. Bone stains yellowish brown, osteoid (new bone) stains green and fibrous tissue (collagen) stains blue.

Resin embedding is also used for evaluating tissue response to metal implants in soft tissue, e.g. vascular stents.

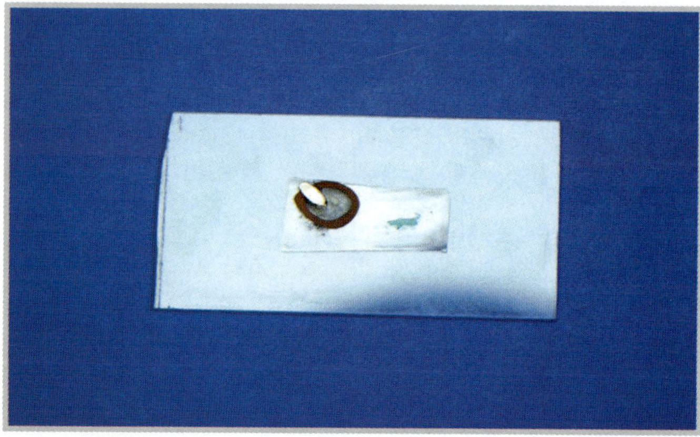

Figure 22 Resin section of bone with implant glued onto a glass slide

2

Implants in Soft Tissue

When a material is placed in any tissue, because the process of implantation itself is an injury, there is destruction of the tissue. The cells in the tissue die and the process is termed necrosis. When cells die there is release of various cell constituents which attract different types of defense cells towards the site of injury. These inflammatory cells are present inside the small blood vessels in the tissue, close to the implant site. The vessels dilate, the cells lining the wall of the blood vessel separate, providing a space between them. The white blood cells comprising neutrophils, monocytes and lymphocytes move out of the bloodstream through these spaces into the adjacent tissue and move towards the site of injury. This directional movement is called chemokinesis. The neutrophils form the first line of defense and through their cell constituents, the cytokines, remove dead tissue. The monocytes from the blood vessels convert to macrophages, the scavenger cells of the body. These cells and the resident macrophages in the extracellular matrix, functionally take up or engulf dead tissue as well as any foreign body. The implant itself being a foreign body, macrophages make every attempt to engulf the implant and when they fail to do so, they coalesce together and form foreign body type of giant cells. These phenomena are known as inflammation. When cell debri due to cell death, are removed, the fibroblasts, the interstitial cells in the extracellular matrix take part in the healing process or repair. The fibroblasts lay down collagen or more of extracellular matrix. New small blood vessels are formed as offshoots of the existing blood vessels, the process known as neovascularization. The tissue around the implant comprising all the migrated cells and new vessels, known as granulation tissue is gradually replaced by collagen deposition or fibrosis around the implant in the form of a layer enveloping or isolating the implant from the surrounding tissue. The histological or microscopic picture seen within 24 hours of implantation is of necrosis and severe inflammation. This is followed within one week by reduced inflammation and gradual formation of a fibrous layer within a month. What follows is the slow transformation of a thick fibrous layer and resolution of a thick capsule to a very thin layer of collagen over a period of few months.

The histological picture gives evidence of the compatibility of the material with the surrounding tissue, i.e. biocompatibility. If the implant or material has components which leach out into the adjacent tissue and if this leaching out occurs continuously, the inflammatory phase is found to continue for a longer time and such materials are termed as toxic or non-biocompatible. Numerous inflammatory cells, particularly macrophages and foreign body type of giant cells are present at the tissue material interface, if the material is not biocompatible.

The same sequences of events take place also with degradable materials, the difference being in the end point of healing. Macrophages enter the material as it degrades, they engulf and destroy the degradable components, forming giant cells to do the same. Release of chemical constituents and ensuing inflammation continue for some time till the entire material is degraded.

Repair follows and tissue architecture is restored to normal. Biodegradable materials which elicit chronic inflammatory response in the beginning but later result in tissue restoration are termed biocompatible and are used in tissue engineering.

Materials are always tested for toxicity along with a biocompatible proved material which has already been found successful in patients without any untoward effects after implantation. Comparison of the tissue response to both the material to be tested and an approved material provides a good method to judge the biocompatibility of a new material.

The different facets of necrosis, inflammation and repair as seen by microscopy can be seen in the following images:

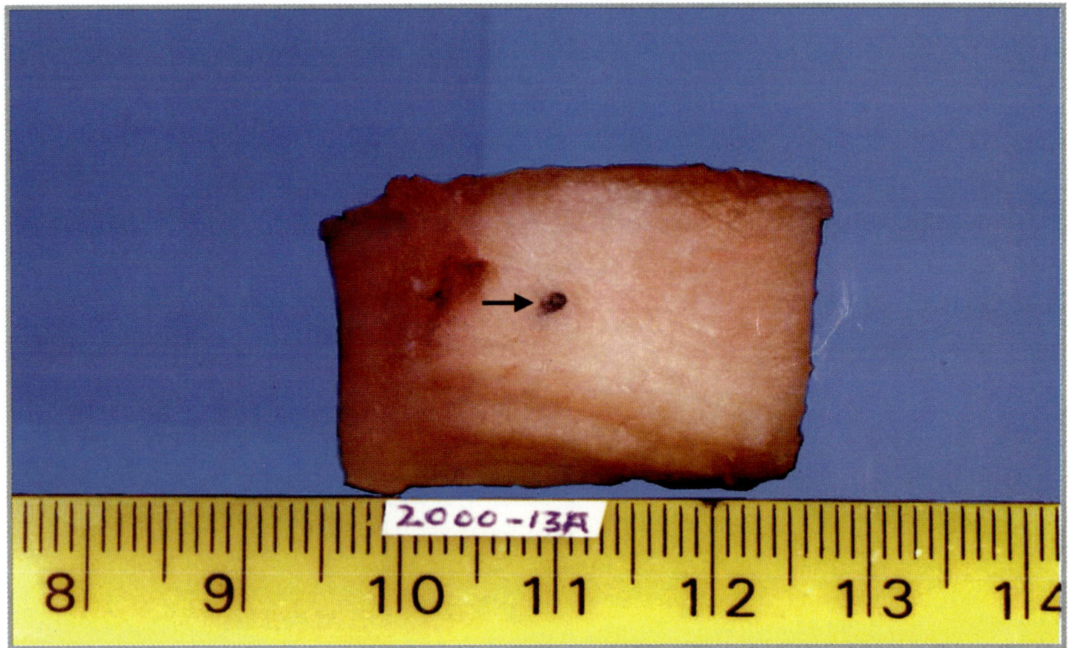

Figure 1 Unfixed piece of skeletal muscle removed with metal implant (↑). Reddish brown muscle

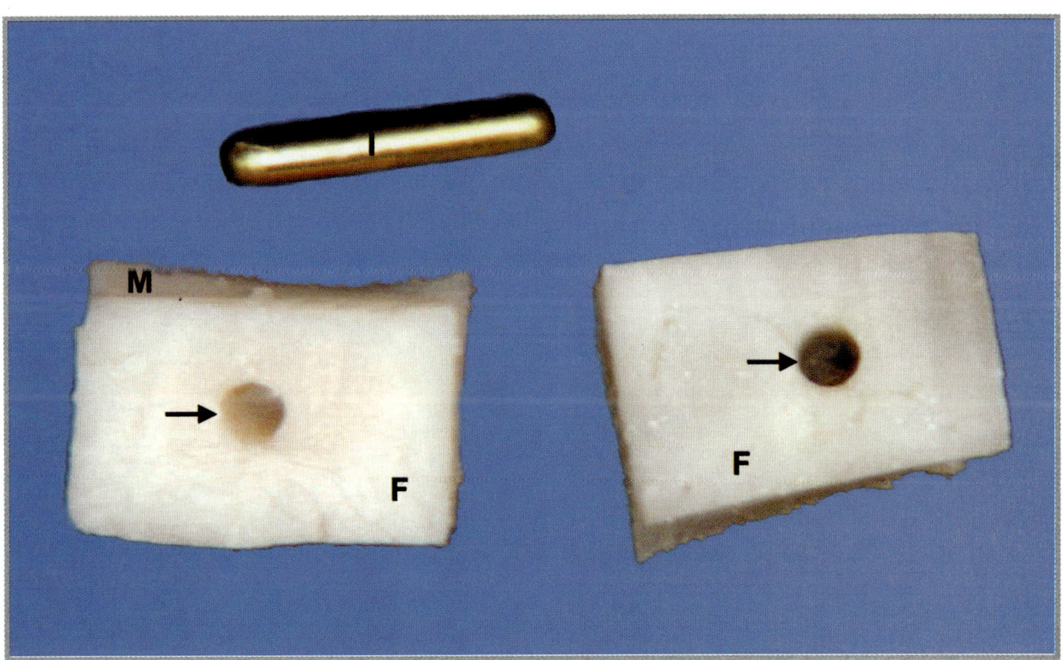

Figure 2 Implant (I) removed from fixed skeletal muscle and well-defined implant site (↑). No grossly evident necrosis, inflammation or hemorrhage. Fascial surface (F) white and glistening. Implant is always placed perpendicular to the fascial surface. Muscle below (M)

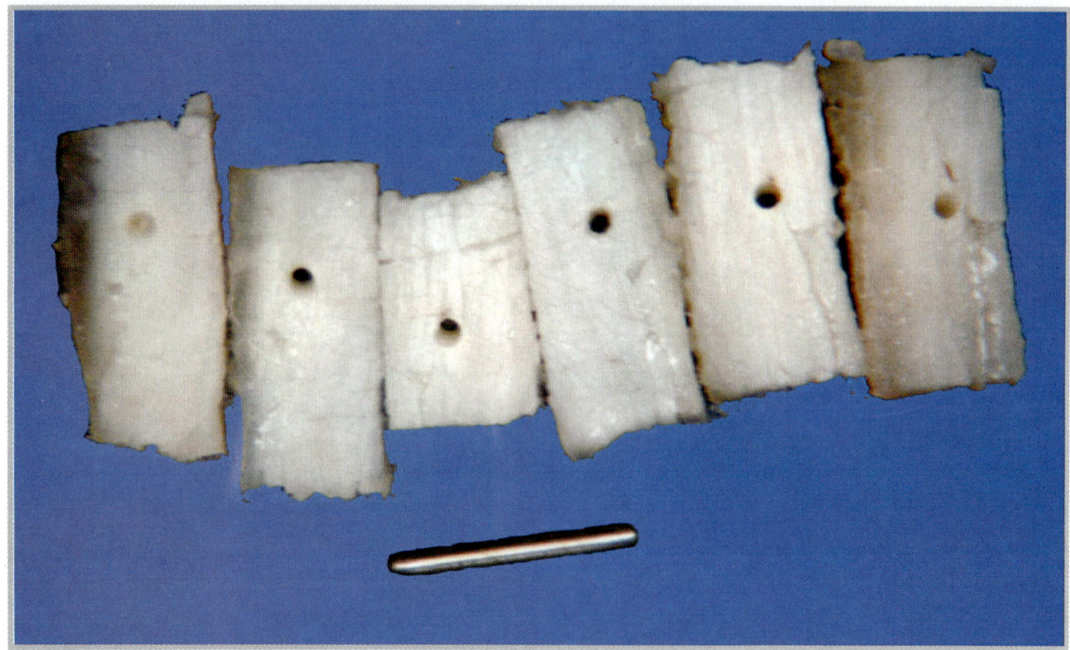

Figure 3 Thin slices cut perpendicular to implant site

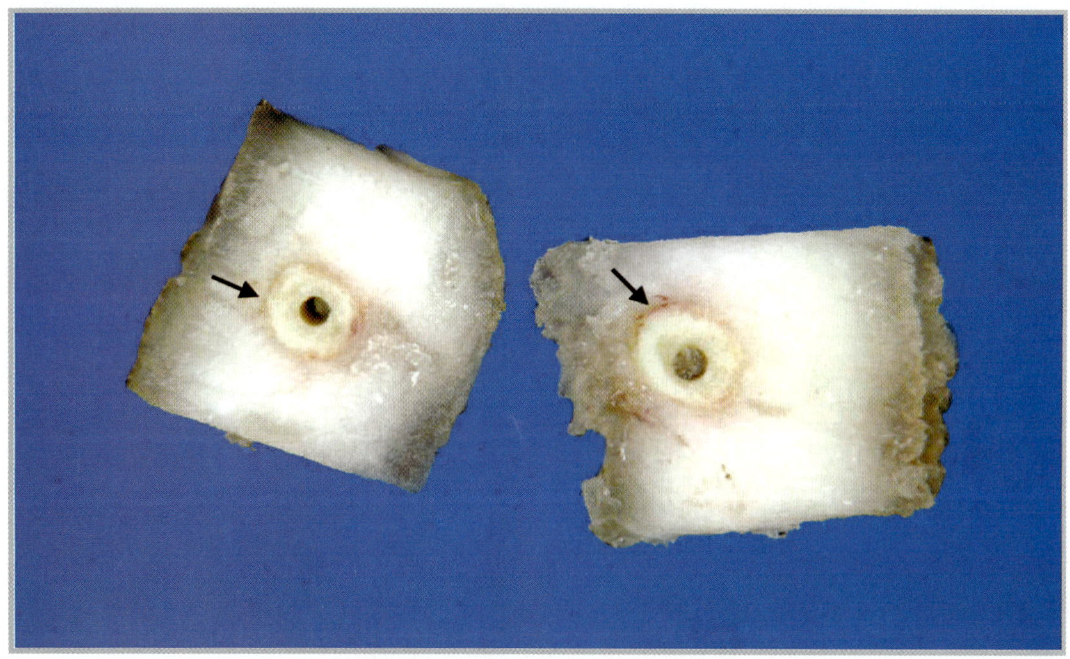

Figure 4 Severe necrosis (↑) around implant site

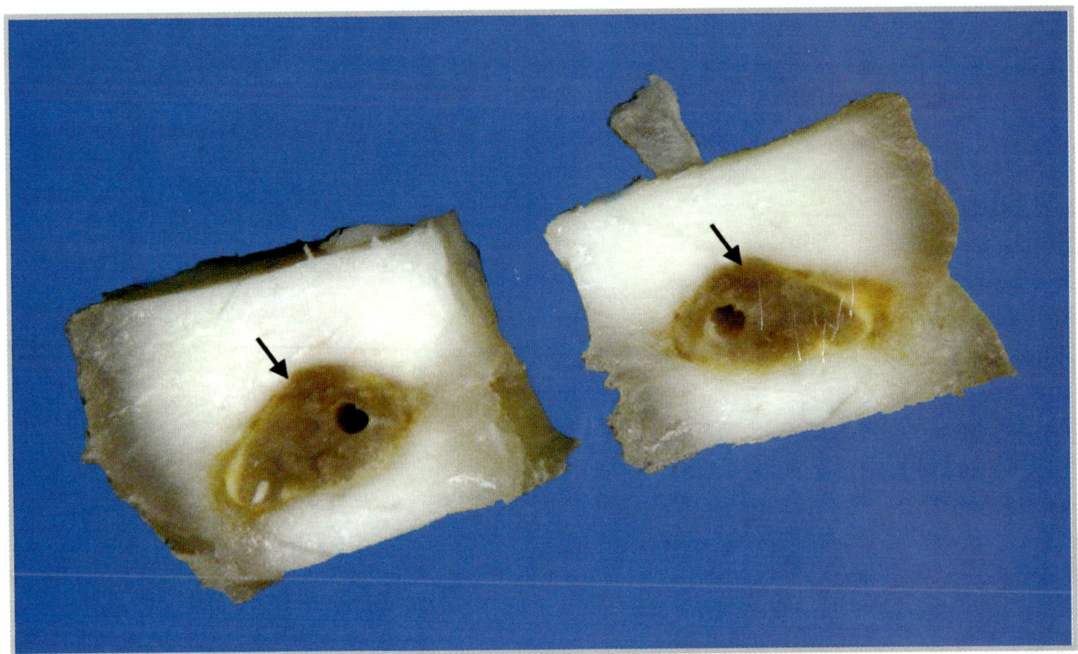

Figure 5 Severe hemorrhage (↑) around implant site

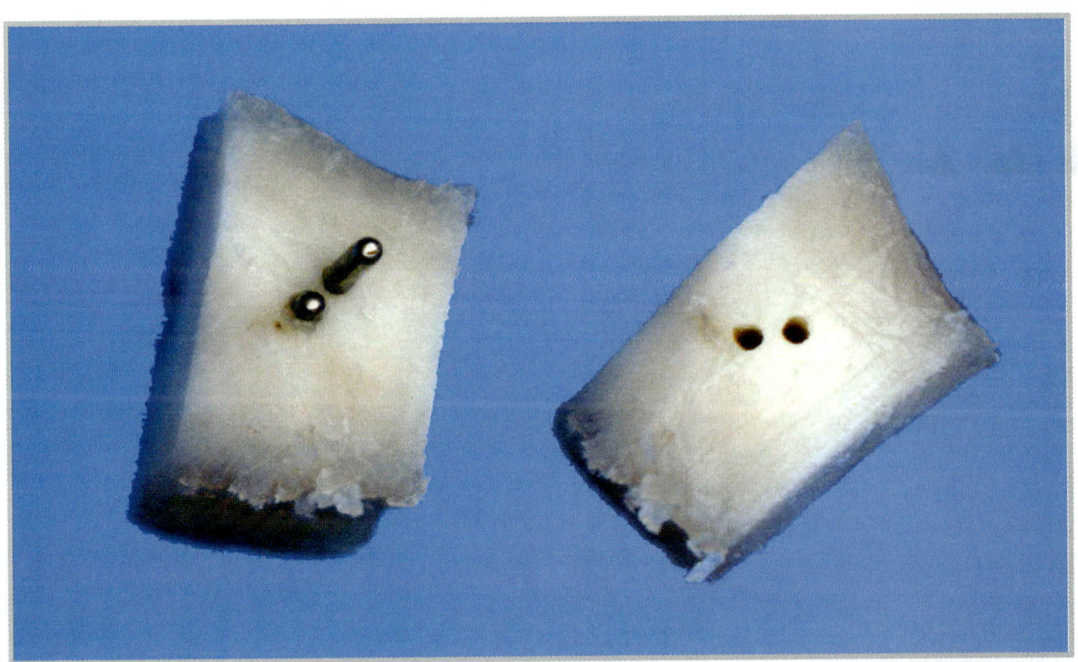

Figure 6 Two implants placed adjacent to each other. Proper evaluation of biocompatibility to individual implants will not be possible due to overlap of tissue response

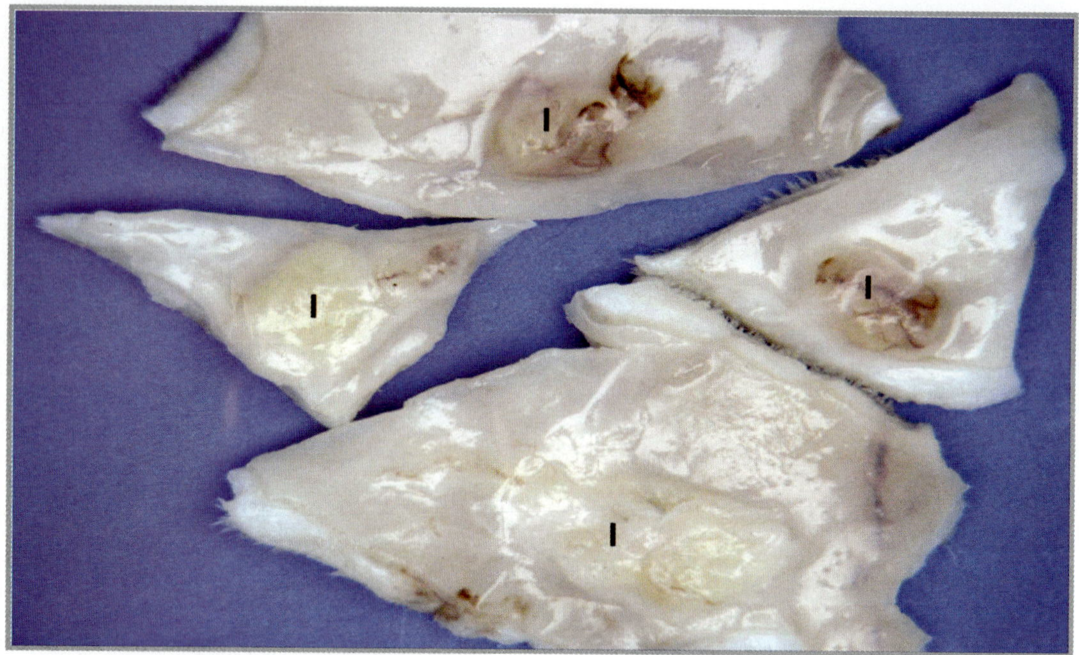

Figure 7 Undersurface of pieces of skin with implants implanted in subcutaneous tissue. Implants (I) covered with soft white tissue

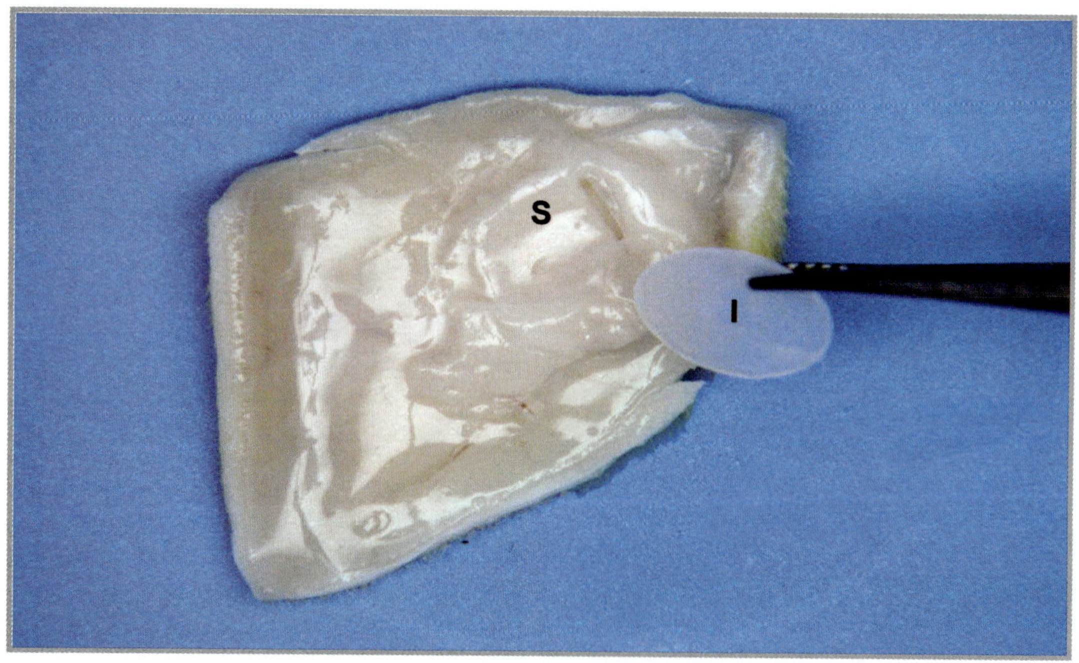

Figure 8 Implant (I) removed from subcutaneous tissue. Implant site (S) as a pocket

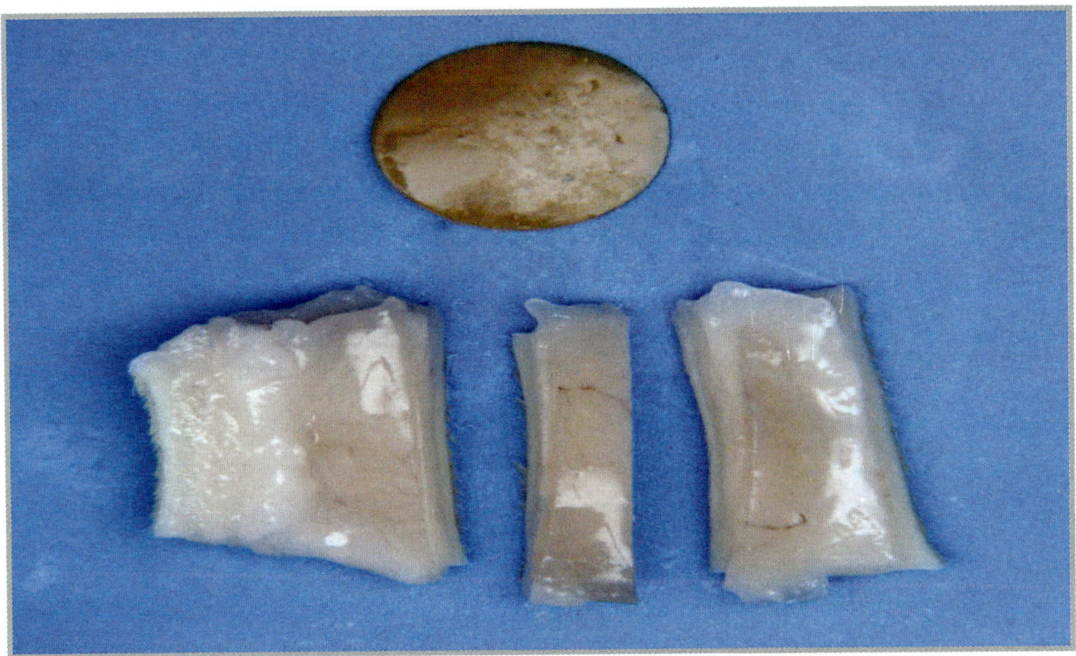

Figure 9 Perpendicular thin slices cut through pocket

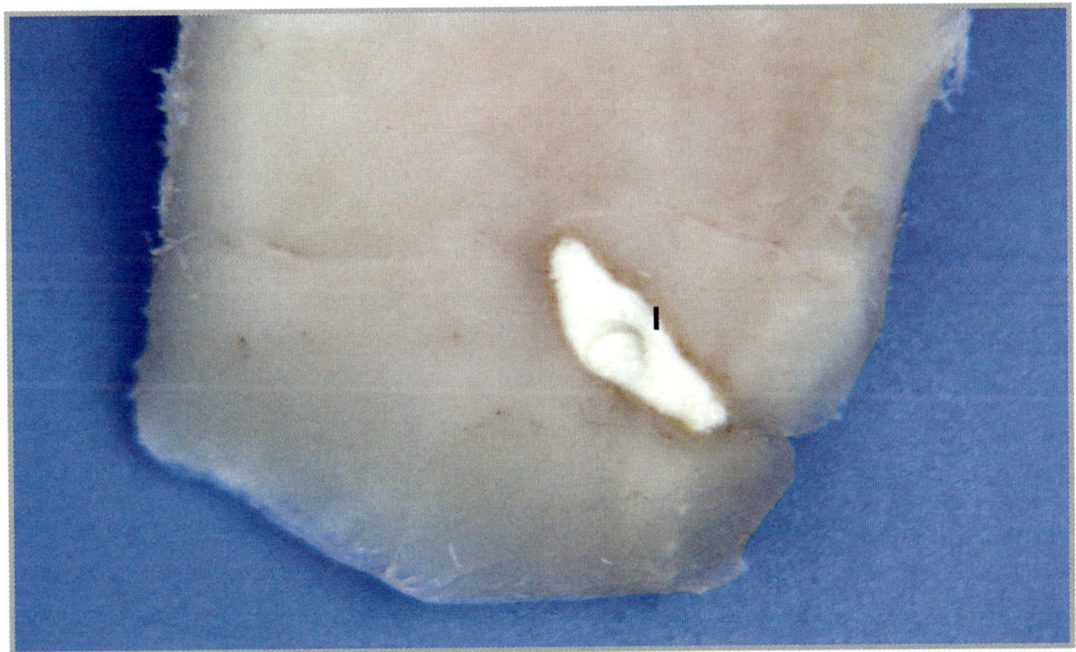

Figure 10 Biodegradable implant (I) in skeletal muscle

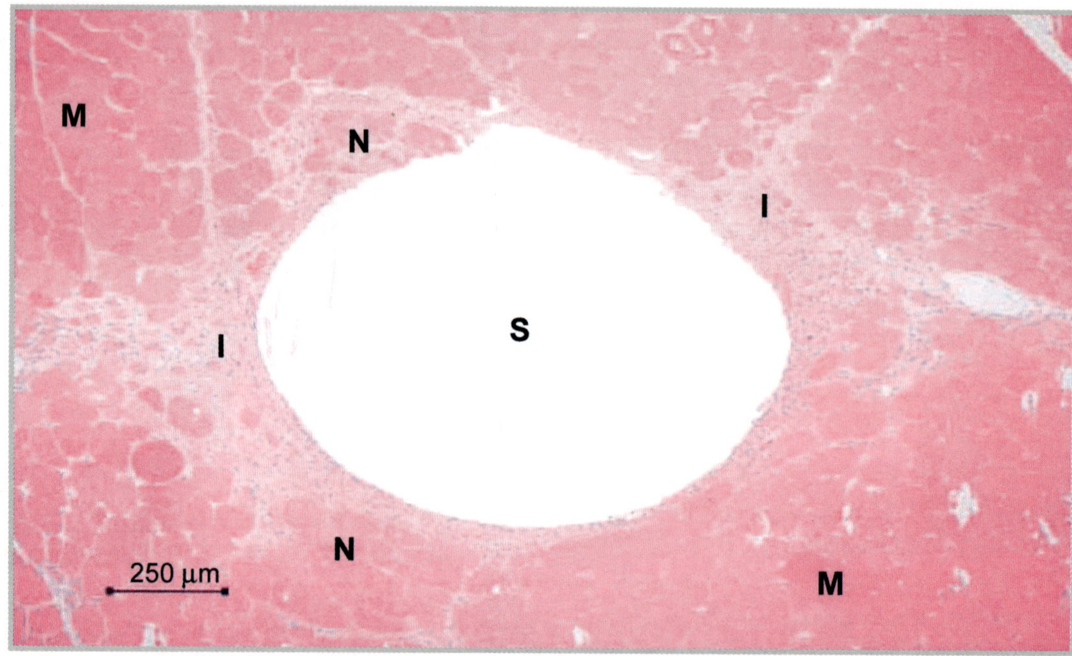

Figure 11 Section of skeletal muscle with implant site. H & E x 4
Implant site (S) in skeletal muscle (M). Necrosis (N) and inflammation (I) is seen adjacent to implant site

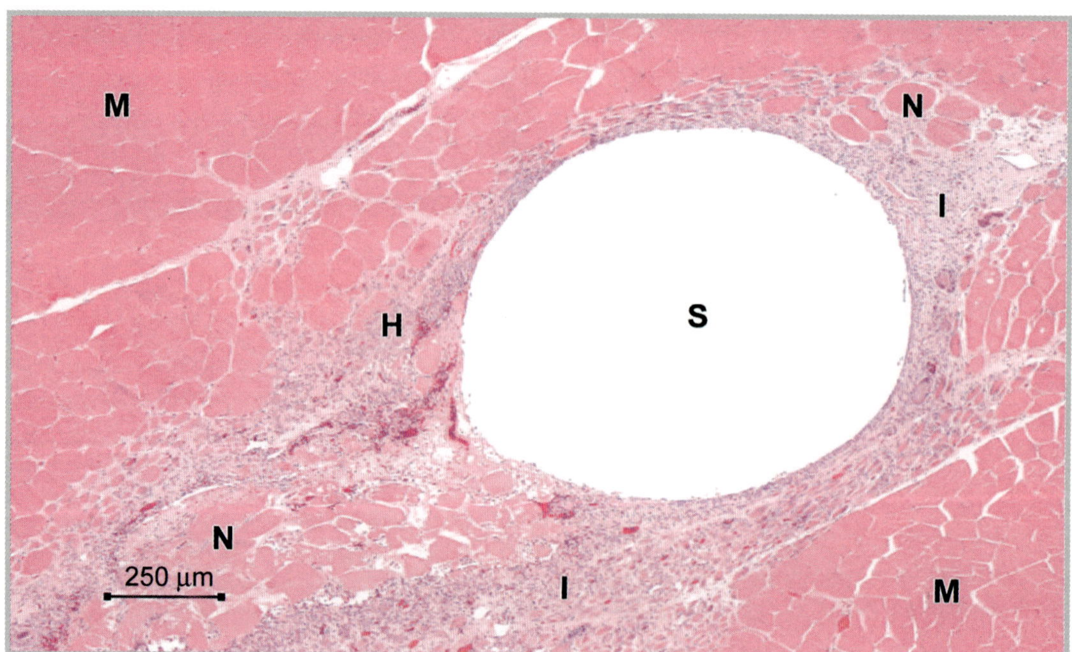

Figure 12 Tissue response to implant. H & E x 4
Necrotic muscle (N), large number of inflammatory cells (I) and fresh hemorrhage (H) seen around the implant site (S). Normal skeletal muscle fibers (M) seen in periphery

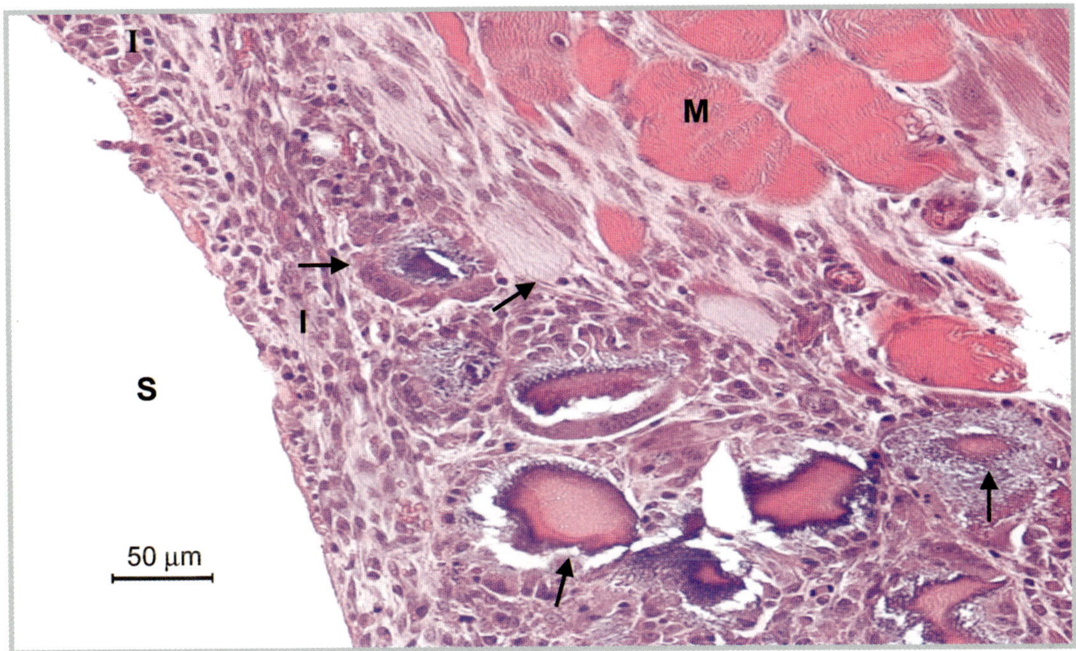

Figure 13 Tissue response to implant. H & E x 20
Necrotic muscle fibers (↑) in different stages of degeneration and different types of inflammatory cells (I) seen around the implant site (S). Normal skeletal muscle fibers (M) seen in periphery

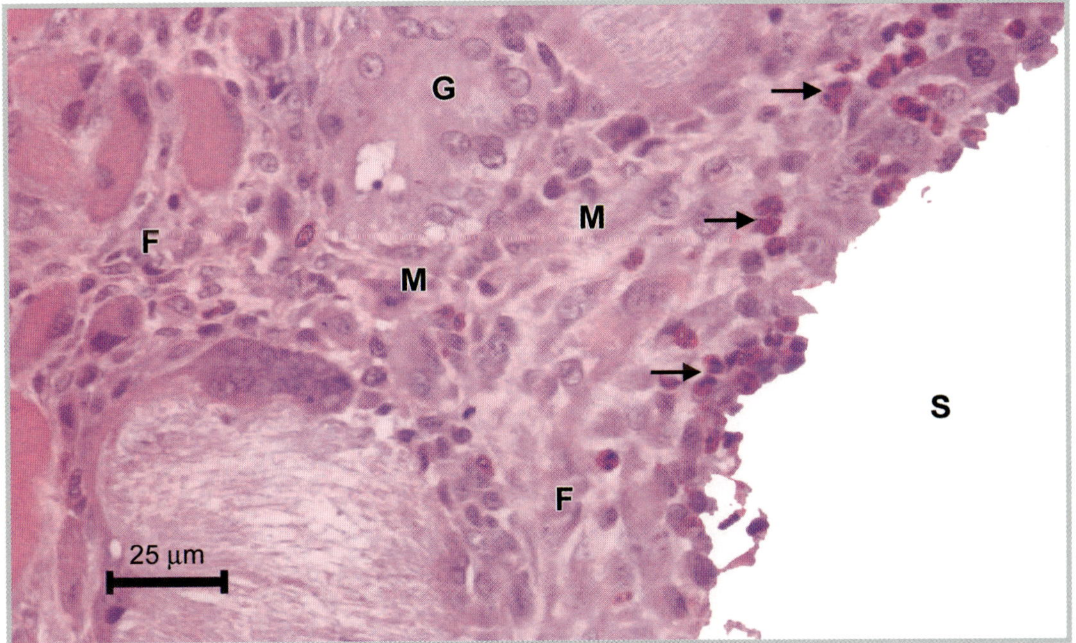

Figure 14 Higher magnification of degenerating muscle fibers H & E x 40
Muscle fiber giant cells (G) with multiple nuclei arranged in periphery. Multinucleated neutrophils (↑) with orangish cytoplasm indicating acute inflammation and large number of macrophages (M) with clear large nuclei and spindle shaped fibroblasts (F) with spindle shaped dark nucleus

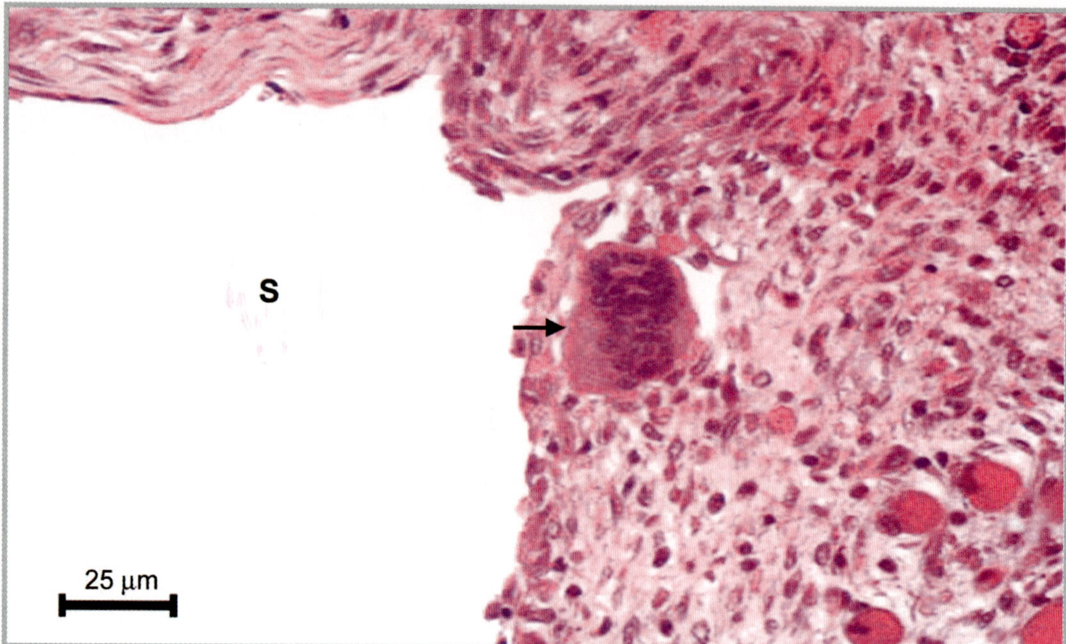

Figure 15 Tissue response to implant. H & E x 40
Large foreign body type of giant cell (↑) with multiple nuclei at implant site (S) — tissue interface

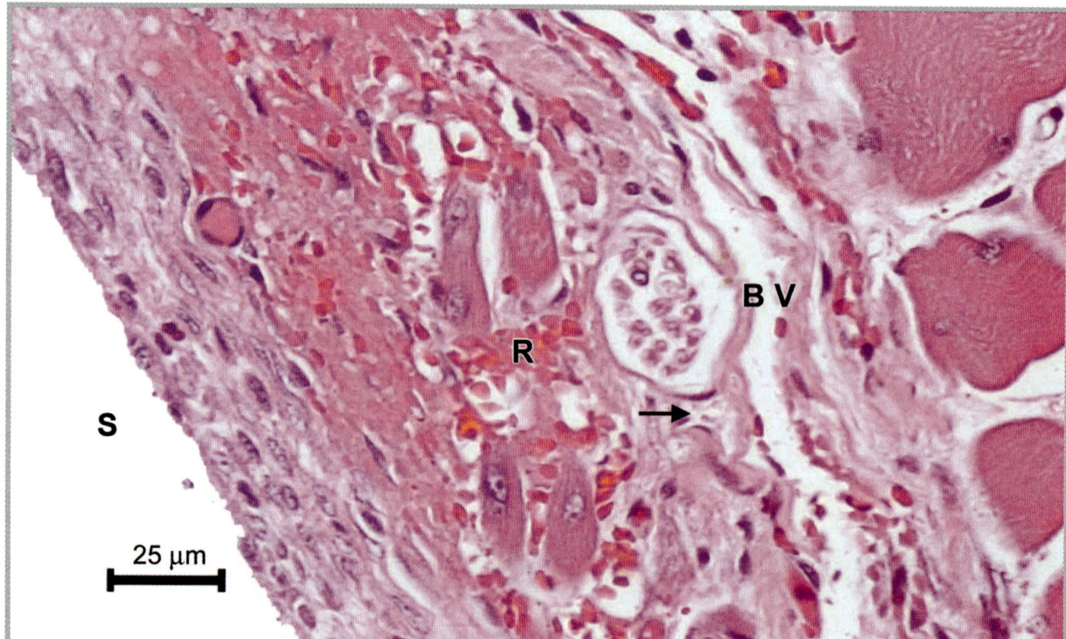

Figure 16 Tissue response to implant. H & E x 40
Red blood cells (R) indicating fresh hemorrhage during explantation, in the extracellular matrix. Small blood vessel (BV) with pericytes (↑) indicating angiogenesis. Pericytes are the external lining cells of small blood vessels. Implant site (S)

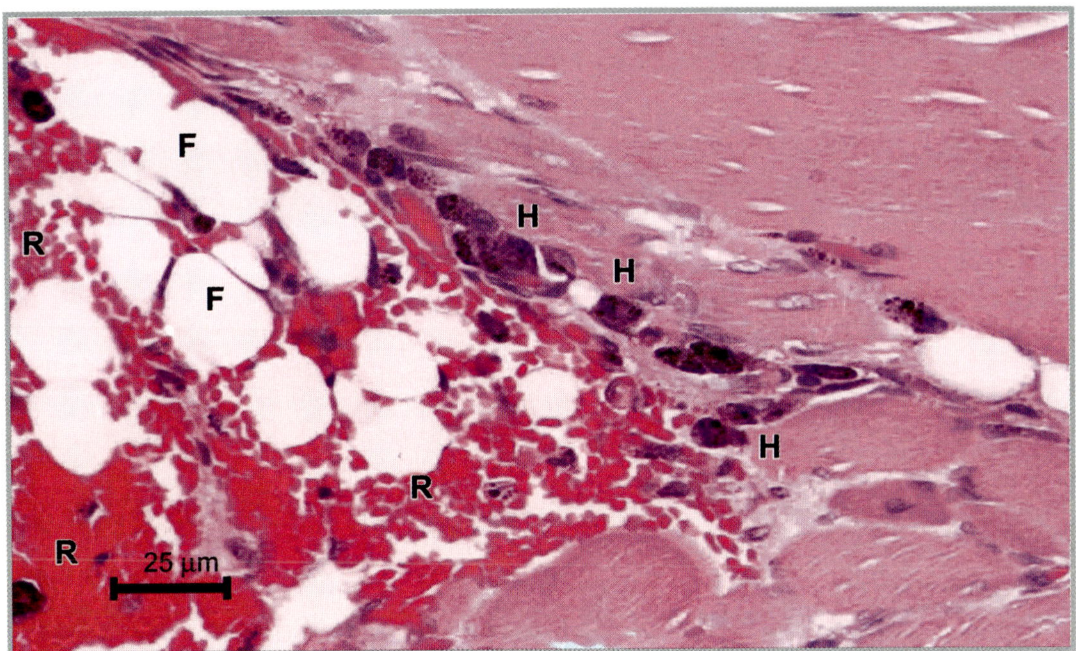

Figure 17 Tissue response to implant. H & E x 40
Hemosiderin laden macrophages (H) indicating old hemorrhage. Fresh hemorrhage (R) and fatty change (F) is also seen

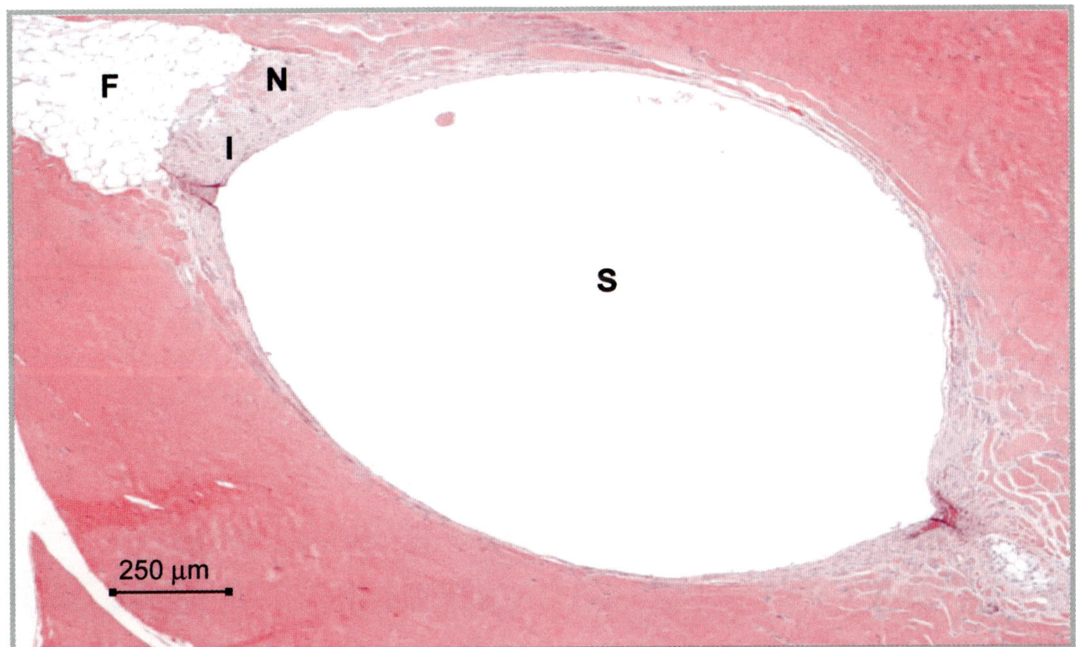

Figure 18 Tissue response to implant. H & E x 4
Fatty change (F) seen in the periphery of necrosis (N) and inflammation (I) around the implant site (S)

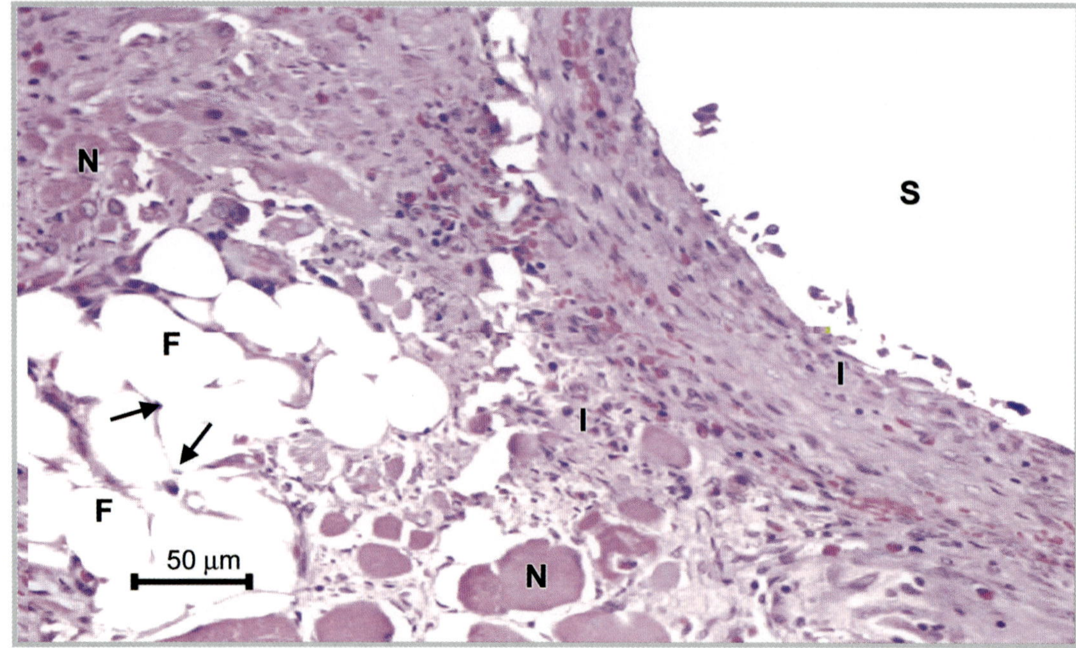

Figure 19 Tissue response to implant. H & E x 20
Fatty change (F) seen in the periphery of necrosis (N) and inflammation (I) around the implant site (S). The fat cell is identified as large clear spaces with small nucleus (↑) in the periphery

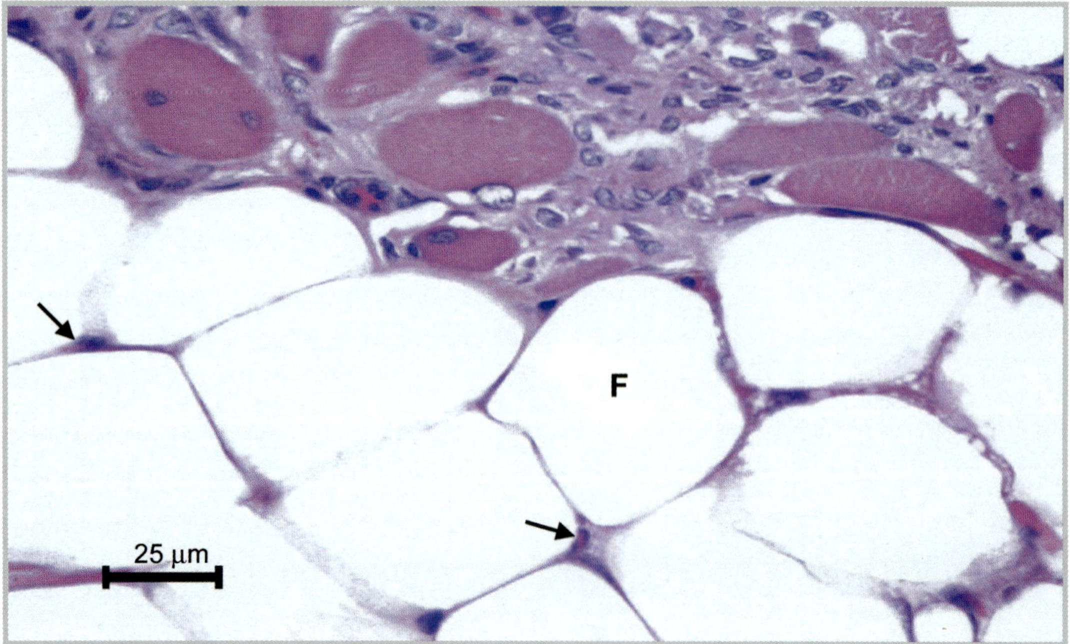

Figure 20 Tissue response to implant. H & E x 40
Higher magnification of fatty change with small nucleus (↑) in the periphery of each fat cell (F). The clear spaces are due to the fat being dissolved in the alcohol during processing of the tissue

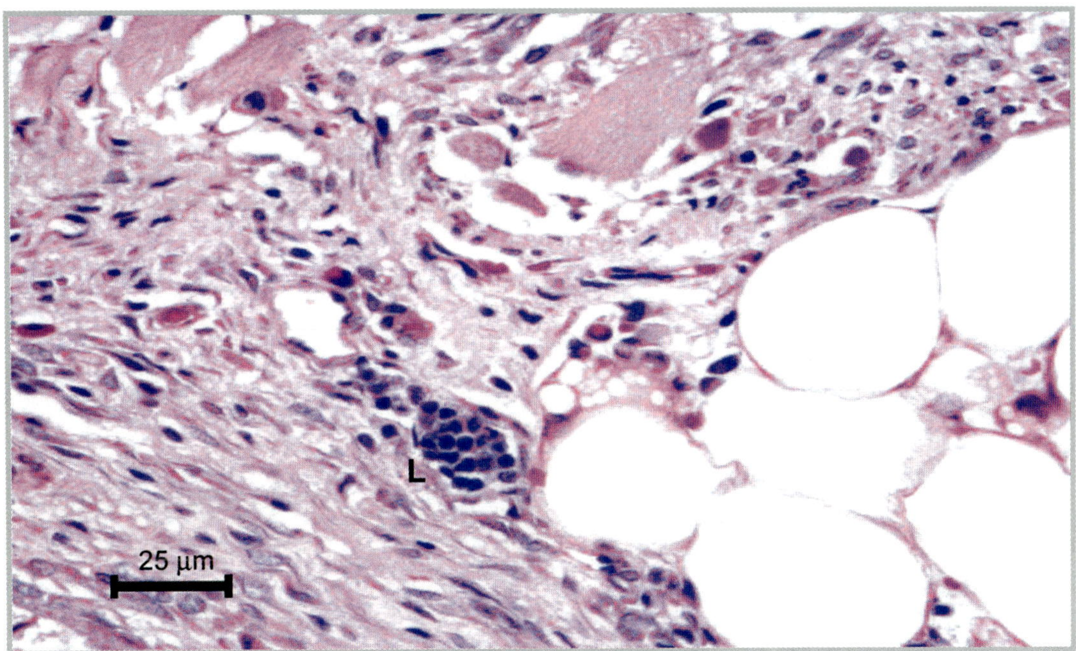

Figure 21 Tissue response to implant. H & E x 40
Collection of lymphocytes (L). Dark nucleus of cells filling-up whole cytoplasm

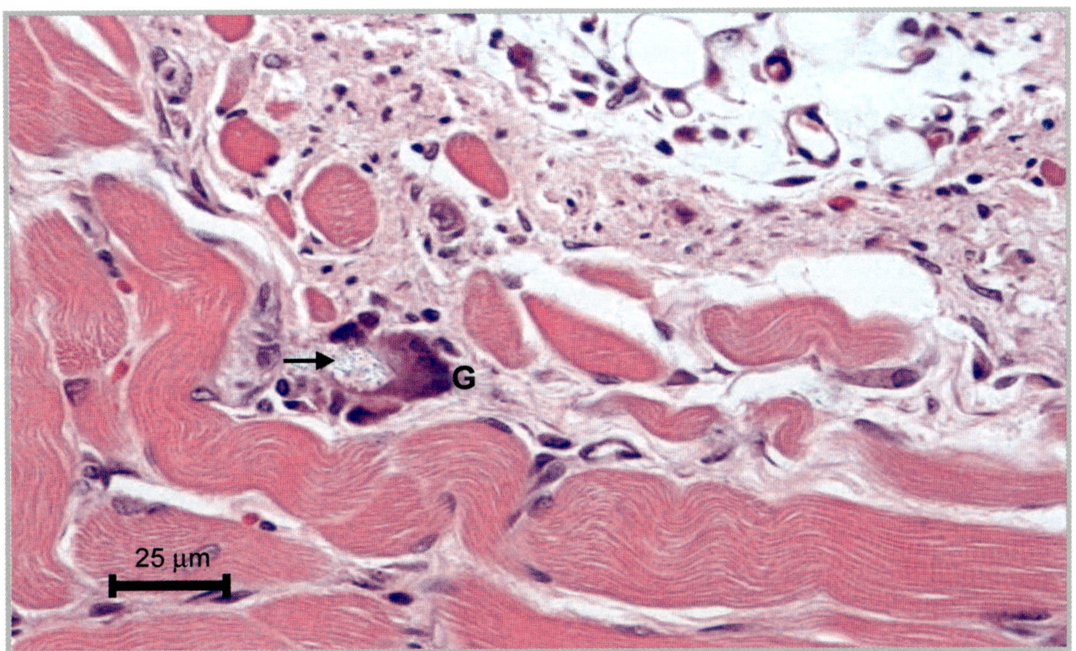

Figure 22 Tissue response to implant. H & E x 40
Giant cell (G) with multiple nuclei and containing foreign body (↑)

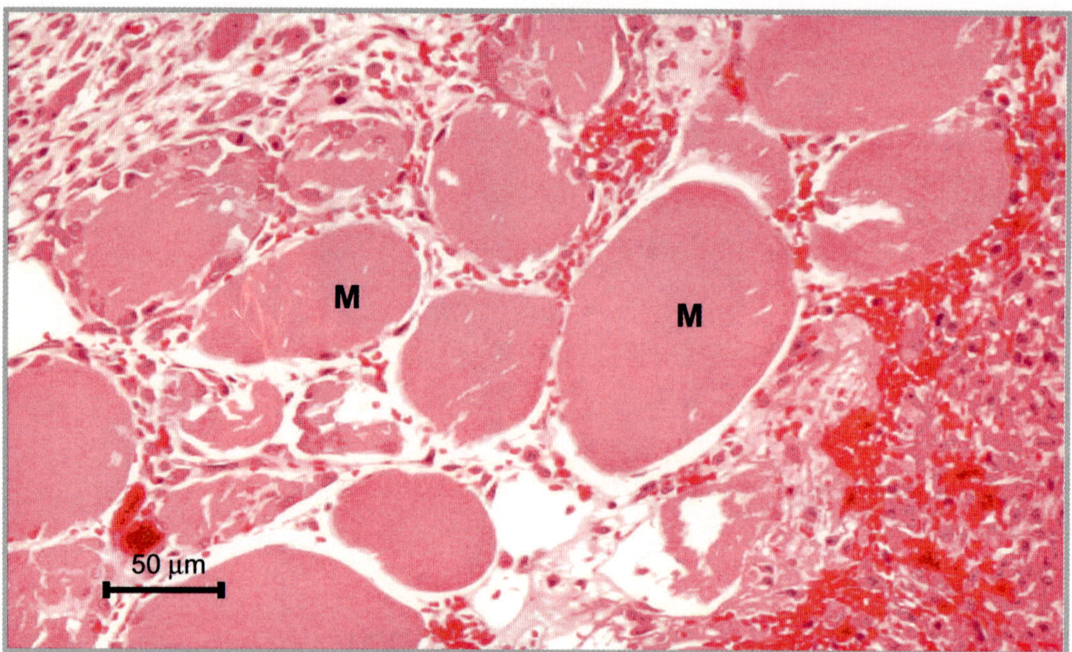

Figure 23A Various facets of necrosis. H & E x 20
Muscle fibers without nucleus (M)

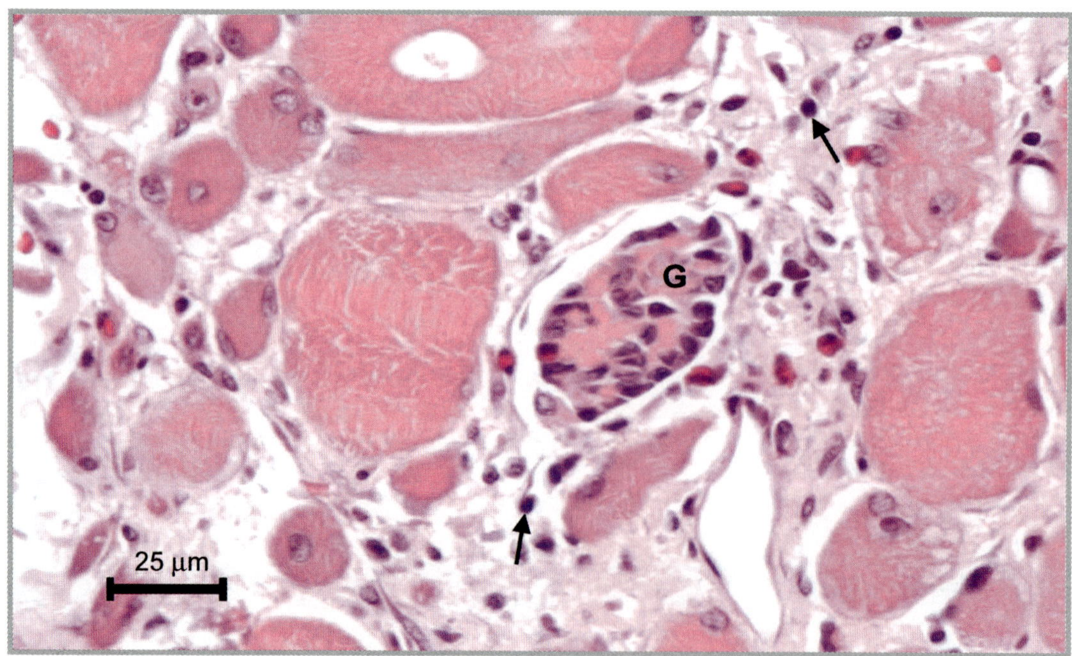

Figure 23B Various facets of necrosis. H & E x 40
Macrophages (↑) and foreign body type of giant cells (G) around individual muscle cells undergoing necrosis

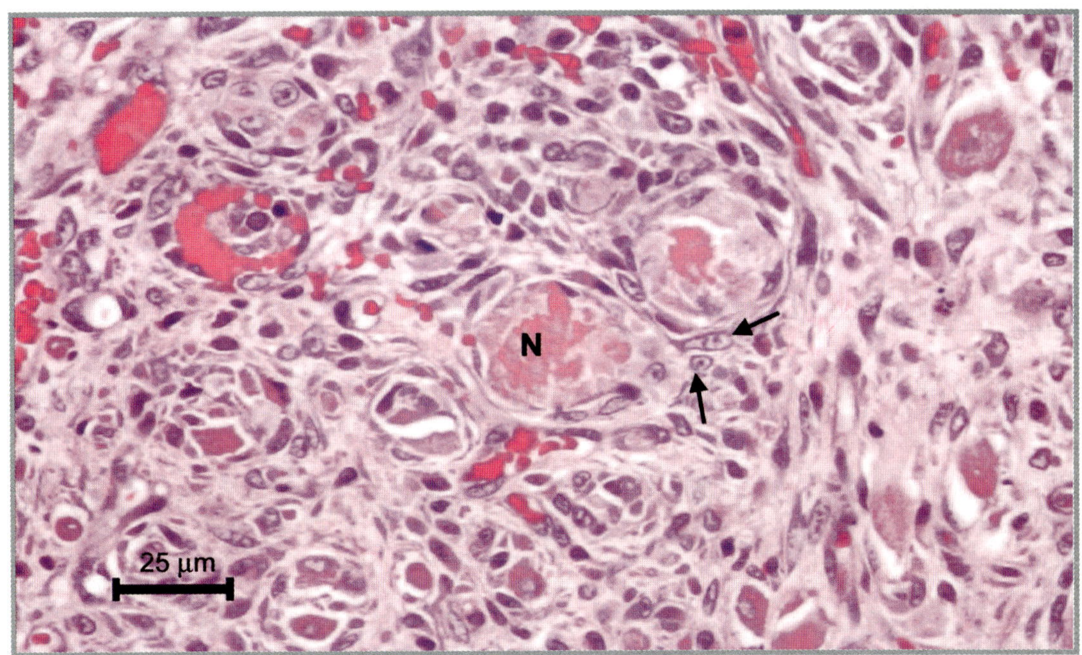

Figure 23C Various facets of necrosis. H & E x 40
Necrotic muscle (N) surrounded by macrophages (↑), both round and spindle shaped

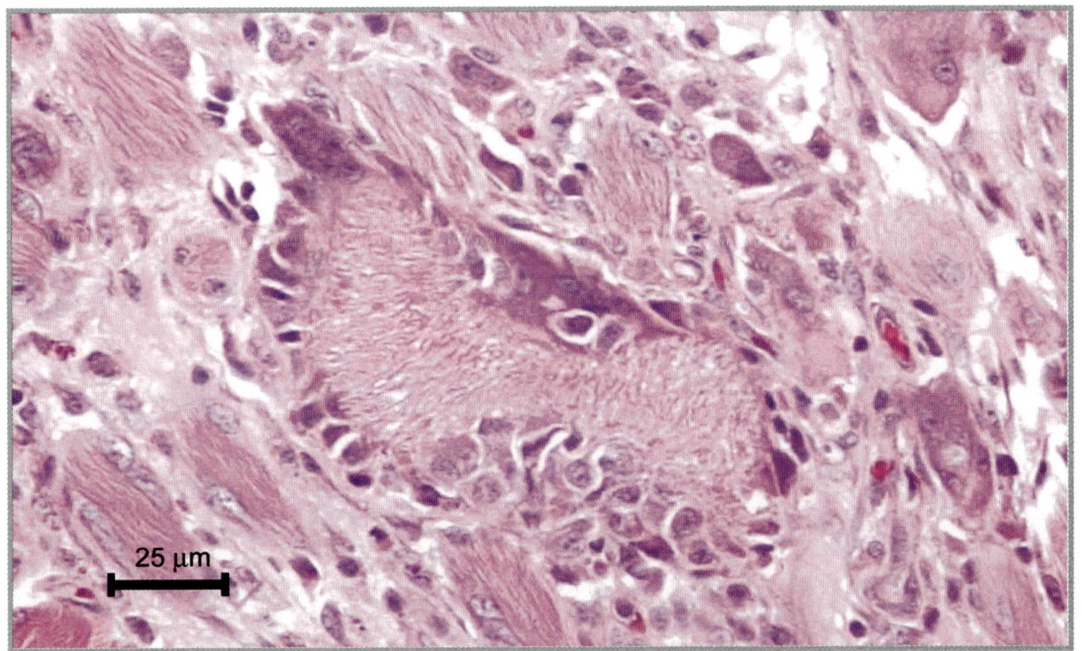

Figure 23D Various facets of necrosis. H & E x 40
Macrophages scavenging degenerating muscle

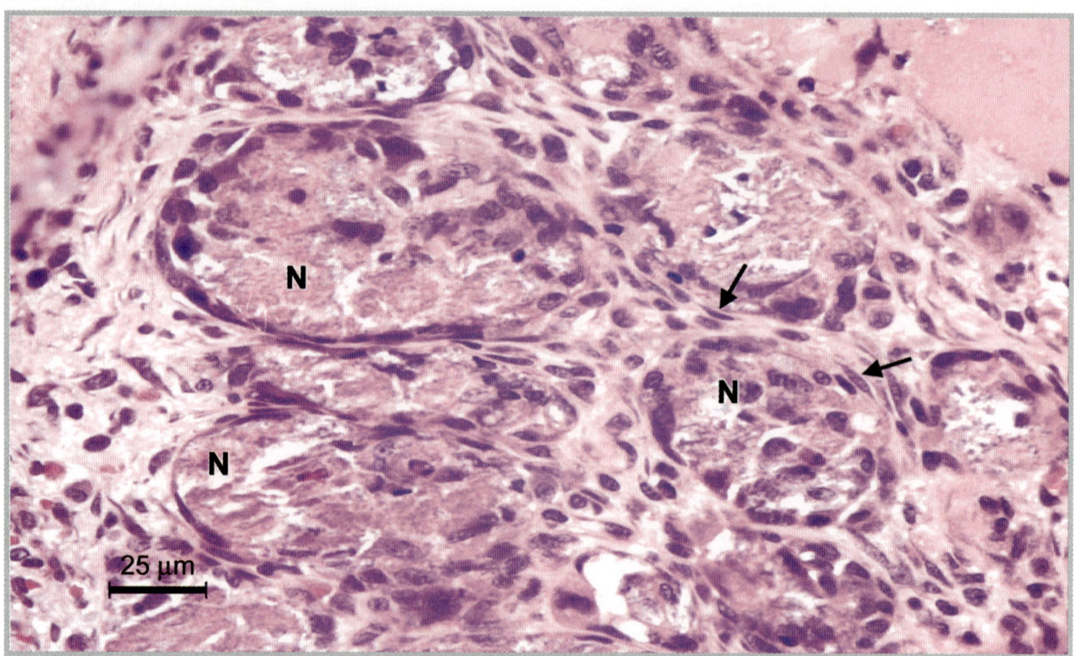

Figure 23E Various facets of necrosis. H & E x 40
Narrow spindle shaped fibrocytes (↑) around necrotic muscle (N)

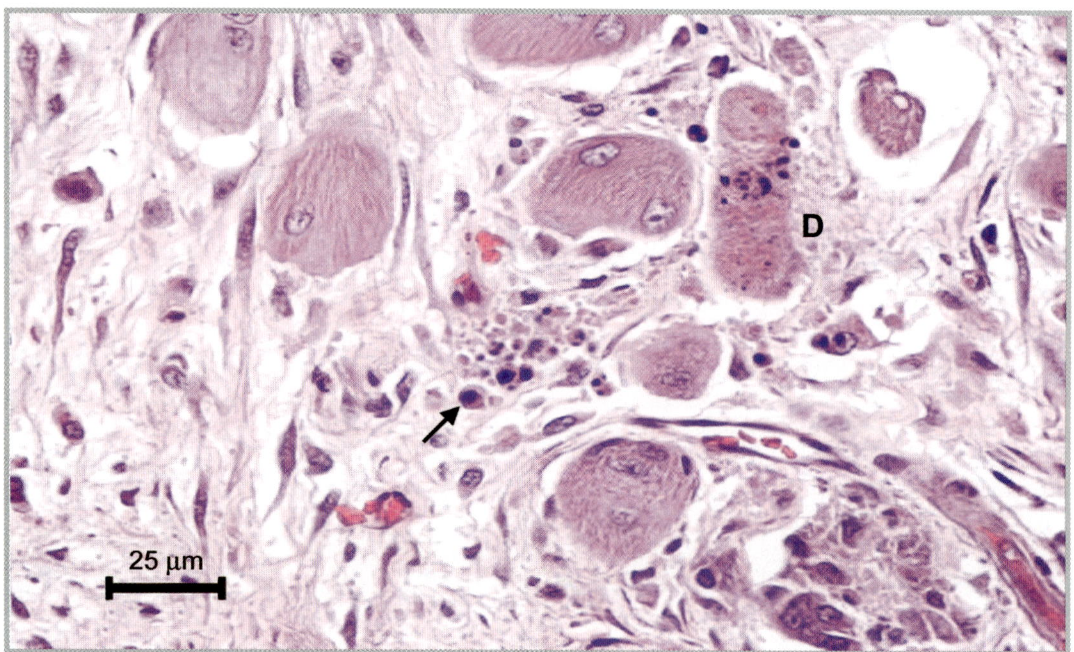

Figure 23F Various facets of necrosis. H & E x 40
Cellular and nuclear debri (D) and apoptotic bodies (↑)

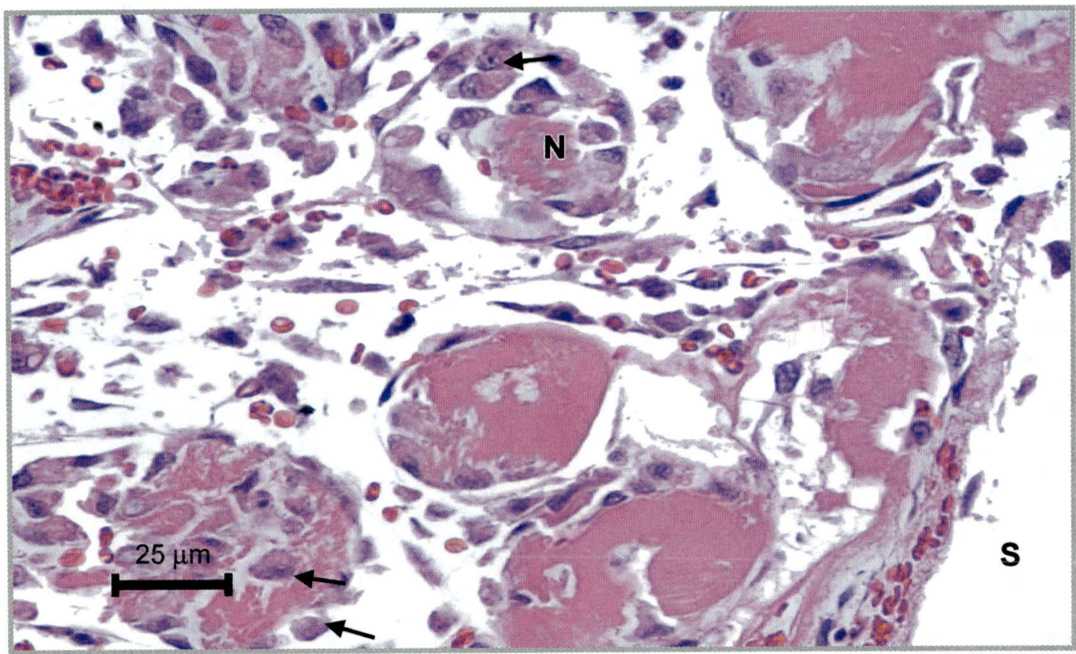

Figure 23G Various facets of necrosis. H & E x 40
Macrophages (↑) around completely scavenged necrotic muscle (N) at implant site (S) muscle interface

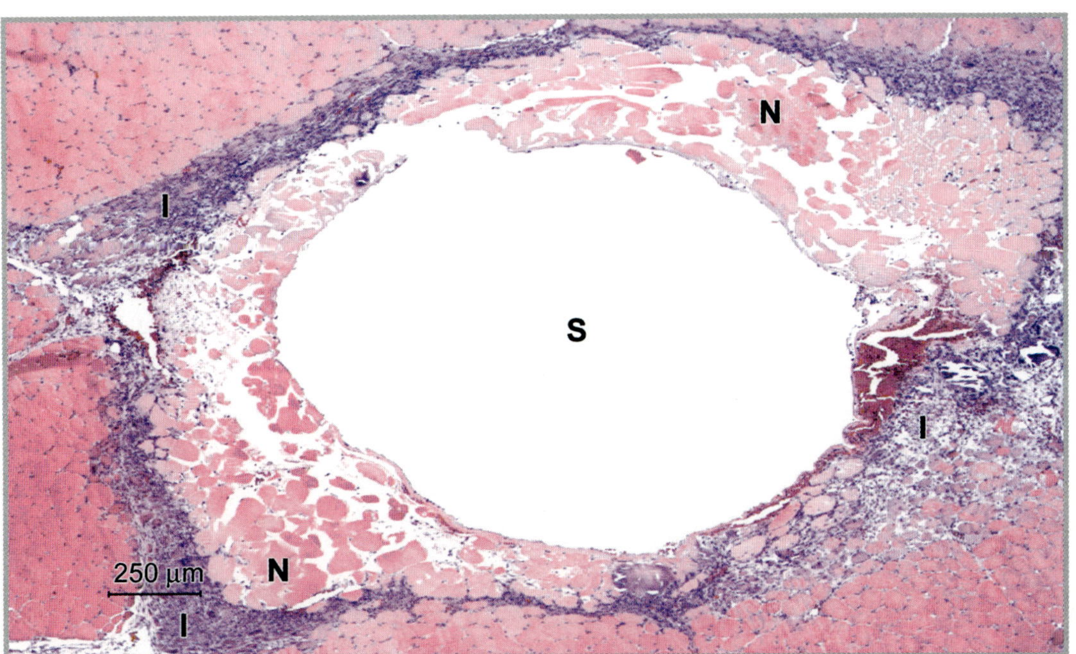

Figure 24 Tissue response to implant. H & E x 4
Severe necrosis (N) and severe inflammation (I) around the implant site (S)

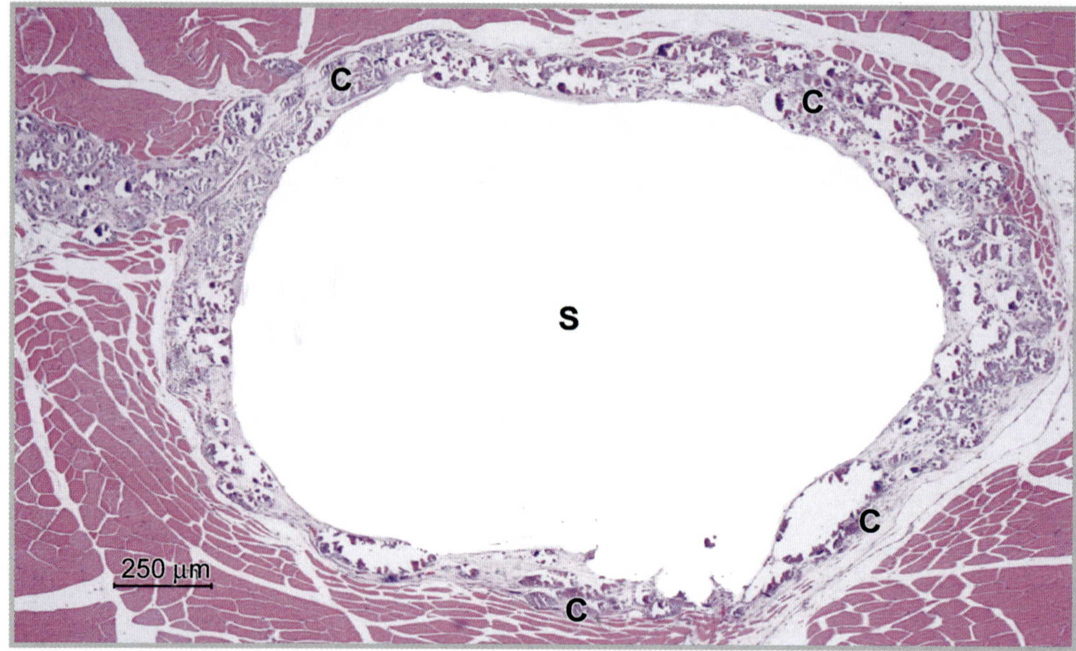

Figure 25 Tissue response to implant. H & E x 4
Deep purple homogenous areas in necrotic tissue indicating foci of calcification (C). Calcification occurs in degenerated or necrotic tissue

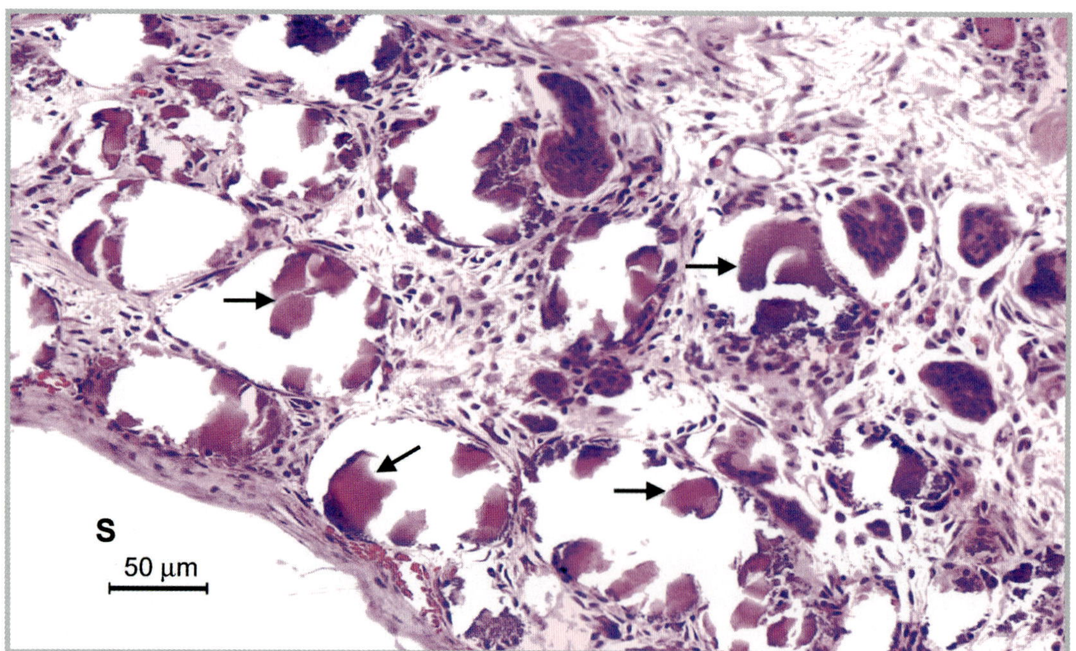

Figure 26A Tissue response to implant. H & E x 20
Higher magnification of calcific foci (↑). Large foreign body type of giant cells are also seen

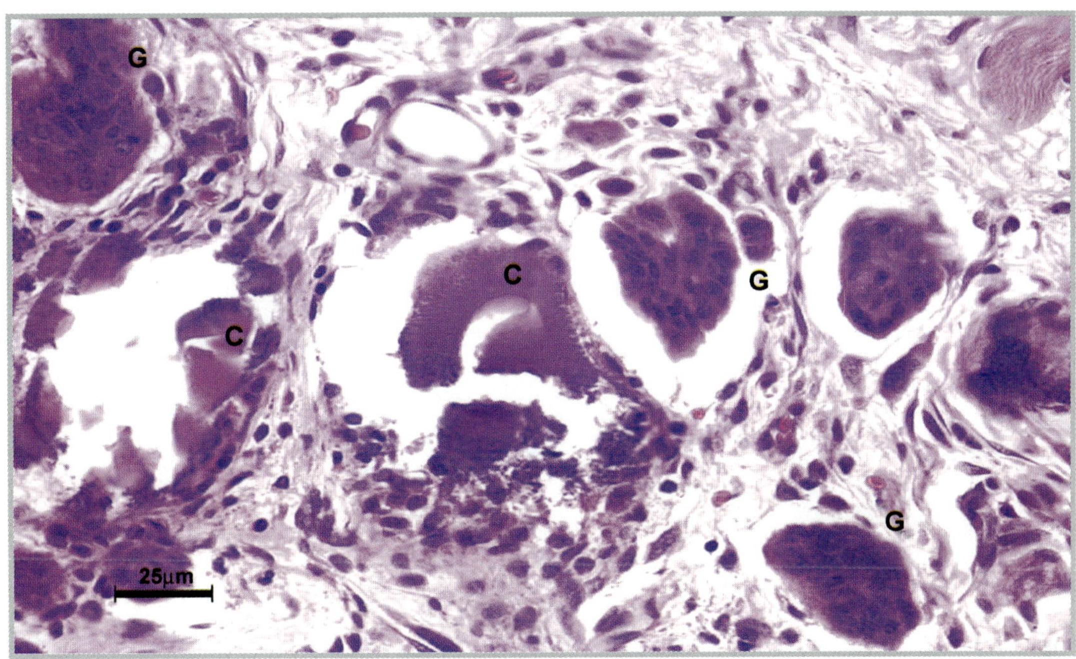

Figure 26B Tissue response to implant. H & E x 40
Large foreign body type of giant cells (G) and calcific foci (C) are seen

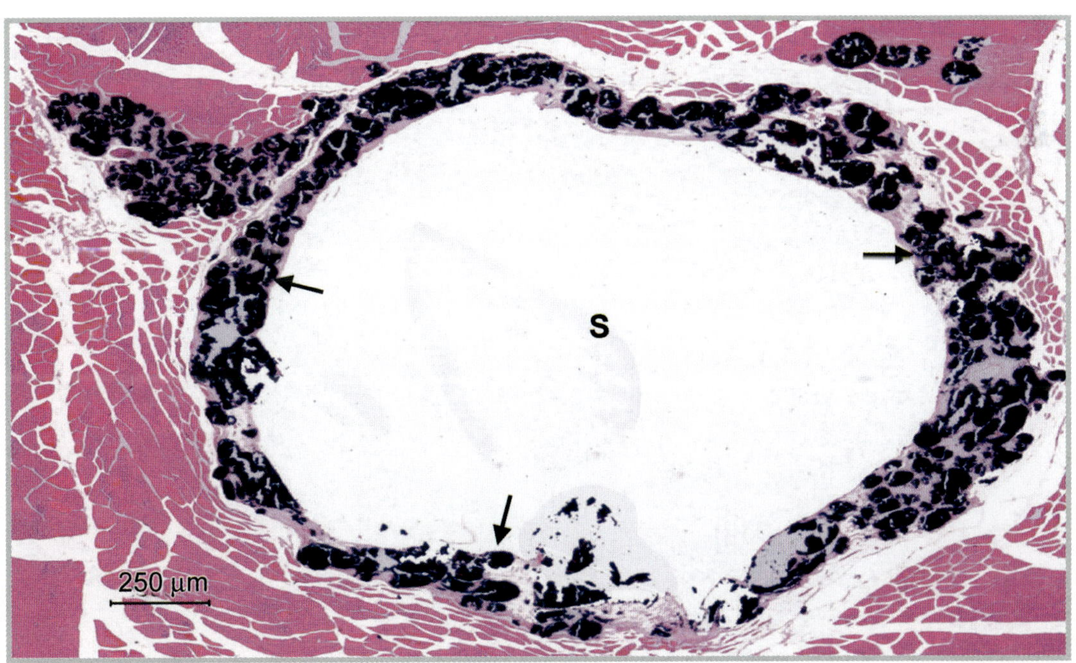

Figure 27A Tissue response to implant. Von Kossa stain x 4
Positive sites of calcification stained black (↑)

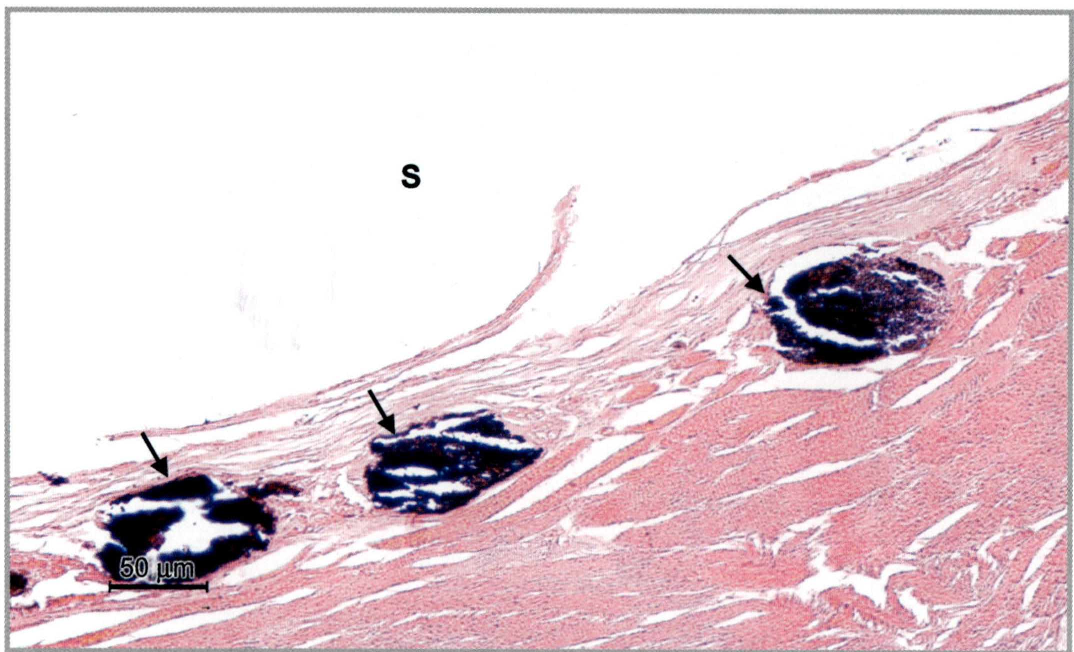

Figure 27B Tissue response to implant. Von Kossa stain x 20
Positive sites of calcification stained black (↑)

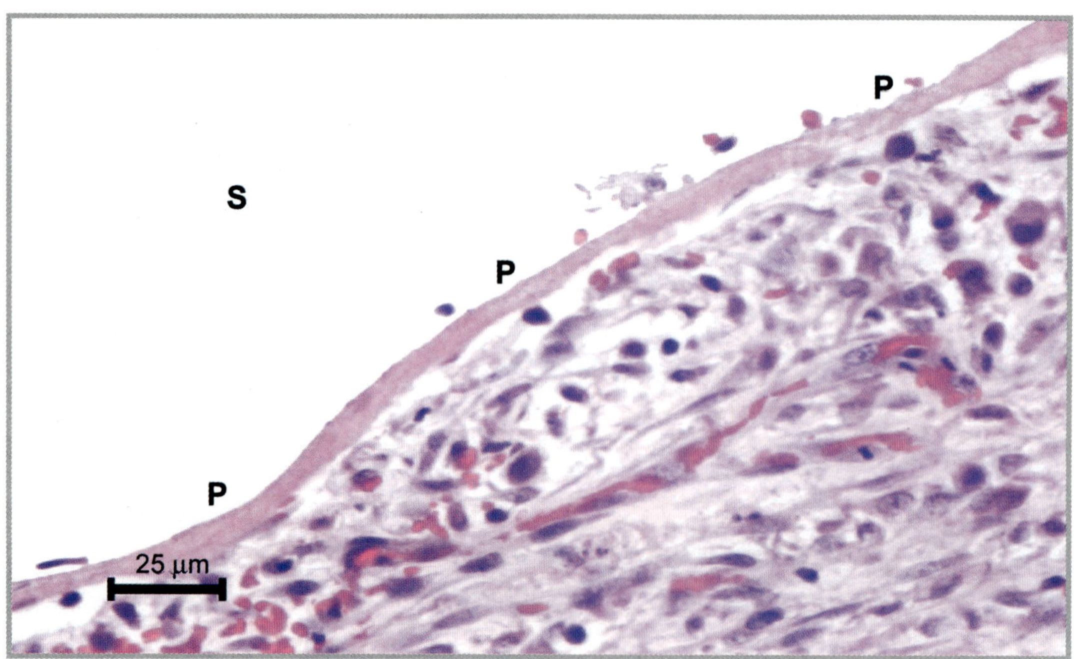

Figure 28 Tissue response to implant. H & E x 40
Thin proteinaceous layer (P) at implant site (S) — tissue interface

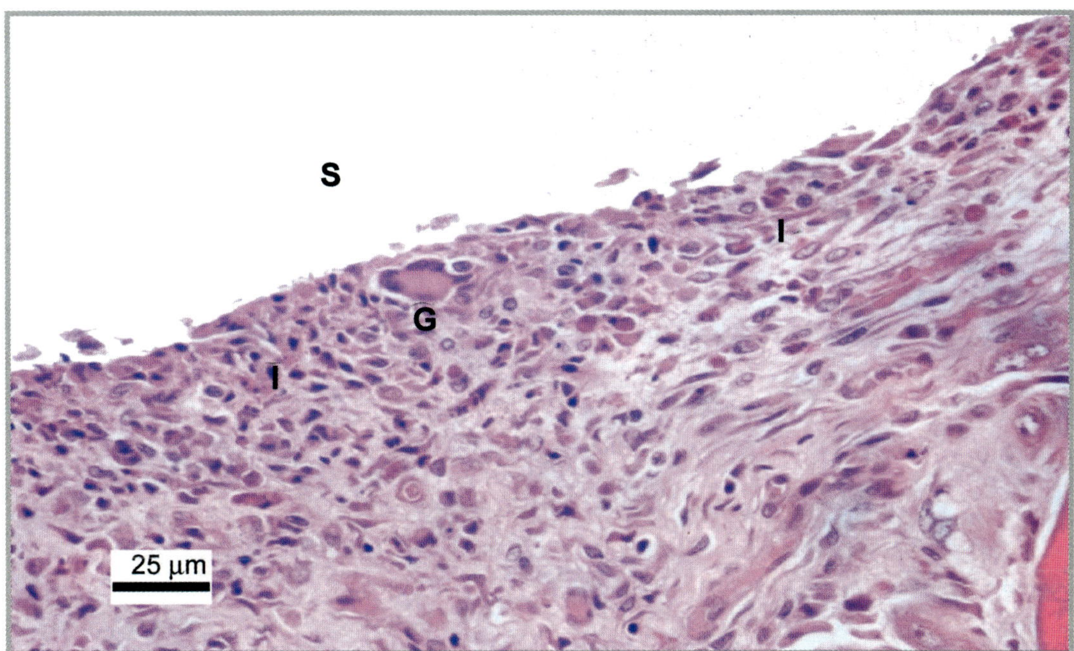

Figure 29 Tissue response to implant. H & E x 40
Inflammatory cells (I) adjacent to implant site (S). Macrophages, lymphocytes, fibroblasts and foreign body type of giant cells (G) are seen

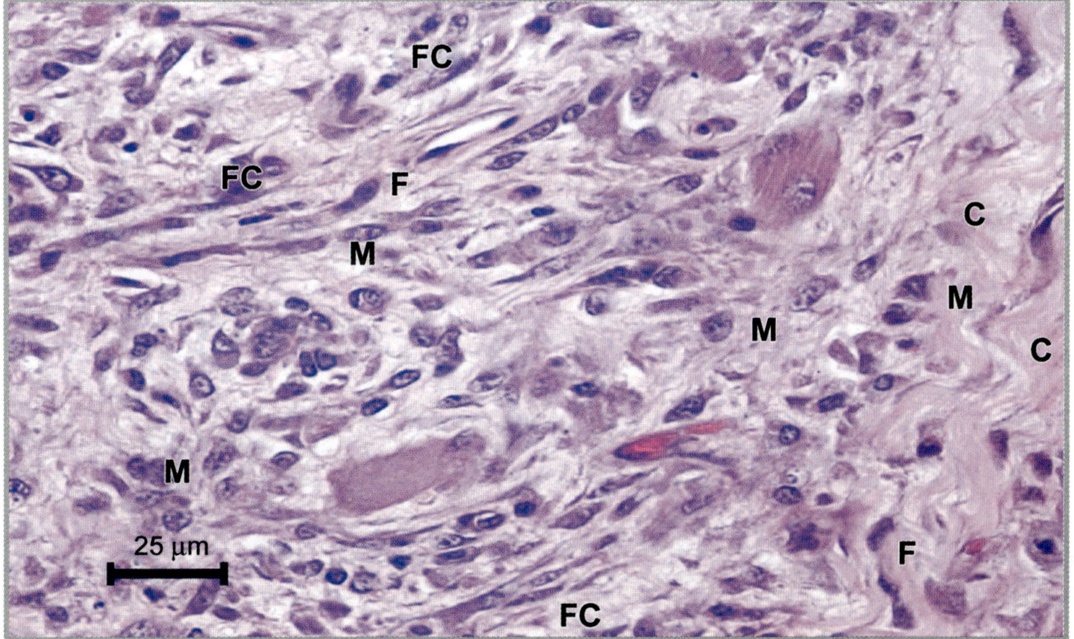

Figure 30 Tissue response to implant. H & E x 40
Macrophages (M) are identified as large cells with clear nucleus with little cytoplasm. Spindle shaped plump cells with a clear nucleus (F) are fibroblasts which mature into fibrocytes (FC) which are narrower with a dark nucleus. Collagen laid down (C)

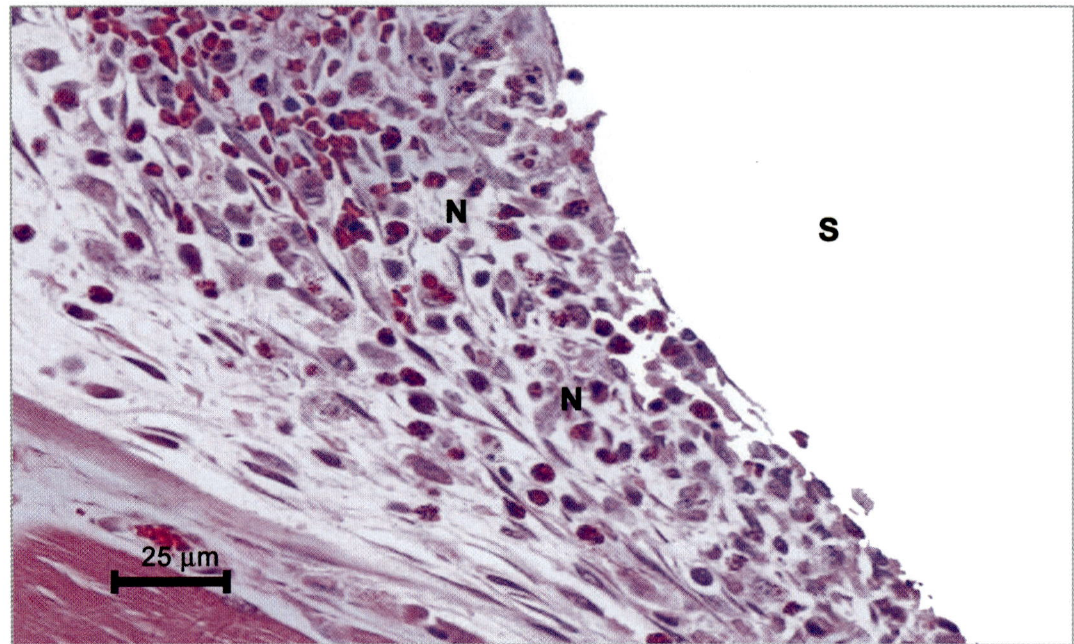

Figure 31 Tissue response to implant. H & E x 40
Inflammatory cells neutrophils (N) adjacent to implant site (S). Cells are deep pink with multilobed dark nucleus

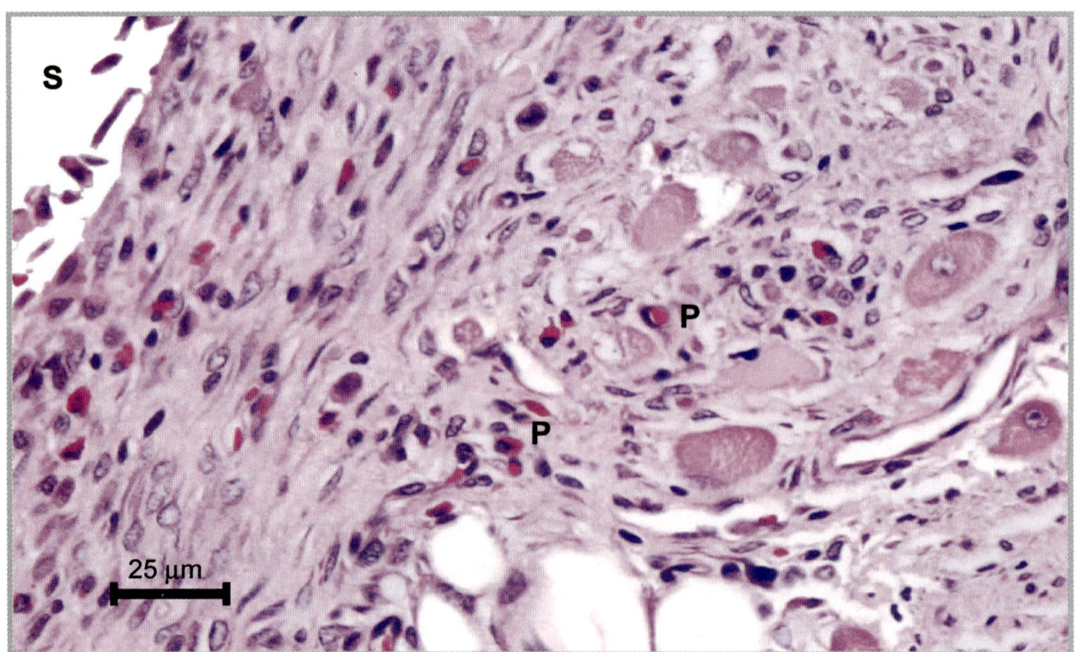

Figure 32 Tissue response to implant. H & E x 40
Plasma cells (P) adjacent to implant site. Cells are deep orange-pink with single dark nucleus which is eccentrically placed

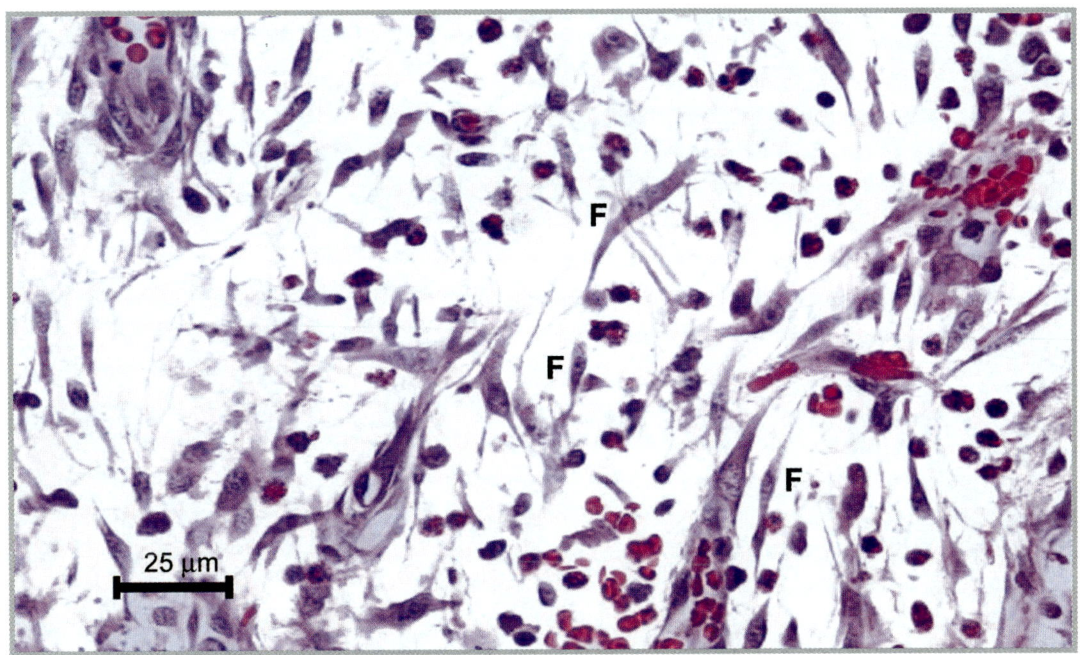

Figure 33 Tissue response to implant. H & E x 40
Active fibroblasts with pseudopods (F) adjacent to implant site

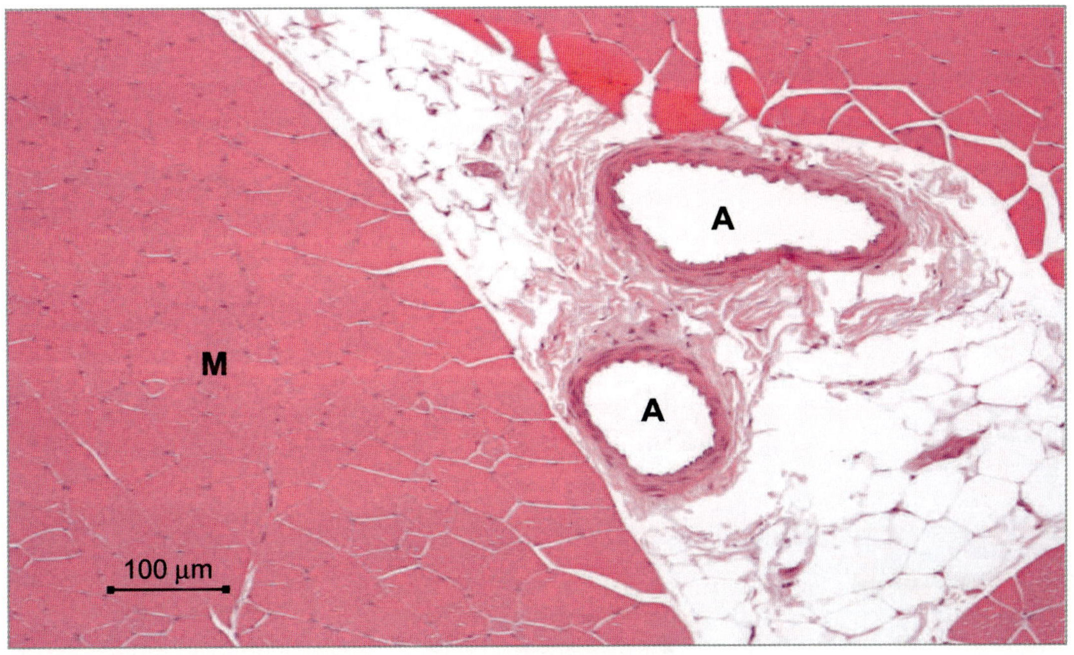

Figure 34 Normal skeletal muscle. H & E x 10
Cross-section of skeletal muscle fibers (M) and arterioles (A)

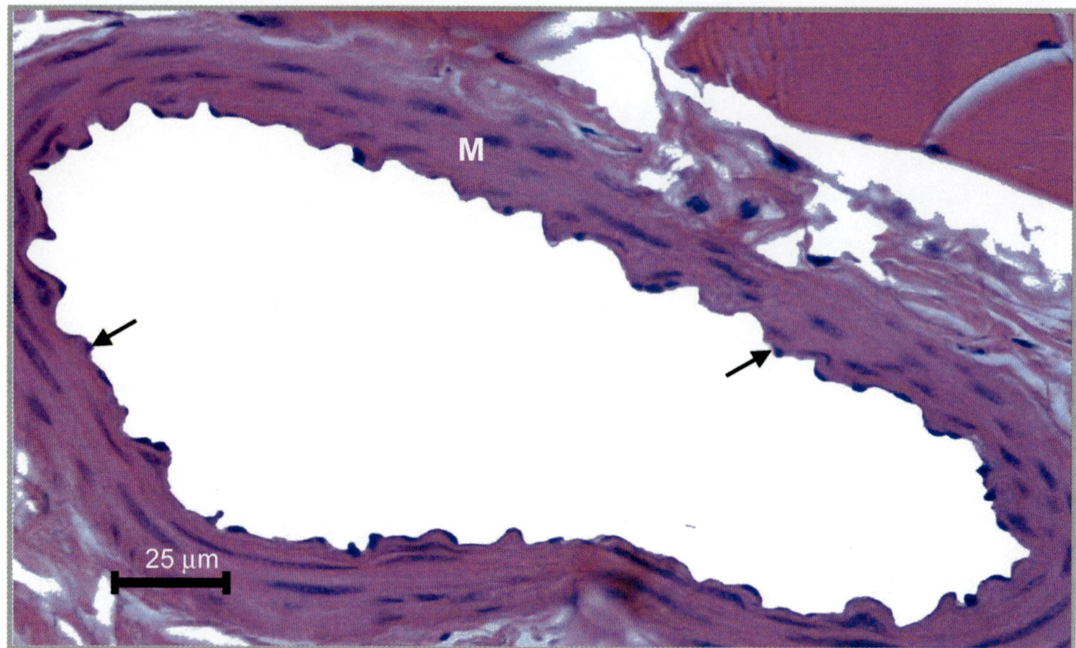

Figure 35 Blood vessels H & E x 40
Arteriole with endothelial cells (↑) in the innermost layer (intima) lining the blood vessel and smooth muscle layer (media) with smooth muscle cells (M)

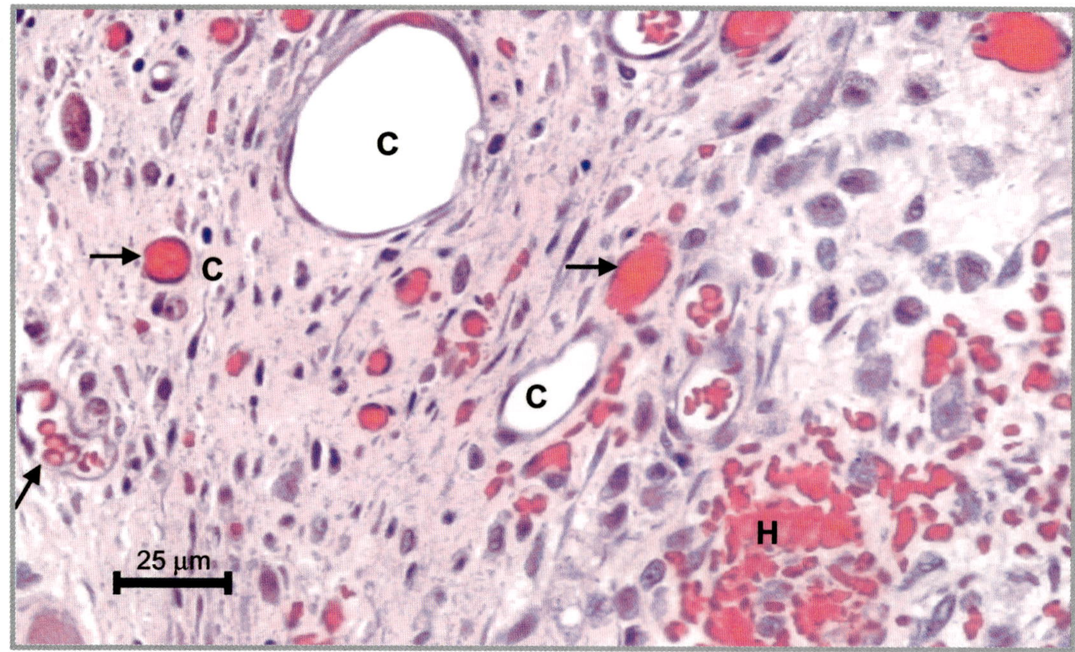

Figure 36A Blood vessels capillaries. H & E x 40
Numerous small new blood vessels (capillaries, C) with flattened endothelial cells. Red blood cells (↑) in the lumen of the capillaries indicating congestion and in the extracellular matrix indicating fresh hemorrhage (H) are also present

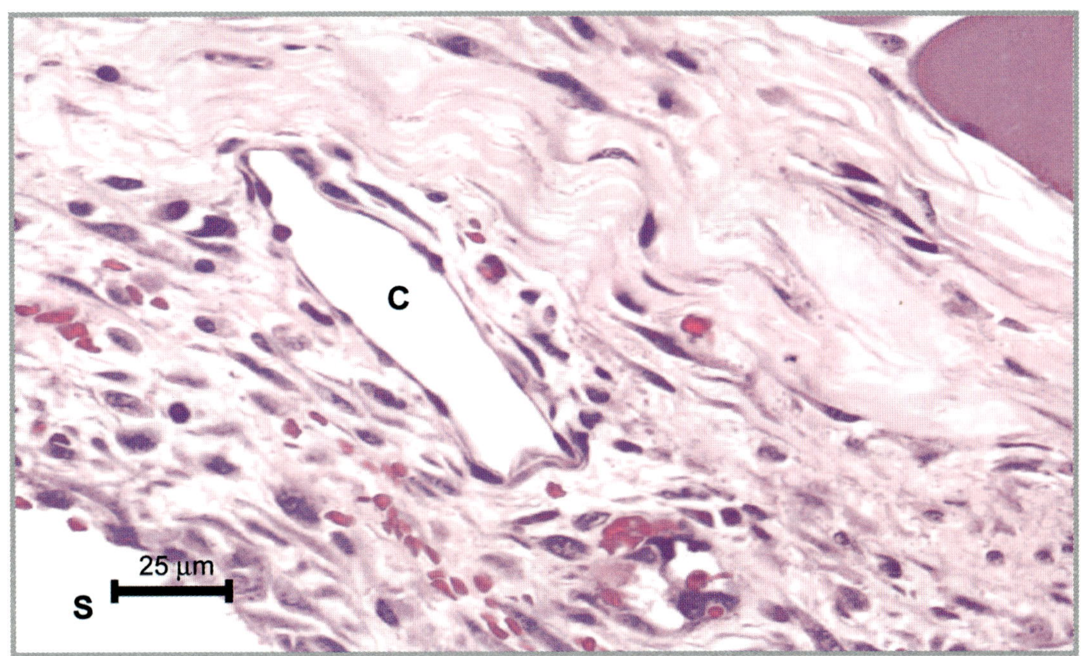

Figure 36B Blood vessels capillaries. H & E x 40
New blood vessels (C) with flattened endothelial cells

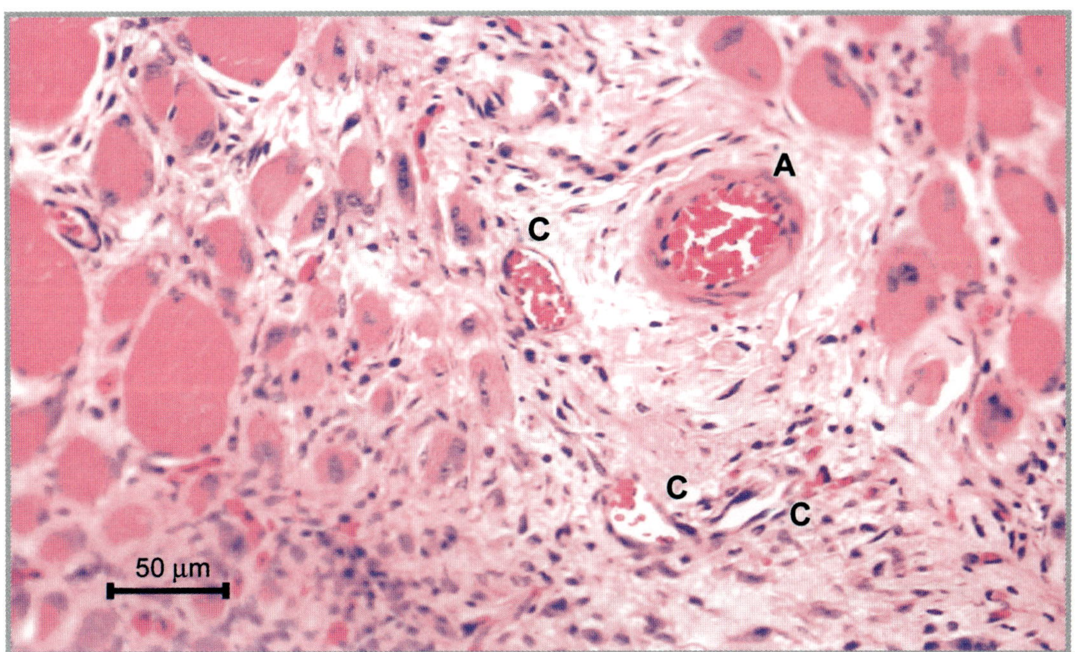

Figure 37 Blood vessels H & E x 20
Arteriole (A) and capillary (C)

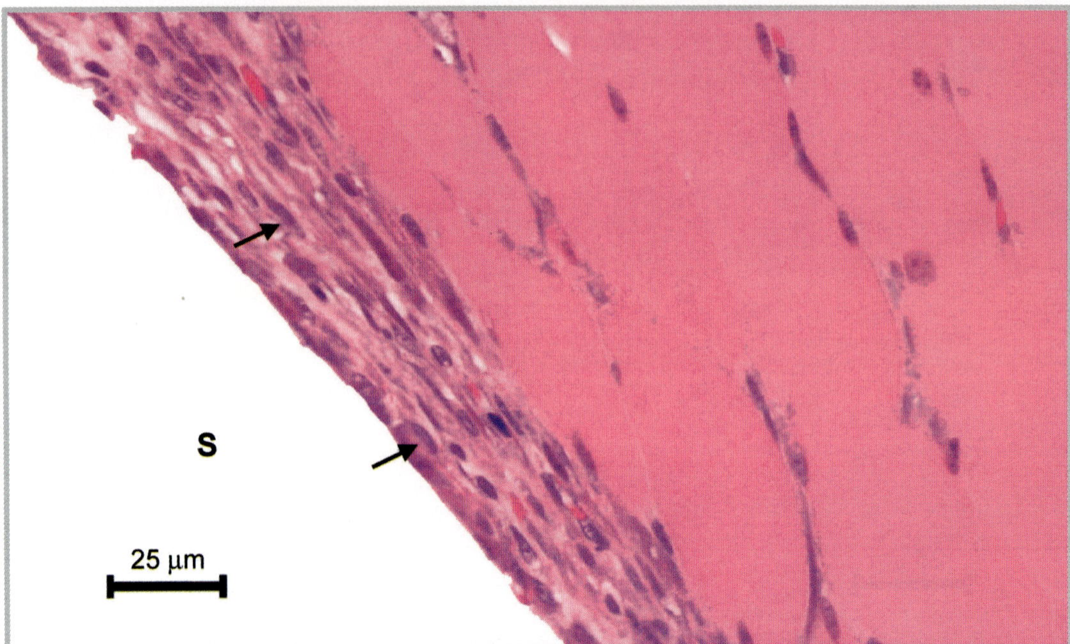

Figure 38 Tissue response to implant. H & E x 40
Thick fibrous capsule with fibroblasts and fibrocytes (↑) adjacent to implant site (S). Note absence of inflammatory cells

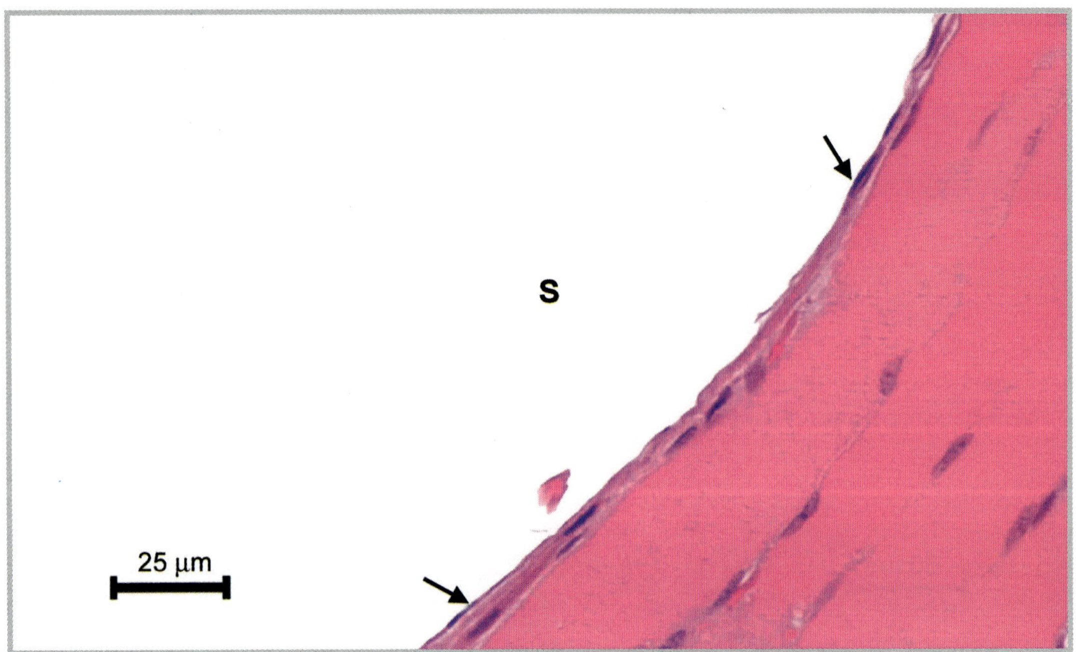

Figure 39A Tissue response to implant. H & E x 40
Thin fibrous capsule with fibrocytes (↑) adjacent to implant site (S)

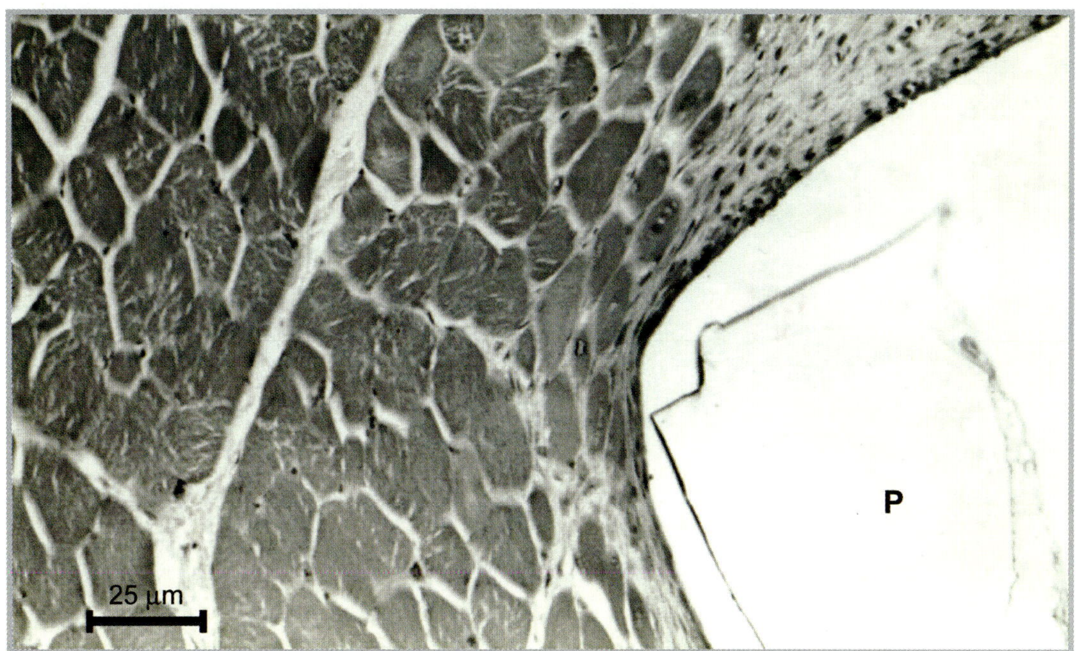

Figure 39B Tissue response to implant. H & E x 40
Cross-section of polymer implant (P). Sections cut along with implant prior to processing

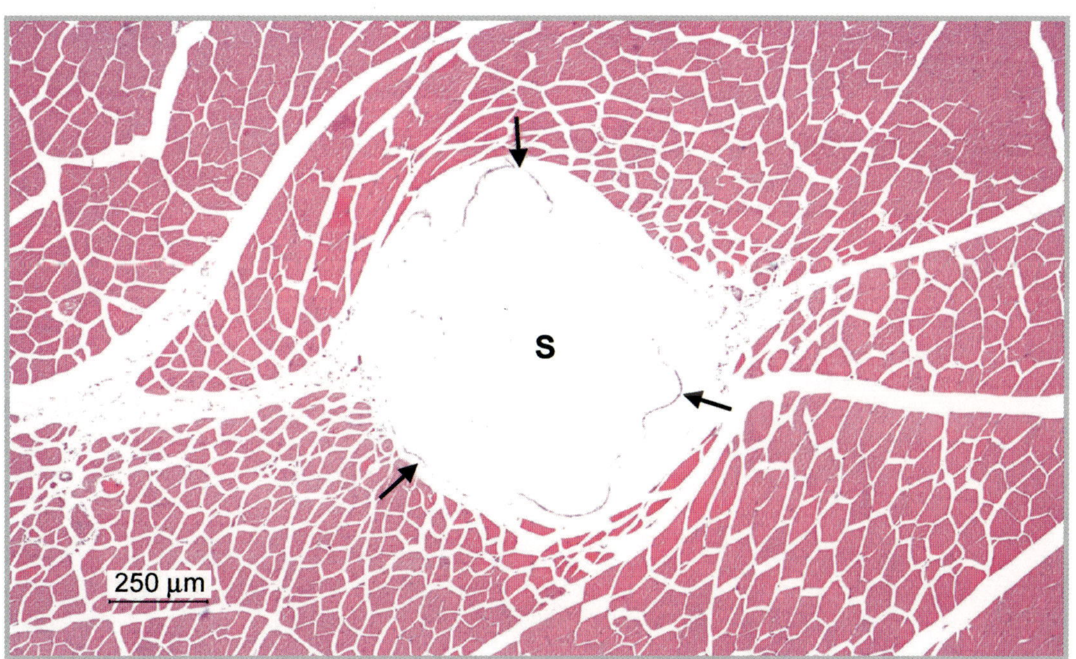

Figure 40A Tissue response to implant. H & E x 4
Thin collagenous capsule (↑) around implant site (S). No fibrocytes seen. Only collagen

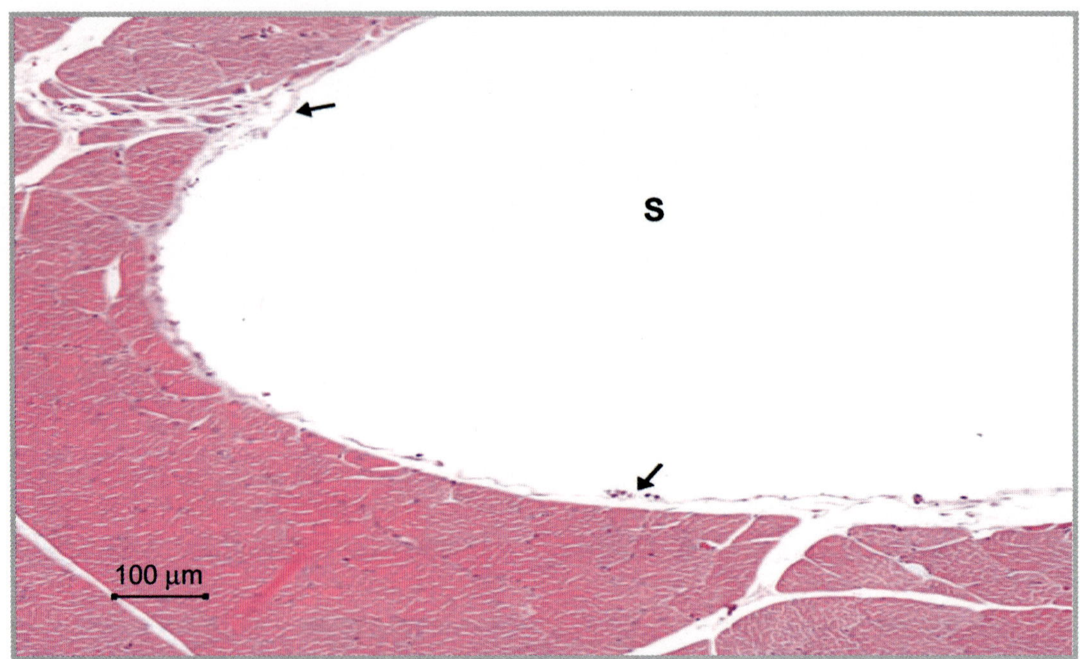

Figure 40B Tissue response to implant. H & Ex 10
Thin collagenous capsule (↑) around implant site (S). No fibrocytes seen. Only collagen

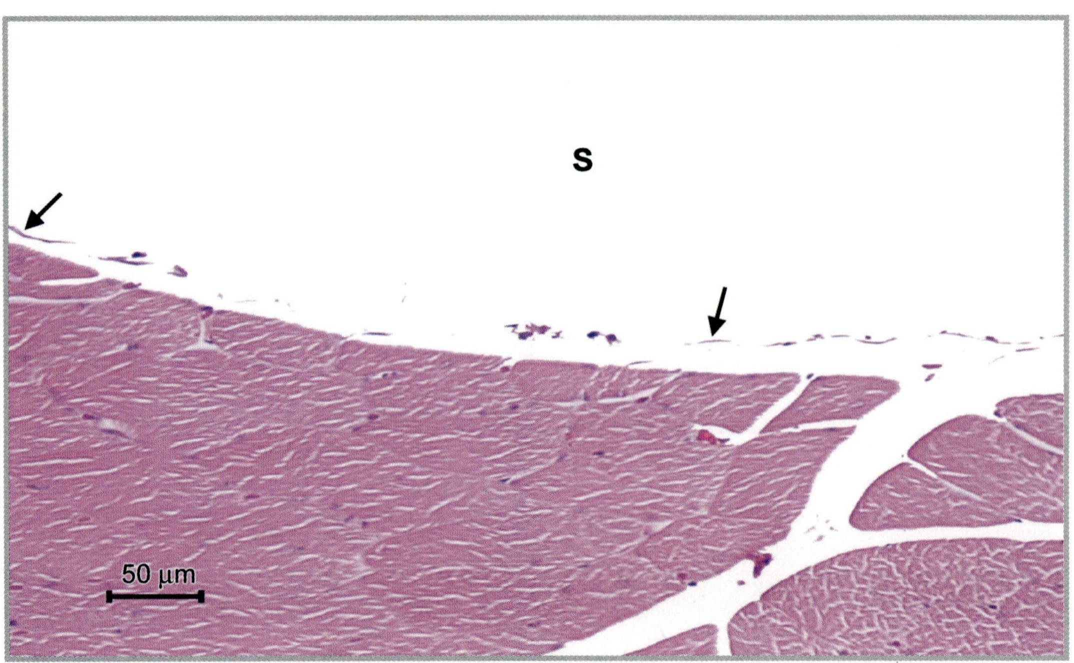

Figure 40C Tissue response to implant. H & E x 20
Thin collagenous capsule (↑) around implant site (S). No fibrocytes seen. Only collagen

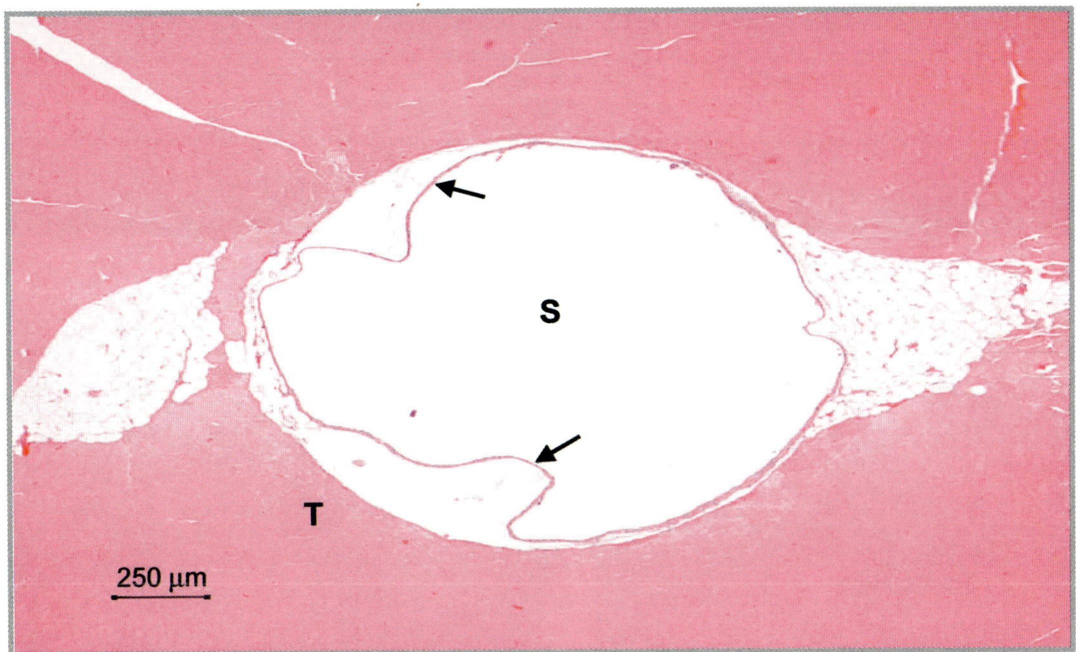

Figure 41 Tissue response to implant. H & E x 4
Thin collagenous capsule (↑) around implant site (S) dislodged from adjacent tissue (T) during removal of implant

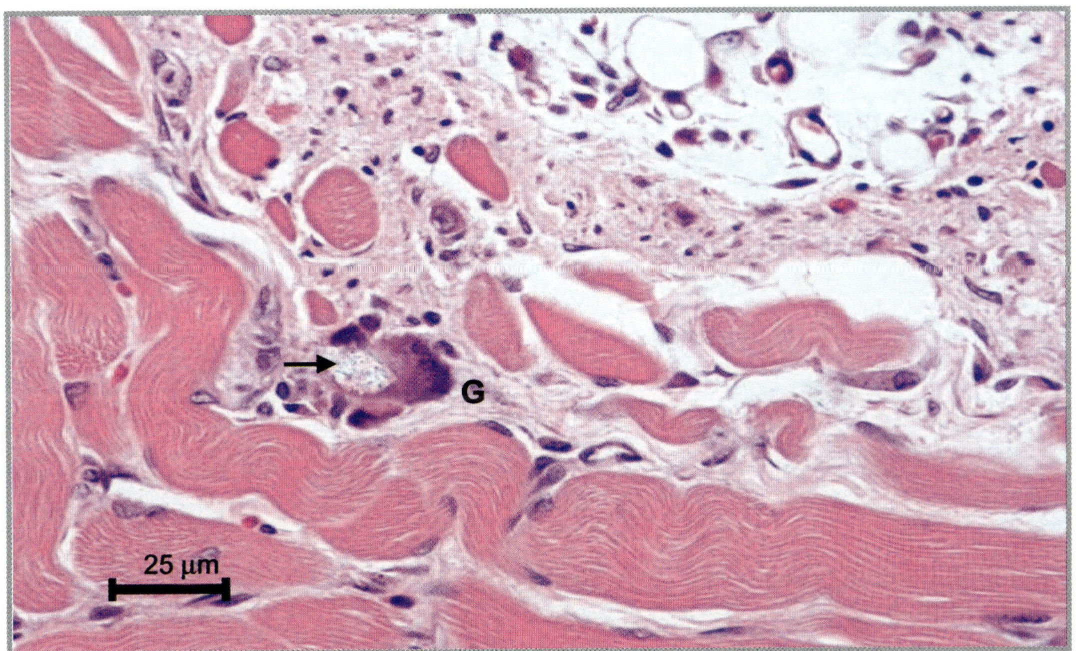

Figure 42 Foreign bodies in tissue adjacent to implant. H & E x 40
Foreign body giant cell (G) containing fragment of polymer implant material (↑)

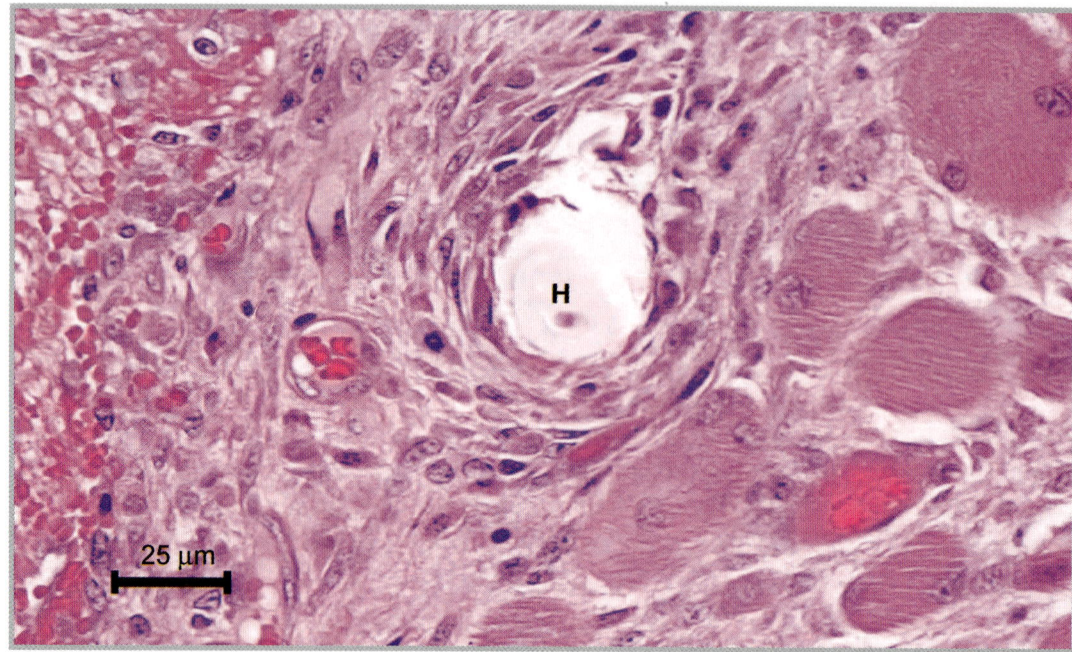

Figure 43 Foreign bodies in tissue adjacent to implant. H & E x 40
Granuloma formation around a cross-section of hair (H) implanted into the surrounding tissue during surgical procedure

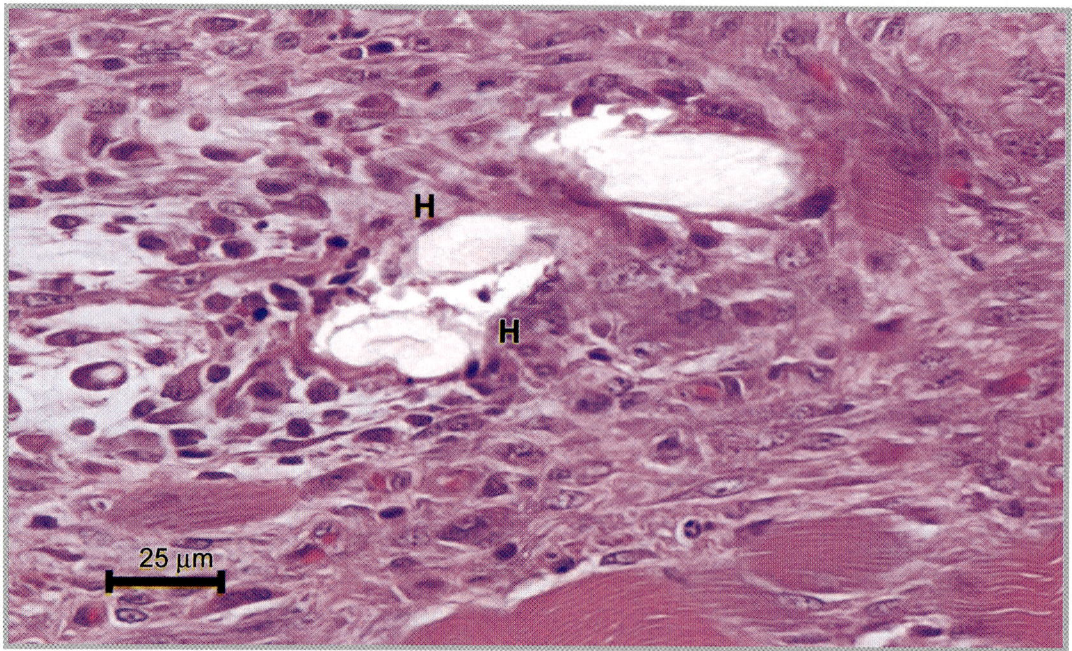

Figure 44 Foreign bodies in tissue adjacent to implant. H & E x 40
Cross-sections of hair (H) implanted into the surrounding tissue during surgical procedure. Evaluation of biocompatibility not possible when such foreign bodies are present due to the inflammatory response they elicit

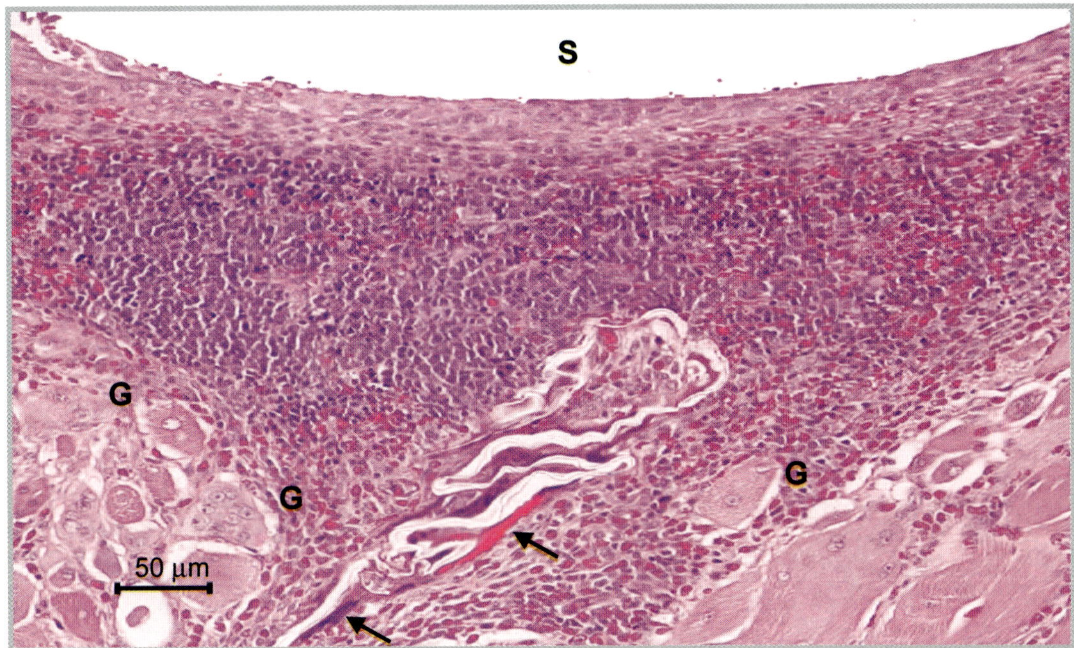

Figure 45A Foreign bodies in tissue adjacent to implant. H & E x 20
Strands of foreign fibers (↑) implanted into the tissue adjacent to implant site (S) during surgical procedure with adjacent inflammation (G)

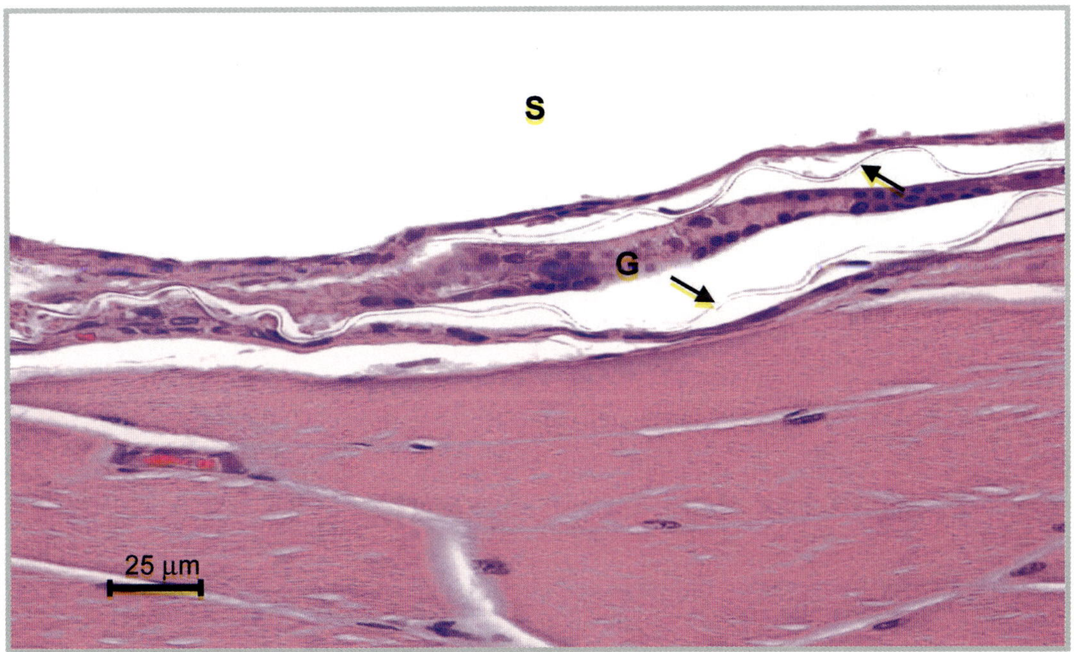

Figure 45B Foreign bodies in tissue adjacent to implant. H & E x 40
Strands of foreign fibers (↑) implanted into the adjacent to implant site (S) during surgical procedure. Inflammation and foreign body type of giant cells (G) are seen

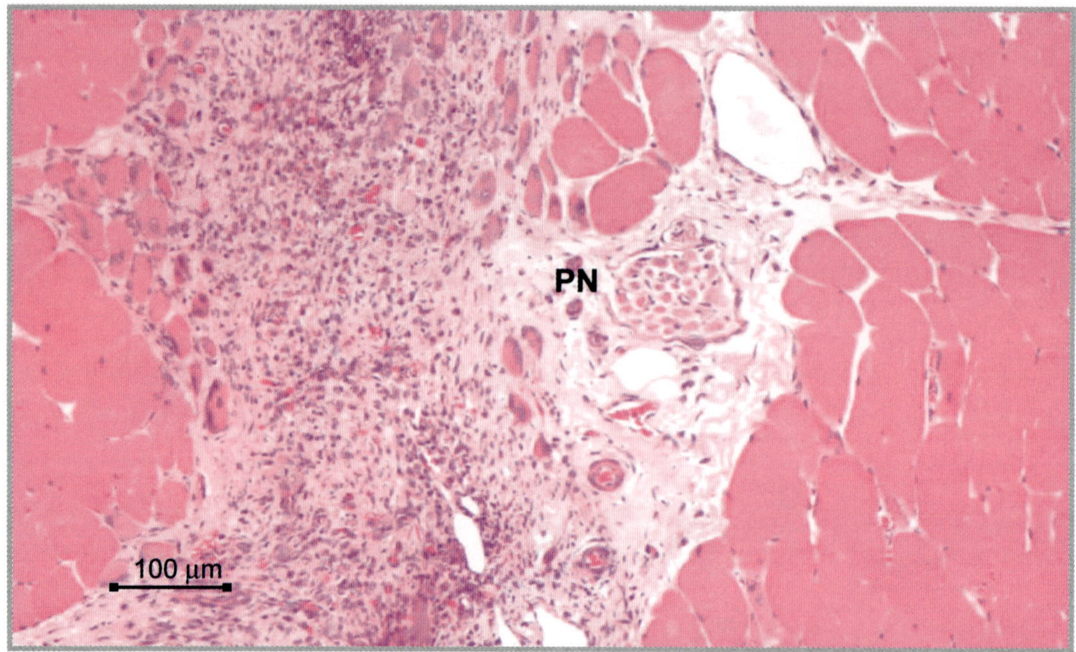

Figure 46A Nerve. H & E x 10
Cross-section of peripheral nerves (PN) in tissue adjacent to implant site

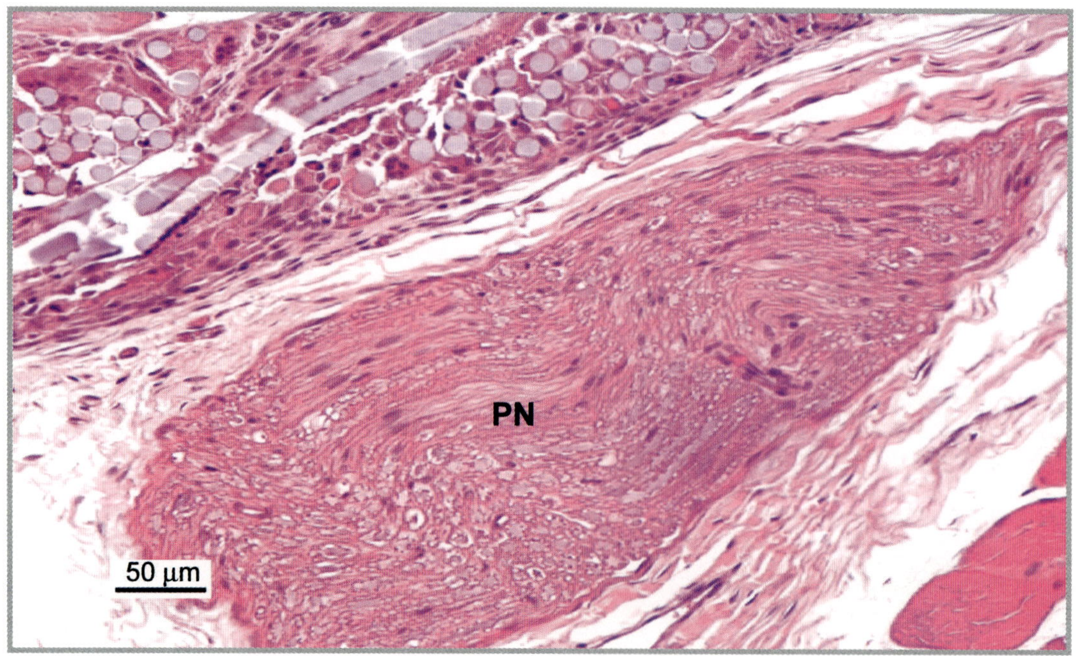

Figure 46B Nerve. H & E x 20
Longitudinal section of peripheral nerves (PN) in tissue adjacent to implant site

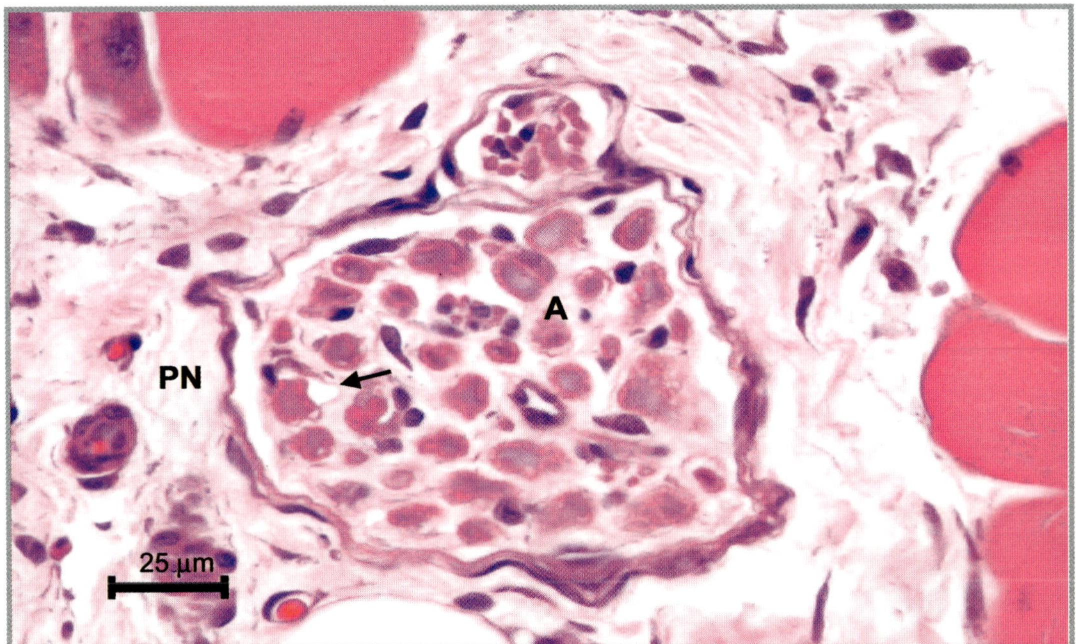

Figure 47 Nerve. H & E x 40
Cross-section of peripheral nerve (PN) with axons (A). The myelin being largely composed of lipid is dissolved during processing leaving an empty space surrounding the axon (↑) with the peripheral ring of Schwann cell cytoplasm

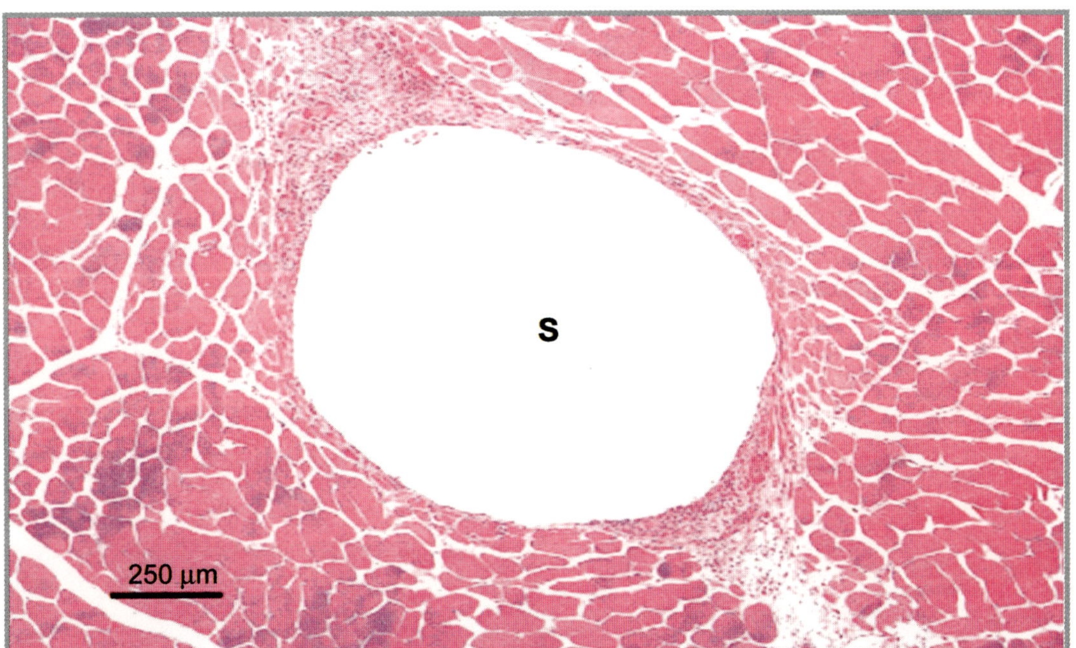

Figure 48A Shapes of implant sites (S) depending on cross-section of the implant. H & E x 4
Circular

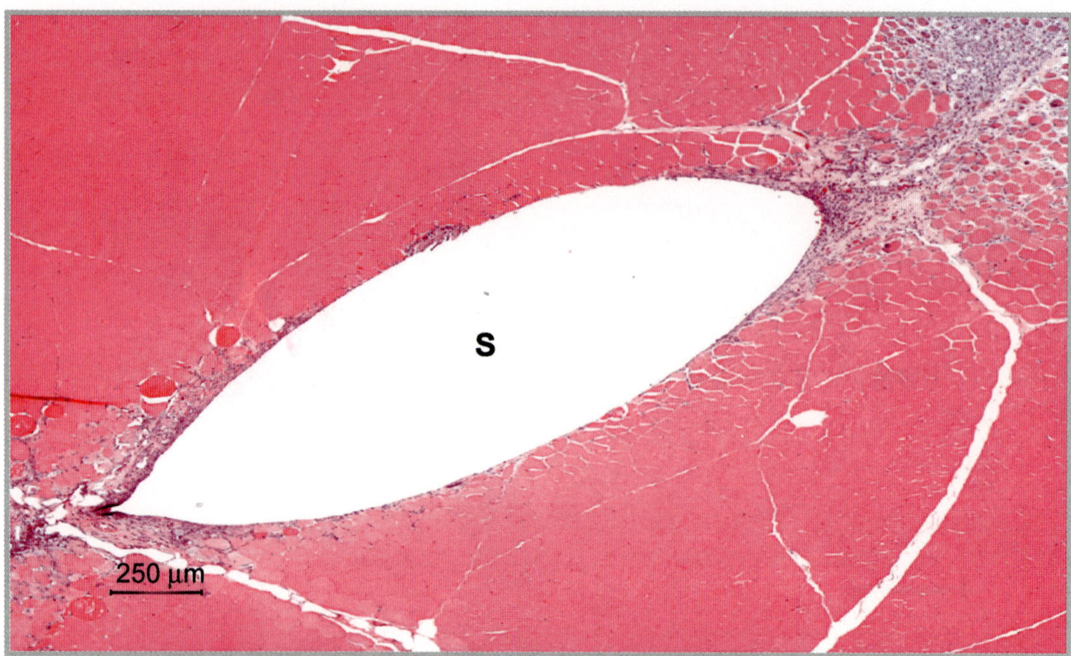

Figure 48B Shapes of implant sites. H & E x 4
Oval

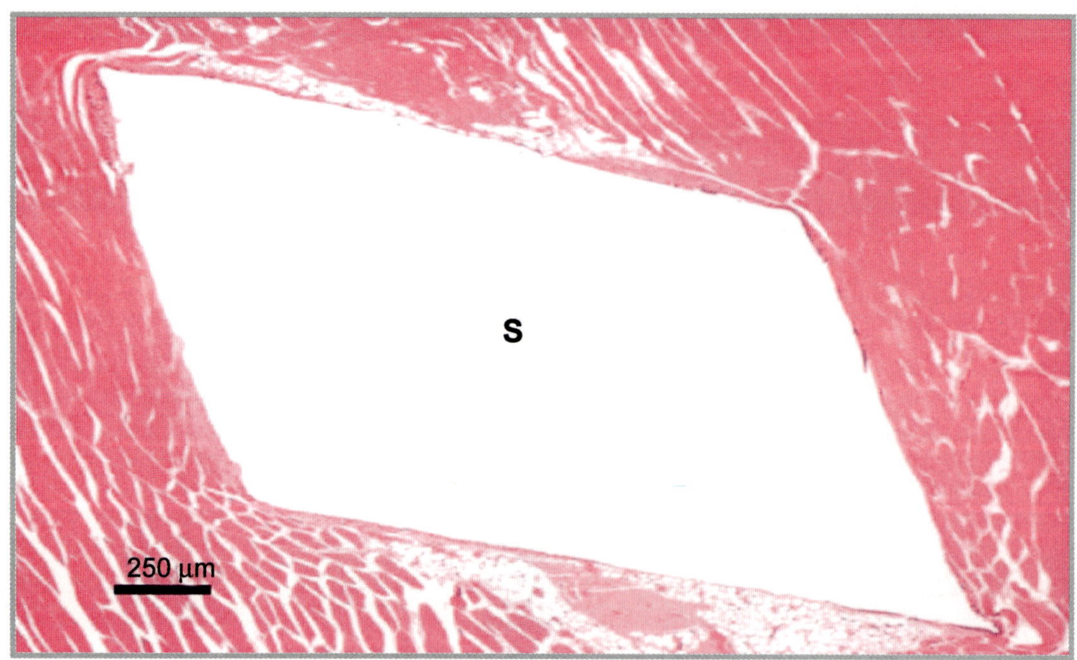

Figure 48C Shapes of implant sites. H & E x 4
Square

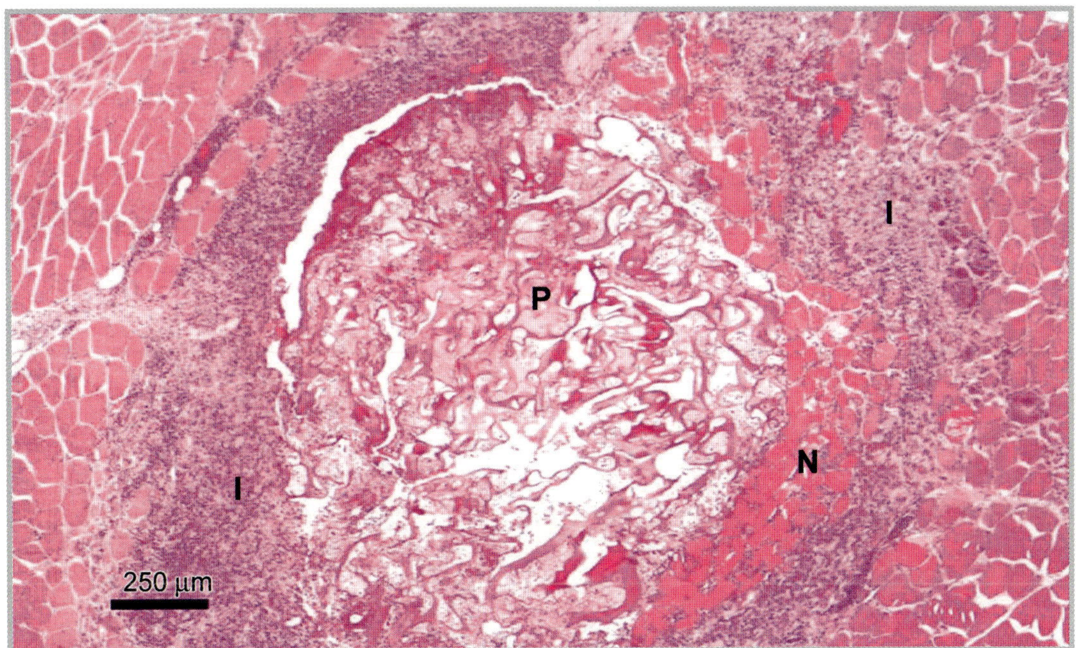

Figure 49A Tissue response to biodegradable implant. H & E x 4
Severe necrosis (N) and inflammation (I) around the implant (P) at one week post implantation

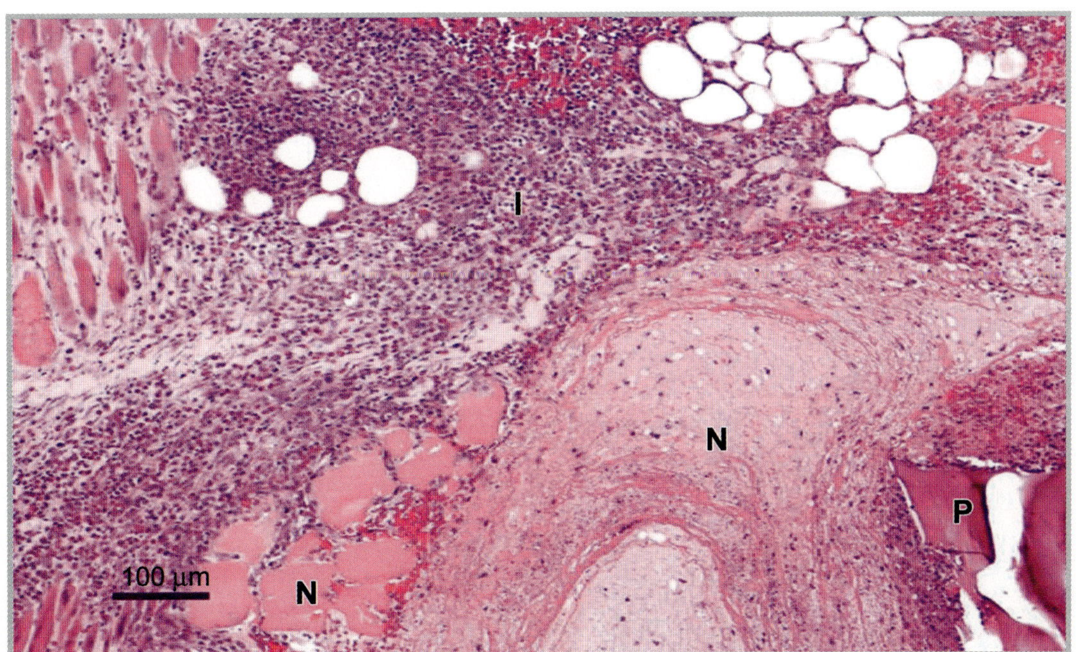

Figure 49B Tissue response to biodegradable implant. H & E x 10
Severe necrosis (N) and inflammation (I) around the implant (P) at one week post implantation

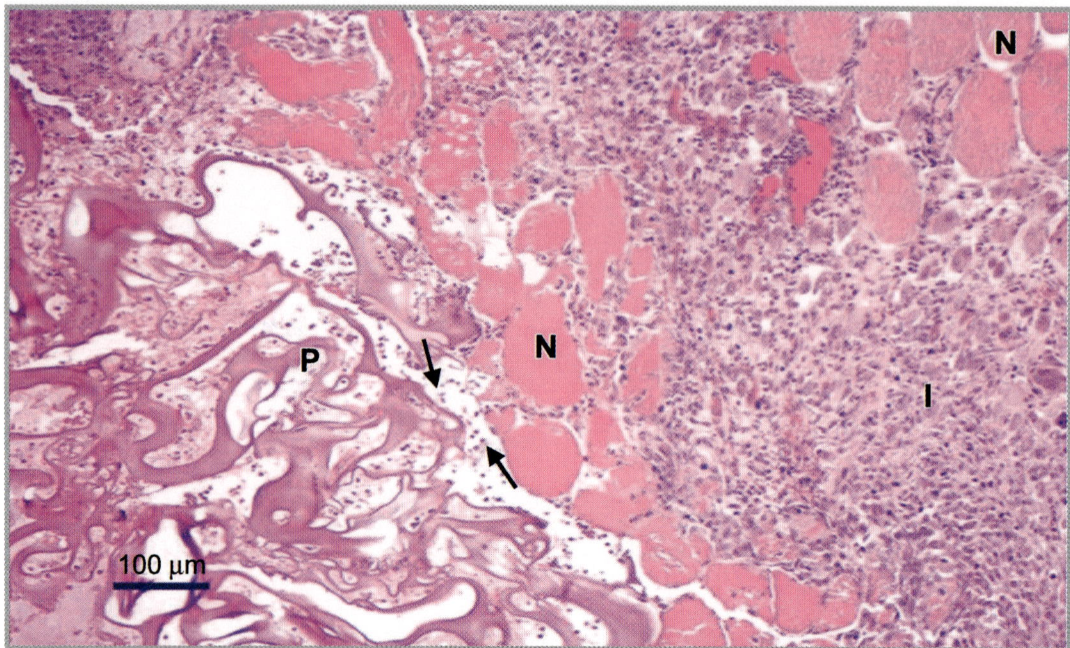

Figure 50 Tissue response to biodegradable implant. H & E x 10
Necrotic muscle fibers (N) and severe inflammation (I) around the implant (P) at one week post implantation. Inflammatory cells (↑) are observed infiltrating the implant

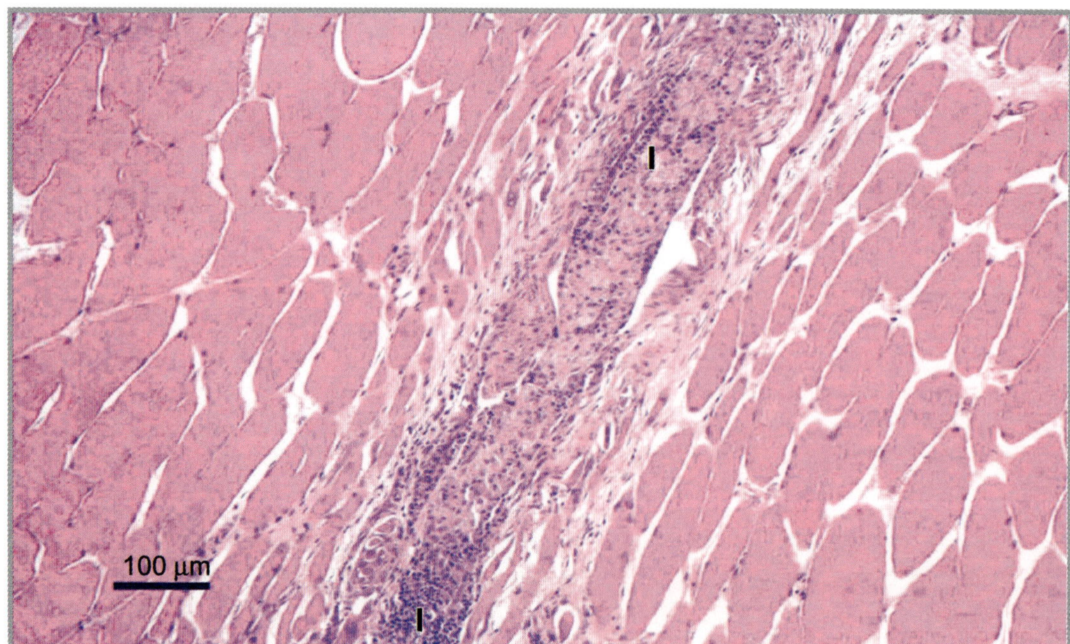

Figure 51A Tissue response to biodegradable implant. H & E x 10
Necrosis and reduced inflammation at the implantation site four weeks post implantation. Only occasional strands of implant noted (I)

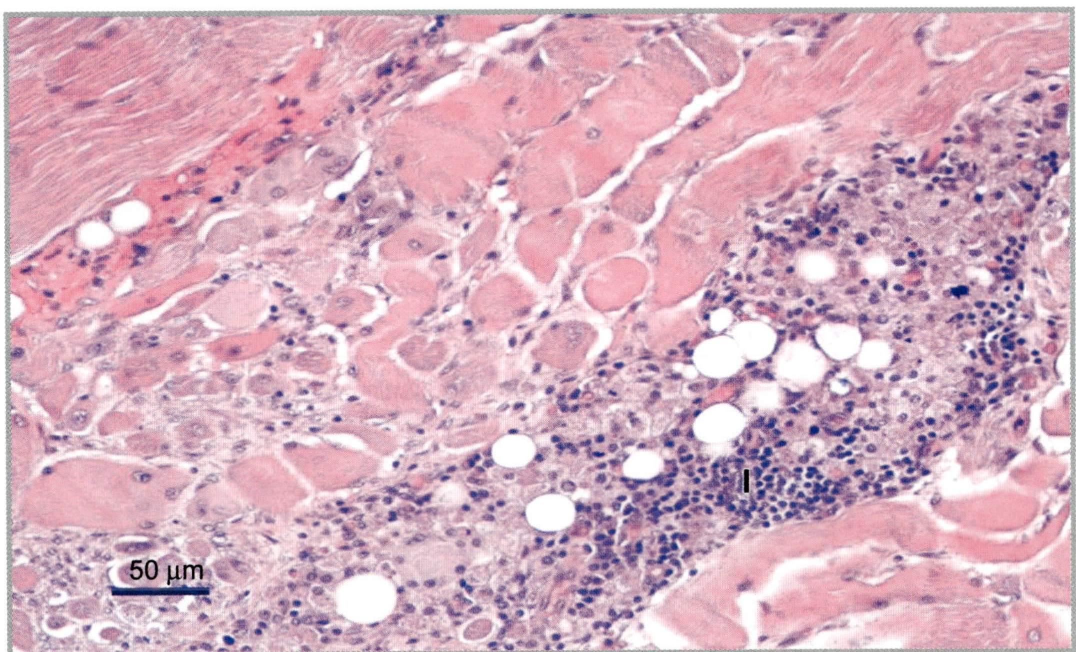

Figure 51B Tissue response to biodegradable implant. H & E x 20
Necrosis and reduced inflammation at the implantation site four weeks post implantation. Only occasional strands of implant noted (I)

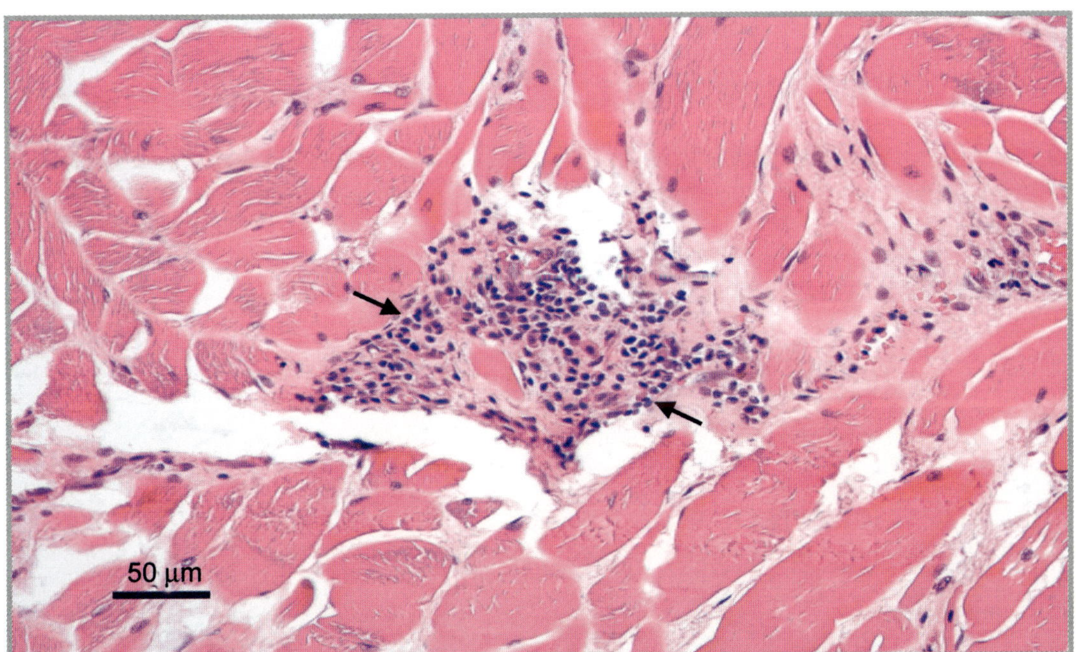

Figure 52 Tissue response to biodegradable implant. H & E x 20
Implant site at twelve weeks post implantation. Implant absent. Occasional inflammatory cells seen (↑)

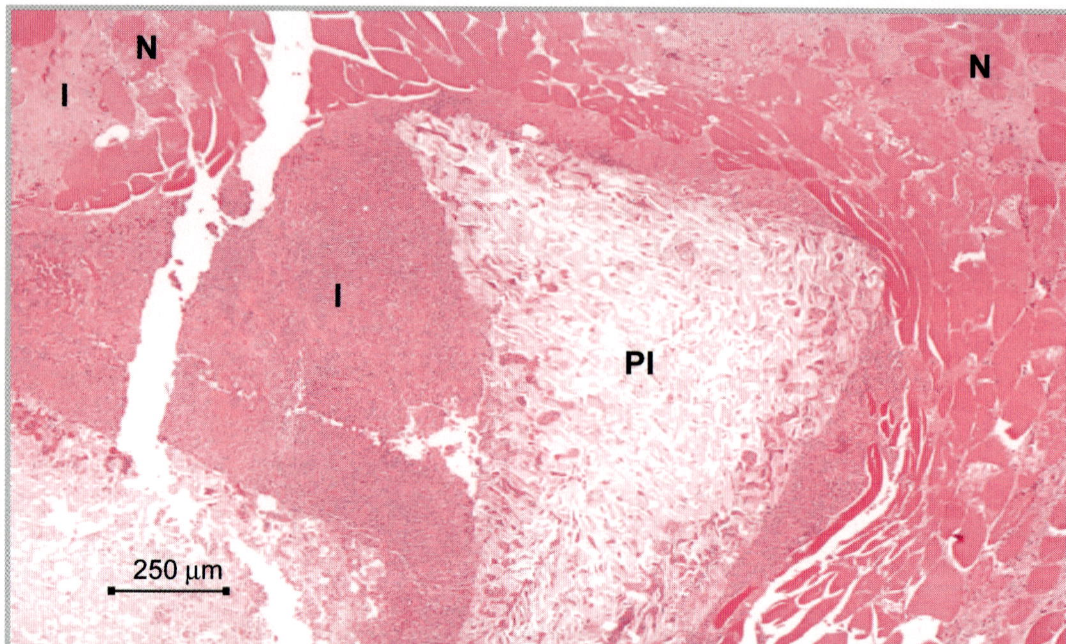

Figure 53A Tissue response to porous biodegradable polymer implant. H & E x 4
Necrosis (N) and severe inflammation (I) around the polymer implant (PI) at one week post-implantation

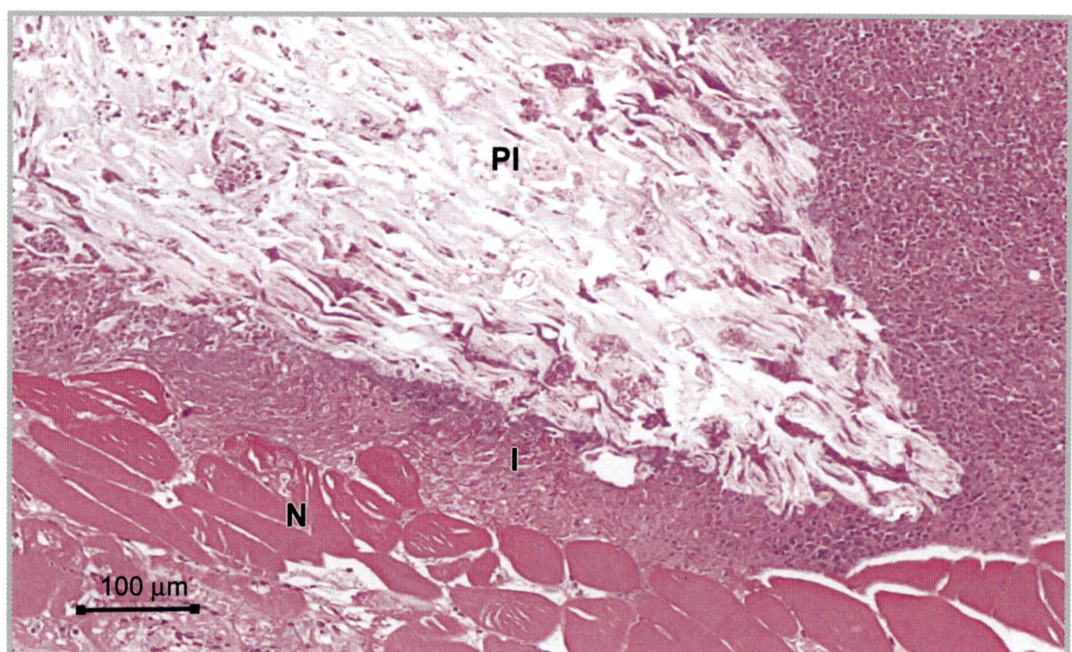

Figure 53B Tissue response to porous biodegradable polymer implant. H & E x 10
Necrosis (N) and severe inflammation (I) around the polymer implant (PI) at one week post implantation

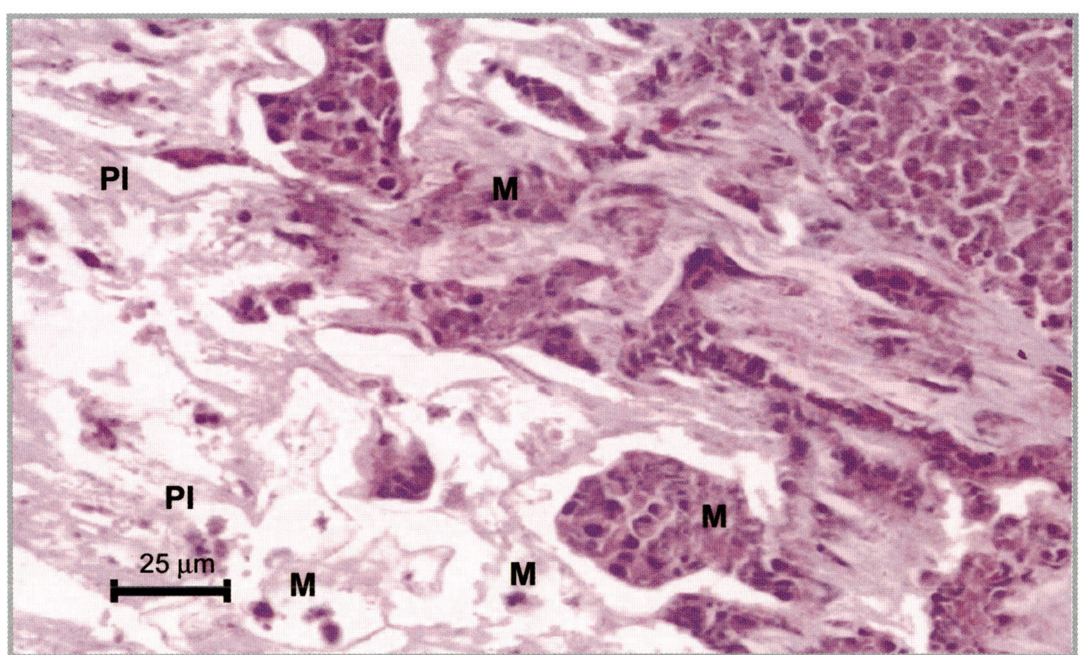

Figure 53C Tissue response to porous biodegradable polymer implant. H & E x 40
Macrophages (M) infiltrating the polymer implant (PI)

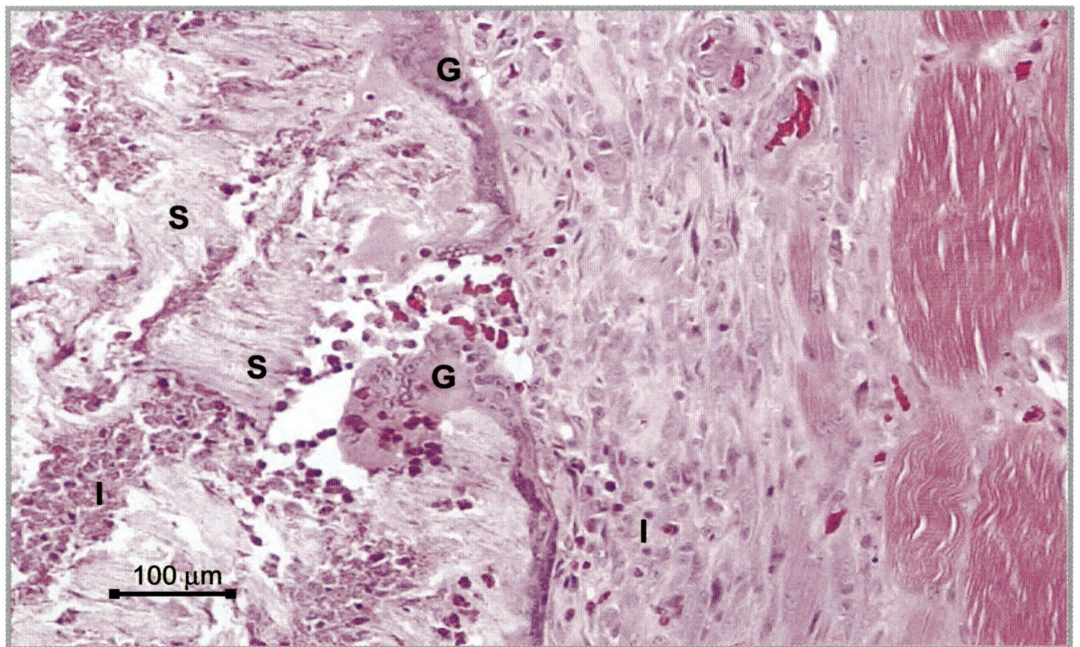

Figure 54A Tissue response to porous biodegradable polymer implant. H & E x 10
Inflammatory cells (I) surrounding and infiltrating the implant. Degradable implant fibers (S) seen with large foreign body giant cells (G)

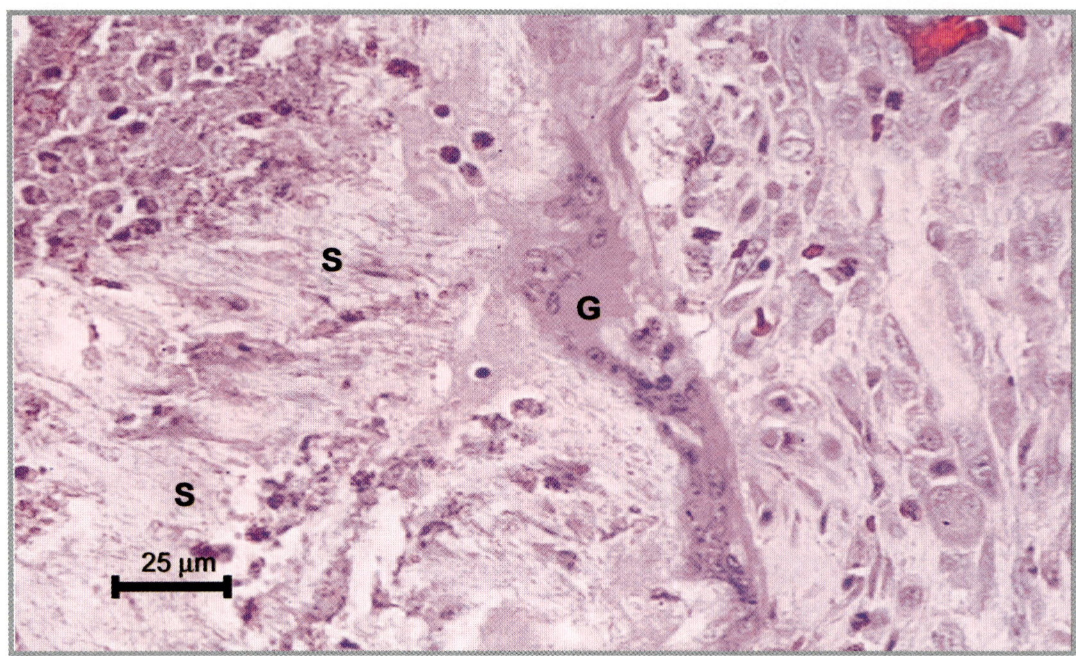

Figure 54B Tissue response to porous biodegradable polymer implant. H & E x 40
Degradable implant fibers (S) seen with large foreign body giant cells (G)

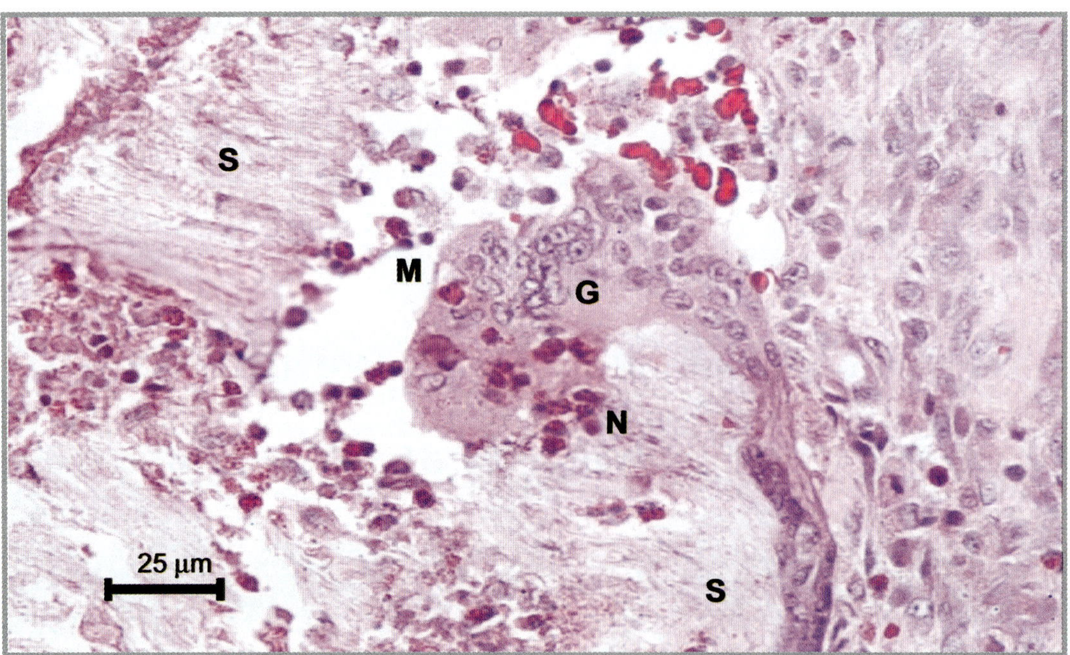

Figure 54C Tissue response to porous biodegradable polymer implant. H & E x 40
Inflammatory cells surrounding and infiltrating the implant. Degradable implant fibers (S) seen with large foreign body giant cells (G), macrophages (M) and neutrophils (N)

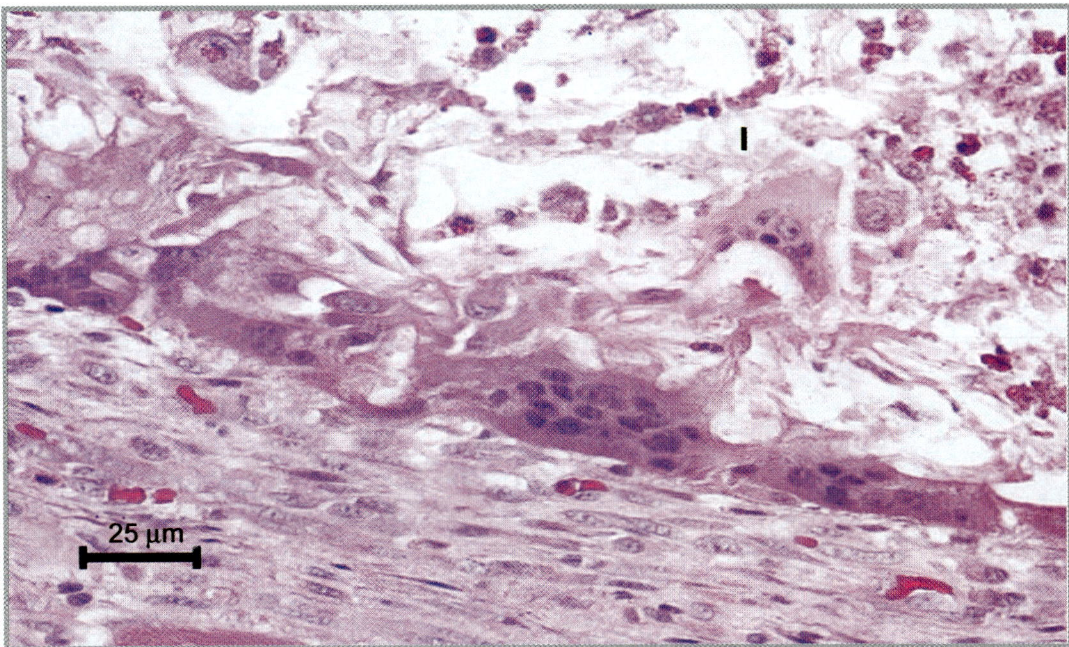

Figure 55A Comparative tissue response to porous biodegradable and bulk non-biodegradable polymer implants at one week post implantation. H & E x 40
Tissue response to a biodegradable implant (I)

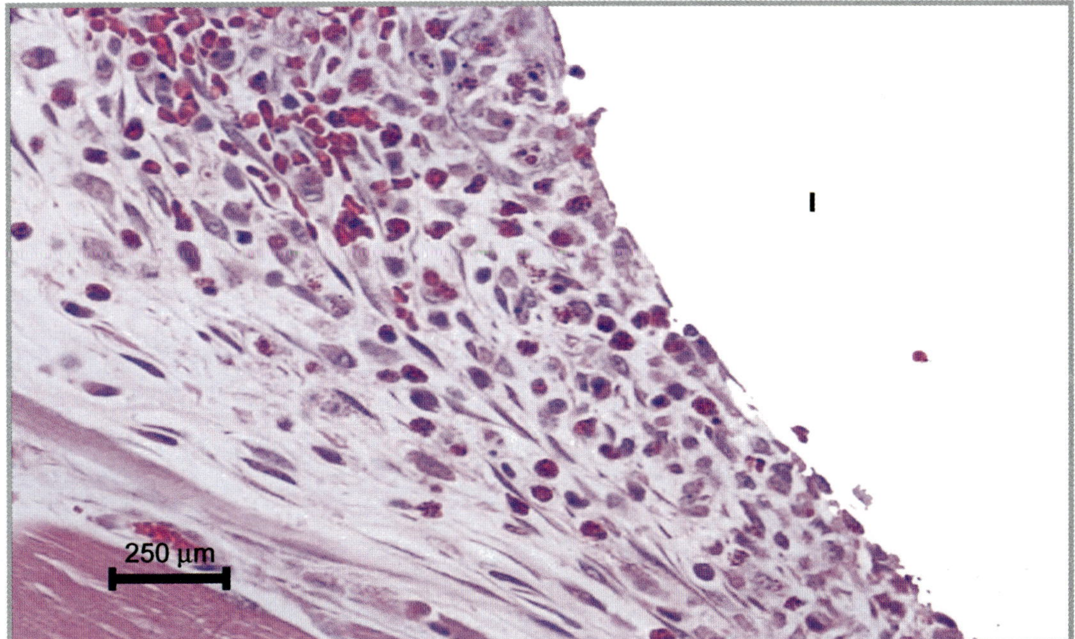

Figure 55B Comparative tissue response to porous biodegradable and bulk non-biodegradable polymer implants at one week post implantation. H & E x 4
Tissue response to a bulk non-biodegradable implant site (I)

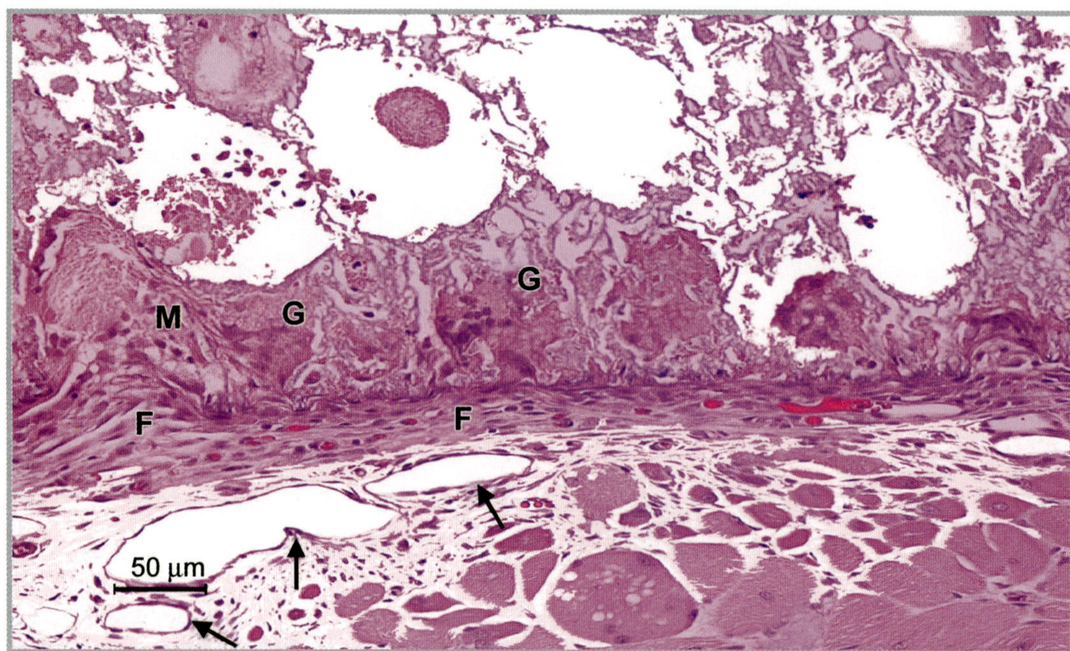

Figure 56 Tissue response to porous biodegradable polymer implant. H & E x 20
Fibroblasts and fibrocytes (F) seen at the porous biodegradable material—tissue interface at four weeks post implantation. Macrophages (M) and foreign body type of giant cells are also present. The thin walled blood vessels (↑) indicate angiogenesis

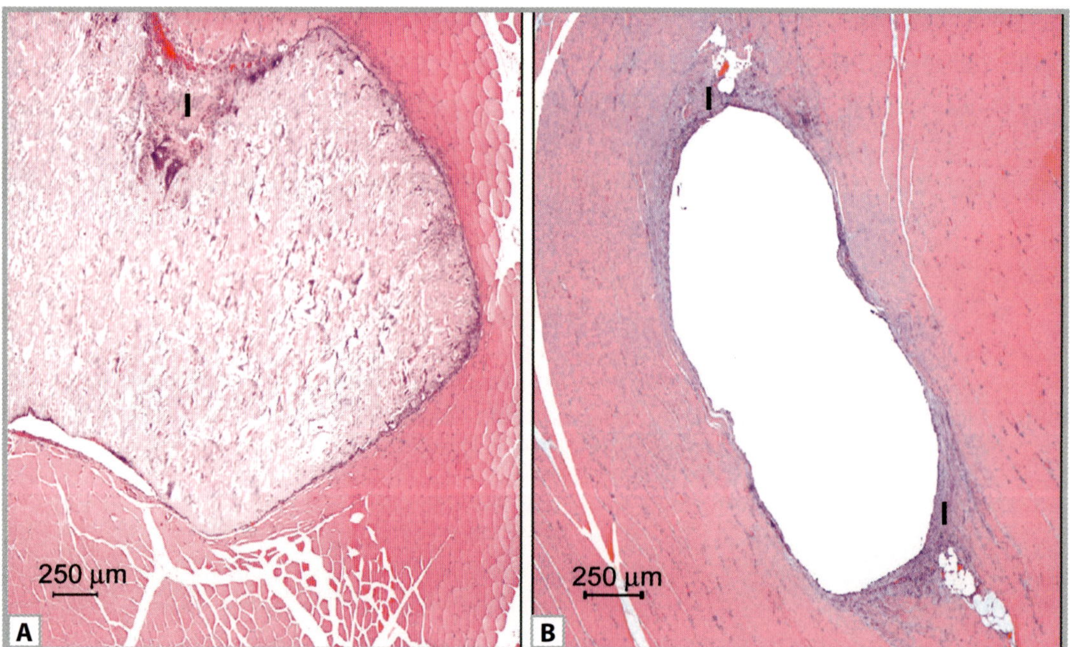

Figure 57 Comparative tissue response to porous biodegradable and bulk non-biodegradable polymer implants at four weeks post implantation. H & E x 4
A. Tissue response (I) to a porous biodegradable implant
B. Tissue response (I) to a bulk non-biodegradable implant site

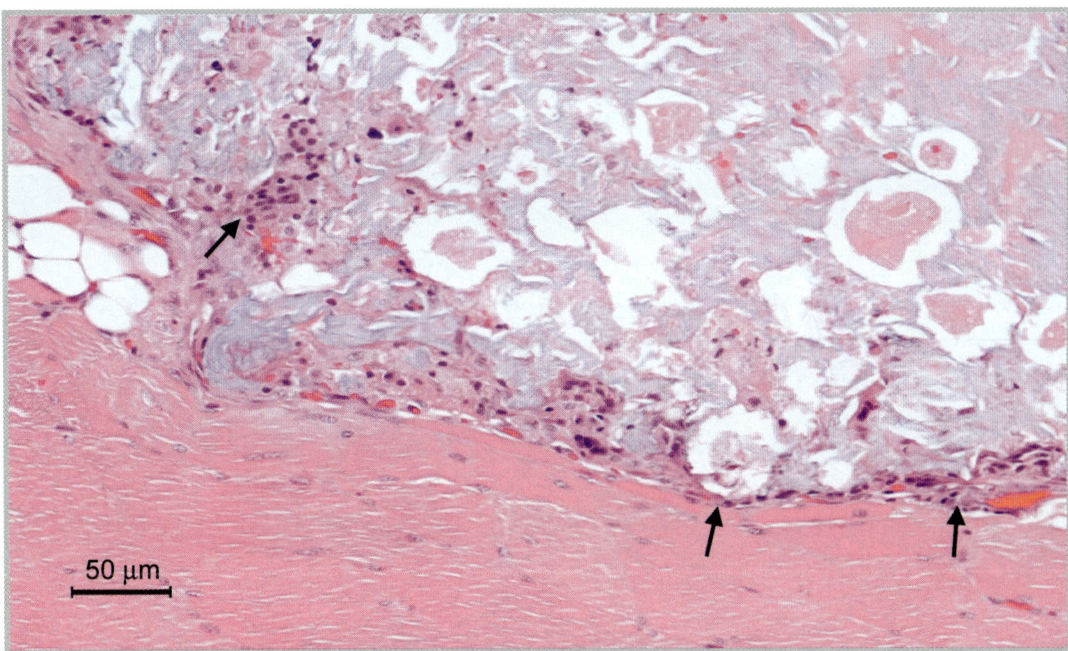

Figure 58 Tissue response to porous biodegradable polymer implant. H & E x 20
Well defined implant at twelve weeks post implantation. Inflammation around the implant has subsided. Few fibrocytes and macrophages are seen at the material-tissue interface (↑). Material has not completely degraded. It is ideal to test the material for longer time periods as there may be burst of degradation leading to an inflammatory response

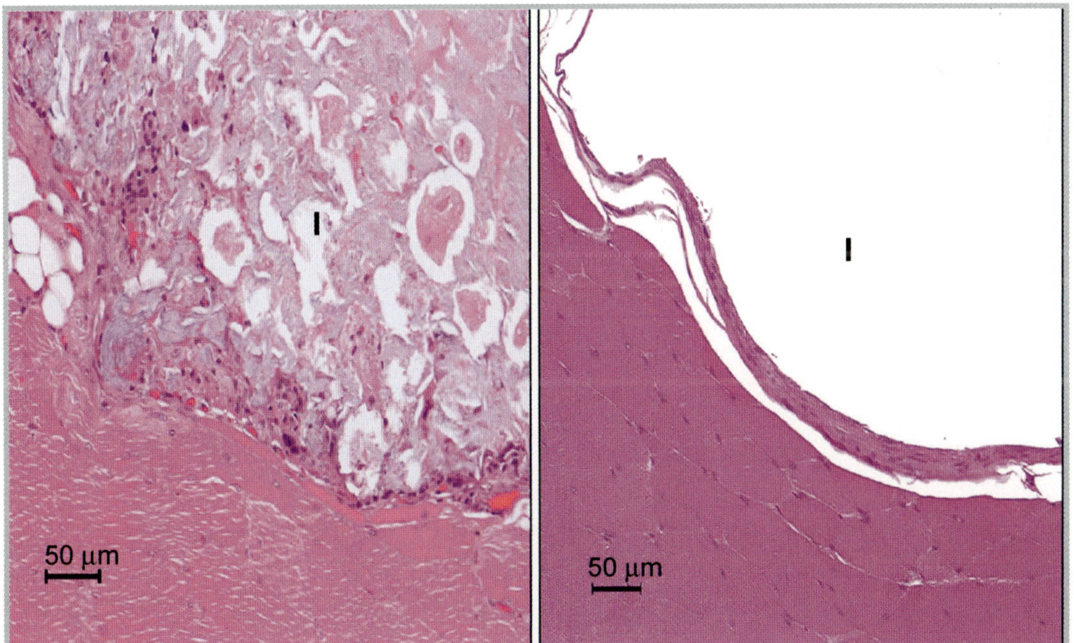

Figure 59 Comparative tissue response to porous biodegradable and bulk non-biodegradable polymer implants at twelve weeks post implantation. H & E x 20

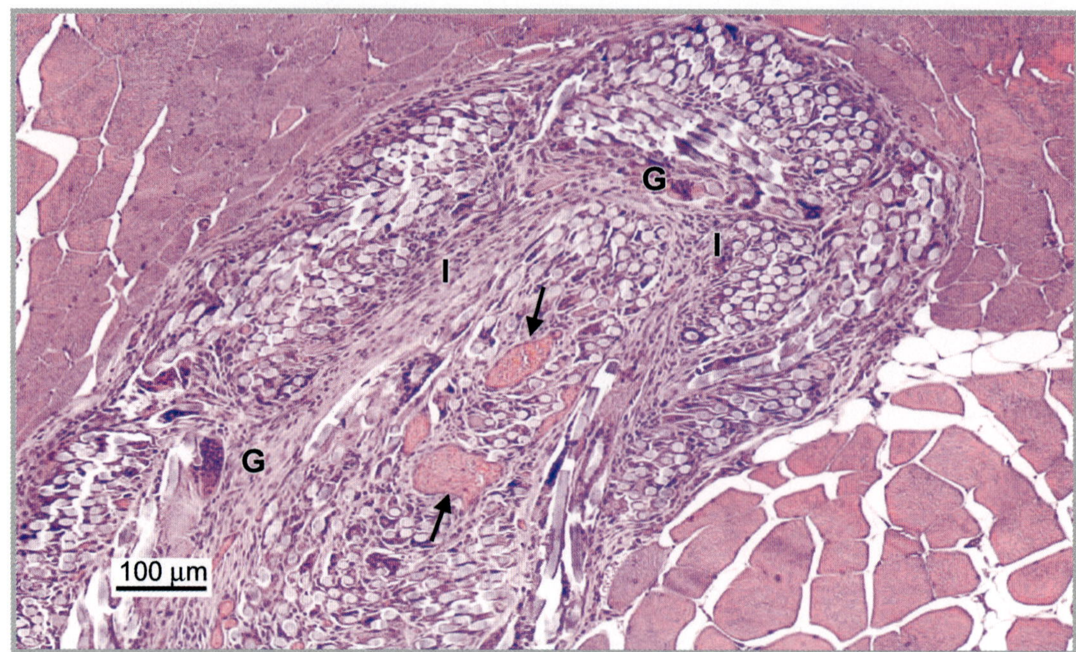

Figure 60A Tissue response to biodegradable polymer implant. H & E x 10
Cross section of the implant at one week post implantation. Inflammatory cells (I), numerous foreign body giant cells (G) and congested blood vessels (↑) are seen

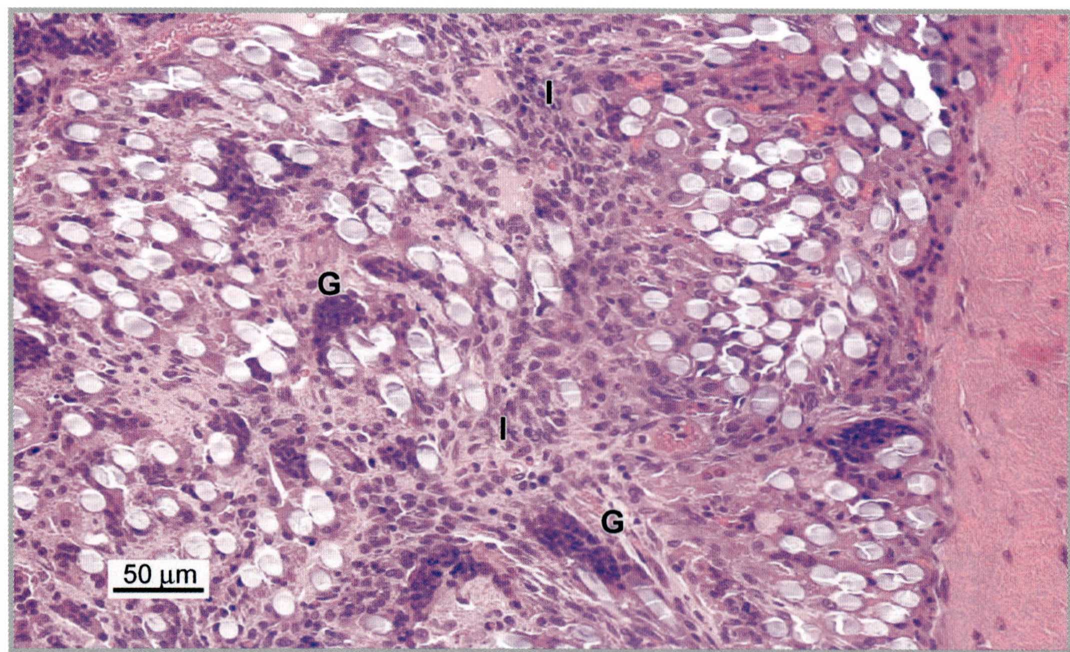

Figure 60B Tissue response to biodegradable polymer implant. H & E x 20
Cross section of fibers of a biodegradable implant implanted for one week in skeletal muscle. Material-tissue interface is well-defined. Inflammatory cells (I), and numerous foreign body giant cells (G) are seen

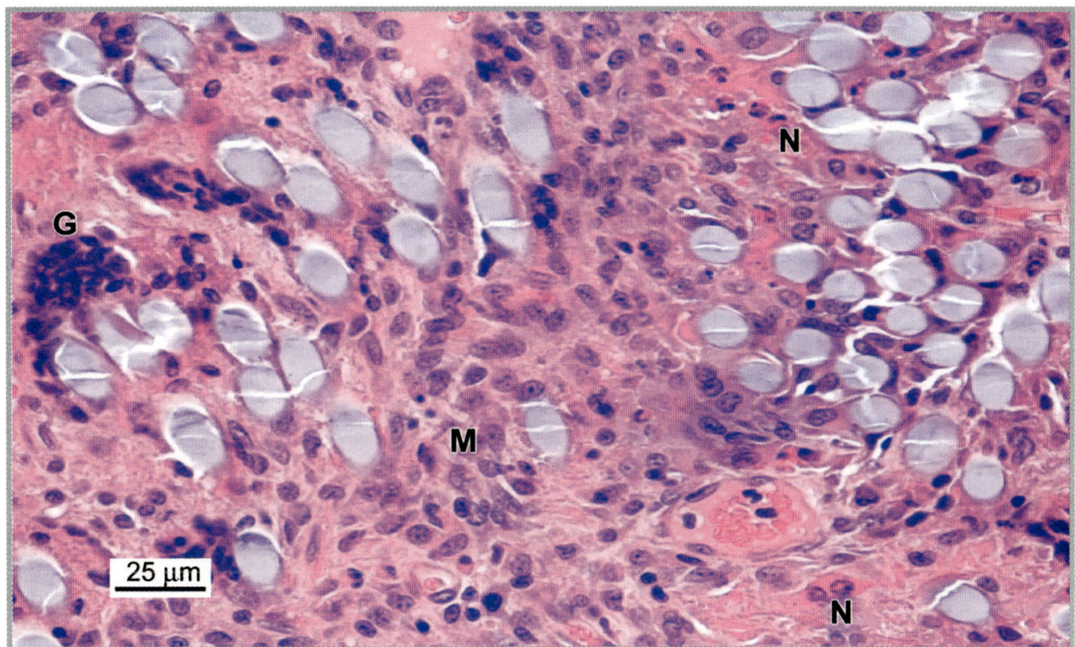

Figure 60C Tissue response to biodegradable polymer implant. H & E x 40
Cross section of fibers of a biodegradable implant implanted for one week in skeletal muscle. Macrophages (M) and neutrophils (N), numerous foreign body giant cells (G) are seen in between fibers of implant one week post implantation

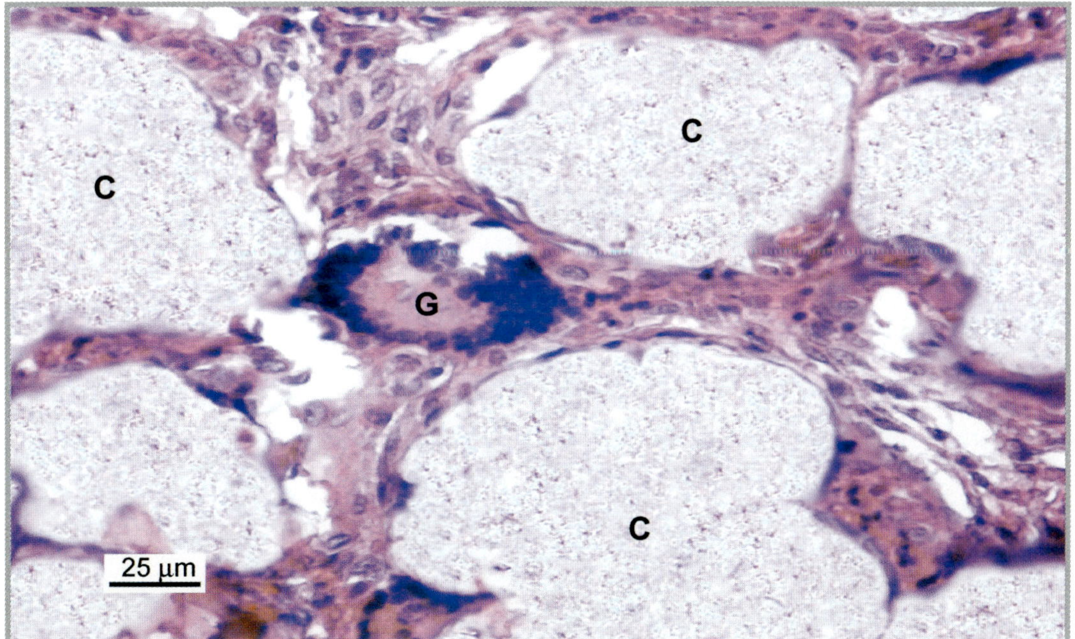

Figure 61 Tissue response to biodegradable implant. H & E x 40
Macrophages, fibrocytes and foreign body type of giant cells (G) in between degrading chitosan capsules (C)

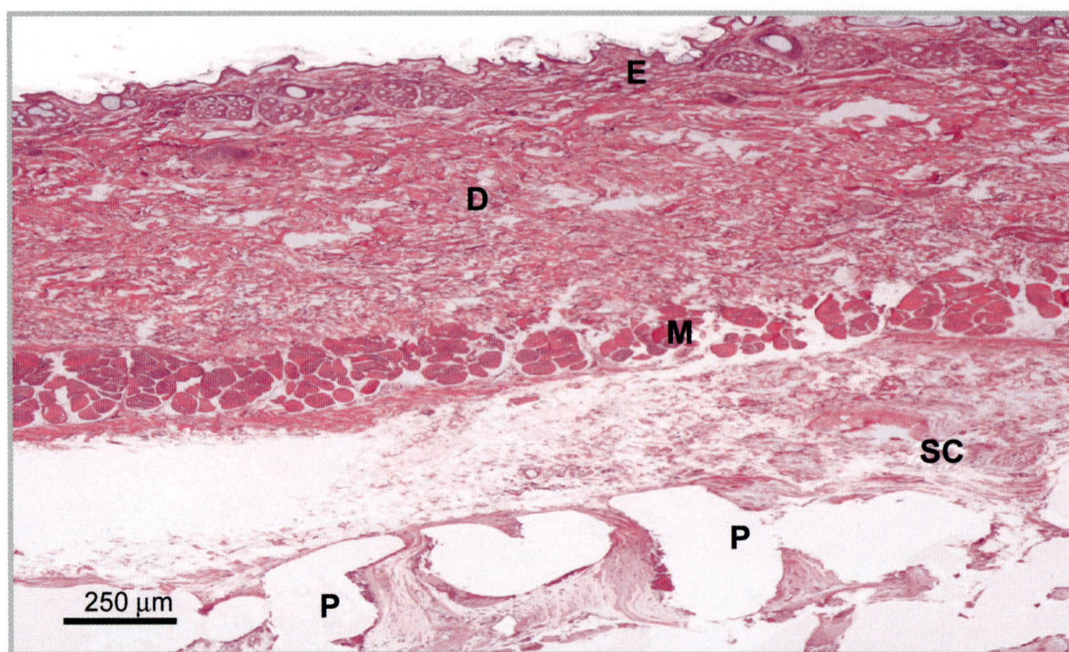

Figure 62 Tissue response to porous polymer implant in subcutaneous tissue. H & E x 4
Section of skin with implant site. Porous polymer (P) implanted in subcutaneous tissue (SC). The subcutaneous tissue is the layer beneath the epidermis with squamous epithelium (E) and dermis (D and thin layer of skeletal muscle (M)

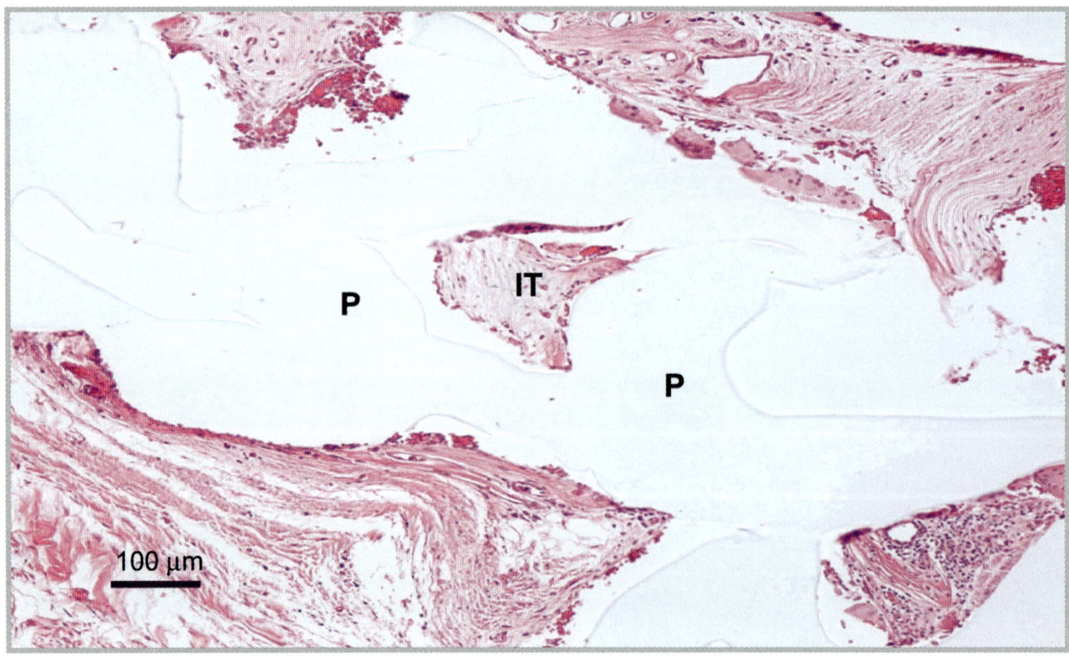

Figure 63 Tissue respone to porous implant in subcutaneous tissue. H & E x 10
Transparent polymer material is seen with tissue response on both sides of implant (P) and infiltrating tissue (IT) in the pores

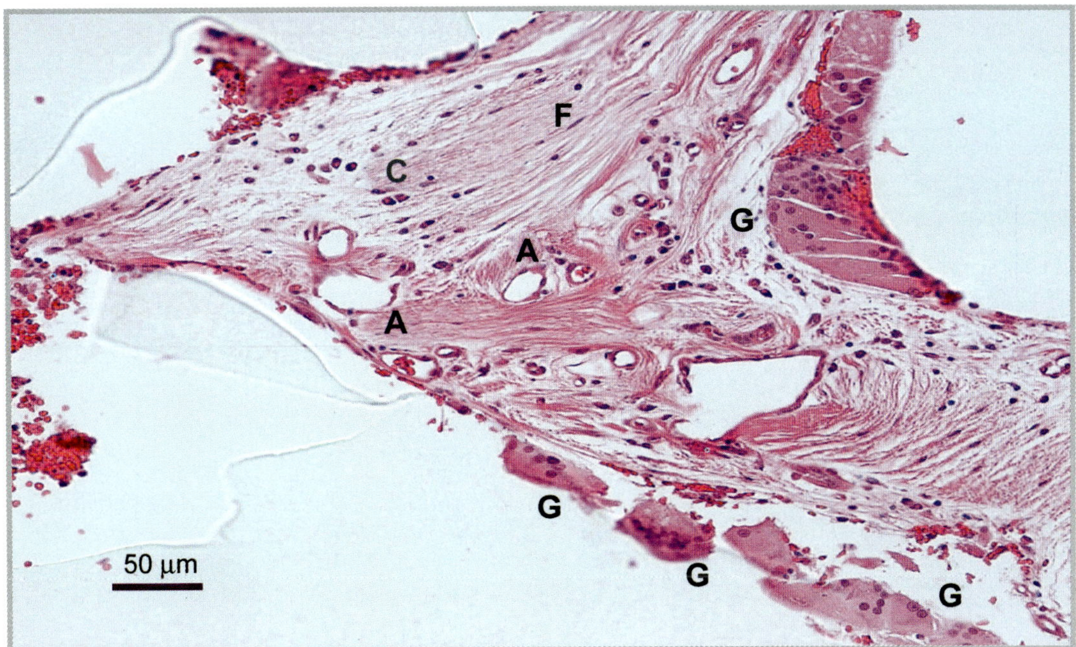

Figure 64 Tissue response to porous implant in subcutaneous tissue. H & E x 20
Inflammatory cells (C), fibrocytes (F), foreign body type of giant cells (G) and angiogenesis (A) are present. Fresh hemorrhage (H) is also seen

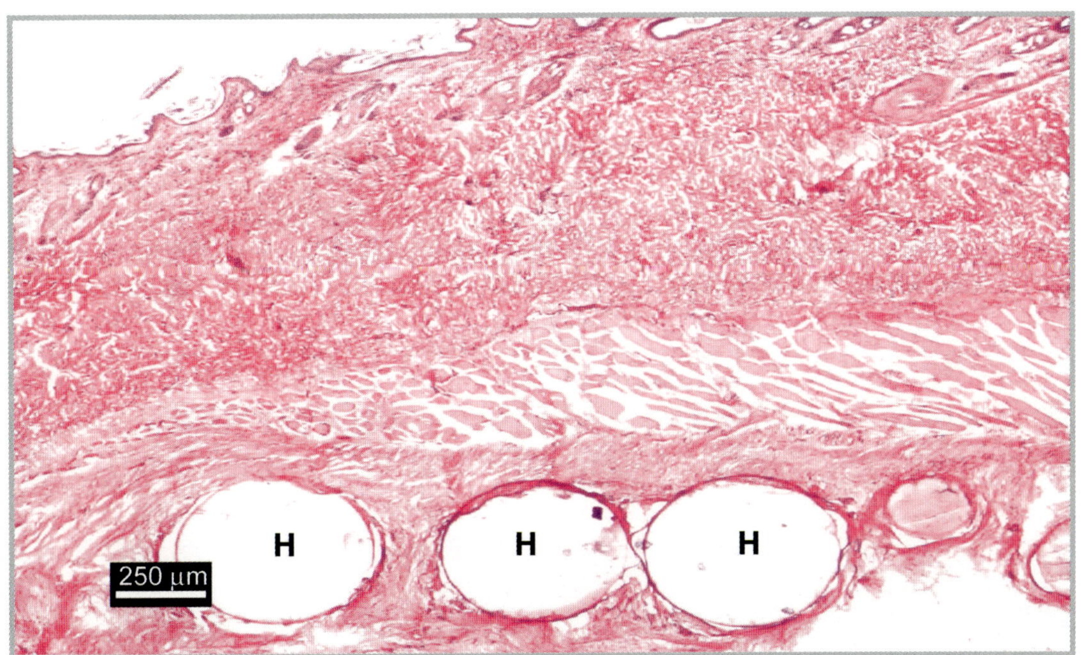

Figure 65A Tissue response to degradable beads in subcutaneous tissue. H & E x 4
Hydrogel beads (H) implanted in subcutaneous tissue in skin

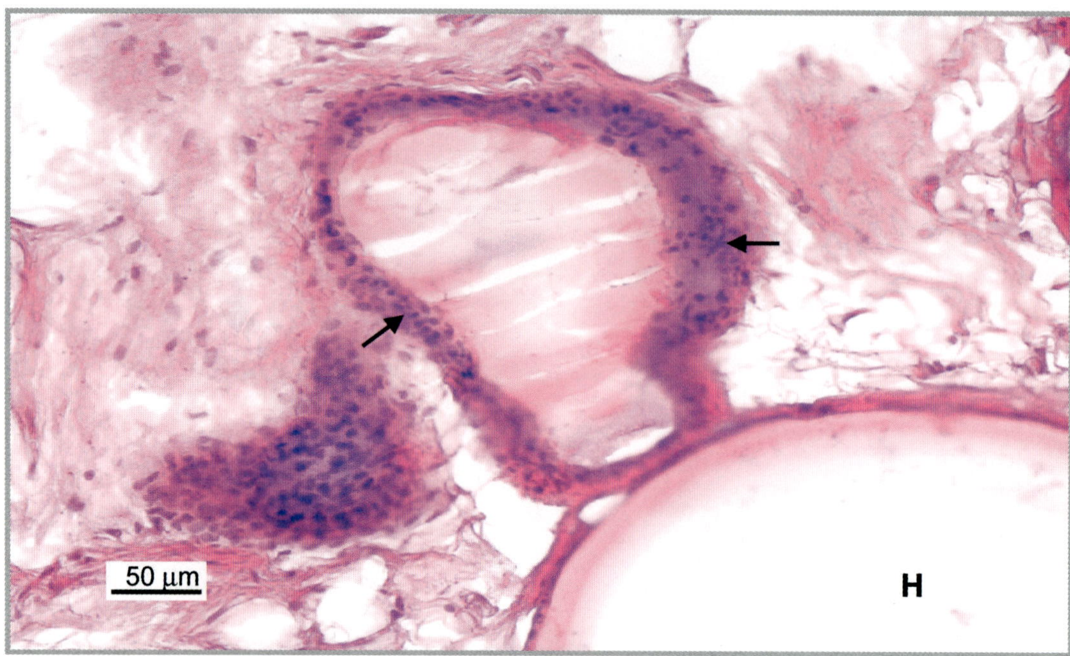

Figure 65B Tissue response to degradable beads in subcutaneous tissue. H & E x 20
Degrading hydrogel (H) surrounded by mononuclear cells (↑)

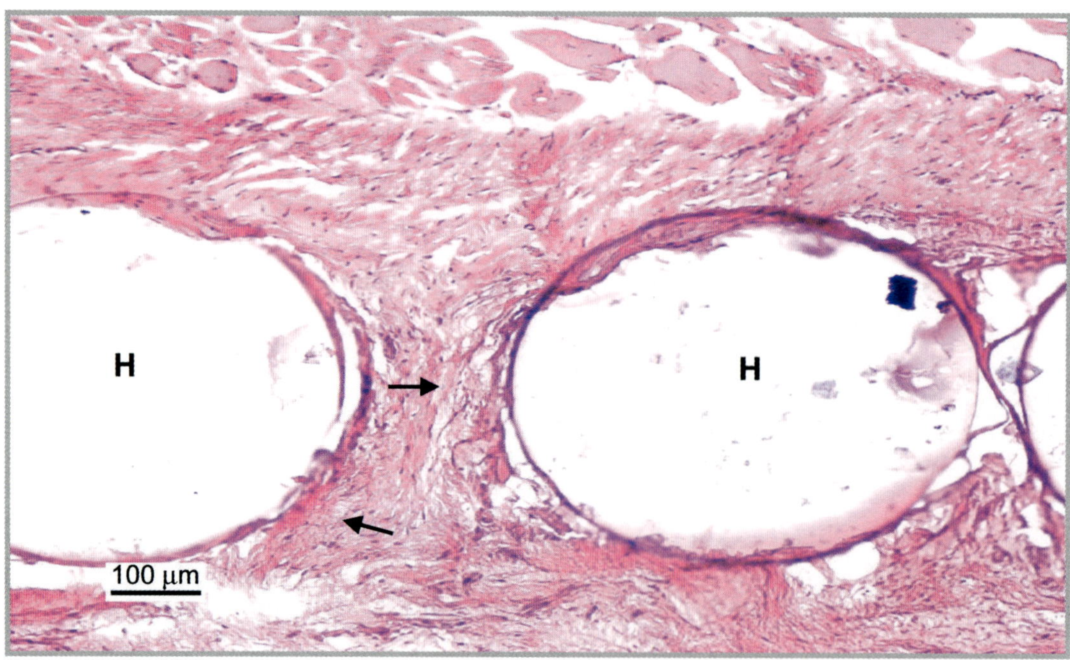

Figure 65C Tissue response to degradable beads in subcutaneous tissue. H & E x 10
Fibrocytes (↑) in between beads

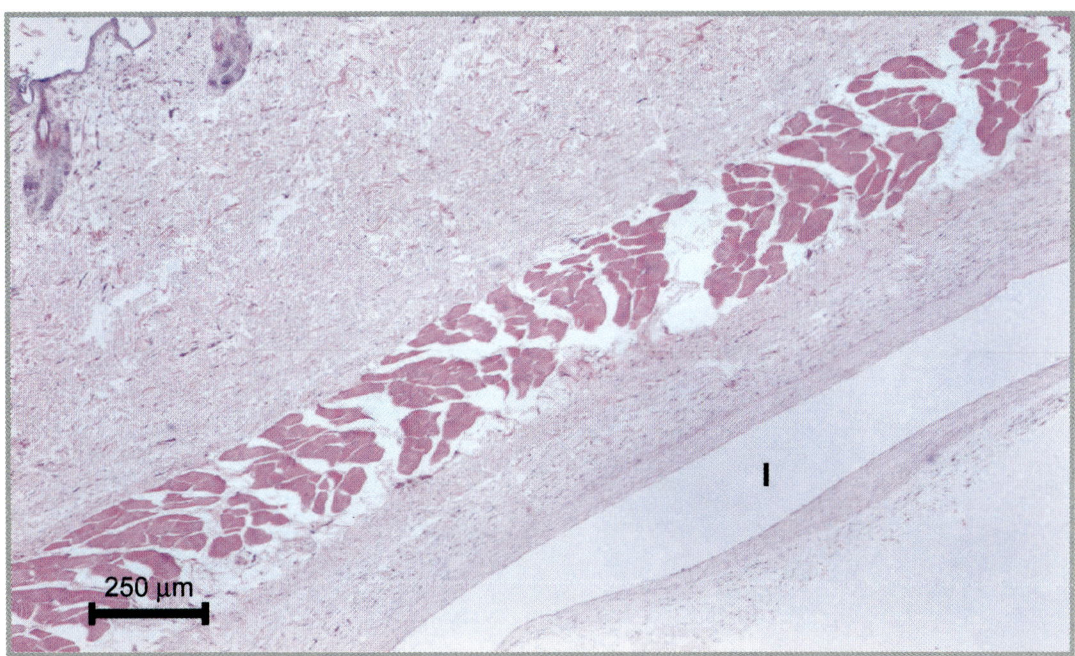

Figure 66A Tissue response to non-degradable implant in subcutaneous tissue. H & E x 4
Section of tissue with implant site (I) in subcutaneous tissue

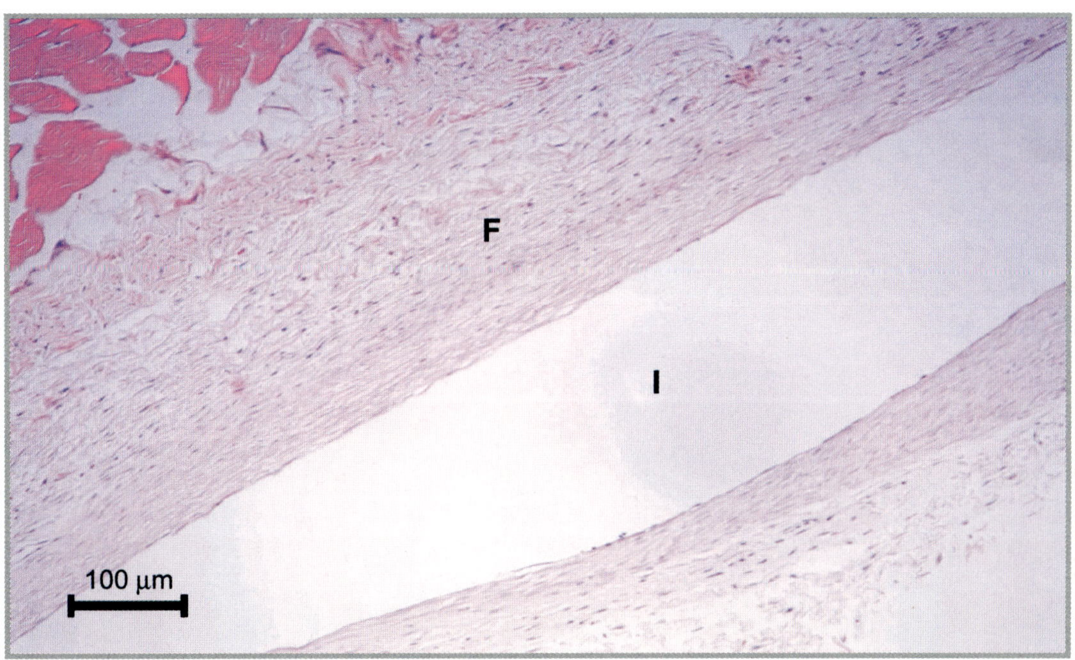

Figure 66B Tissue response to non-degradable implant in subcutaneous tissue. H & E x 10
Section of tissue with implant site (I) in subcutaneous tissue. Fibrous capsule (F) with fibrocytes around the implant site (I)

3

Implants in Bone

When implants are placed in bone, the sequence of events are very much similar to those seen in soft tissue and in response to a fracture in bone. Necrosis is followed by acute and chronic inflammation and the process ends in healing with fibrosis and deposition of new bone around the implant. Following the entry of inflammatory cells, namely the neutrophils, macrophages and lymphocytes, fibroblasts and osteoblasts are present. The osteoblasts lay down osteoid matrix which is then calcified and converted into new bone. The bone deposited initially, has no pattern and is known as woven bone. It is further remodeled by matrix deposition by osteoblasts and bone removal or resorption by cells known as osteoclasts. These osteoclasts are multinucleated. Areas of bone resorption can easily be identified as resorption bays. Woven bone is gradually layered into laminae and forms lamellar bone. This lamellar bone is deposited in concentric rings around canals called Haversian canals which contain capillaries and nerve fibers. Canal with the concentric lamellar bone is called a Haversian system. The new bone then resembles the host bone on either side of the implant. However, a neat demarcation can always be seen between new and host bone, due to the plane of section cutting.

The most important factor in good bone implant interaction is the nature of tissue at the implant interface. Is it fibrous tissue or bone? The future functional stability of the implant depends predominantly on this interface. In the case of metal implants like steel and titanium, there is always a thin layer of fibrous tissue with collagen between the material surface and adjacent healed new bone. However, in the case of ceramic implants which contain hydroxyapatite or calcium phosphate which are normal constituents of bone, new healed bone is always in direct contact with the material and also replaces it as the ceramic gets resorbed with time. Ceramic implants being brittle are not suitable for load bearing prosthesis like hip or knee prosthesis. However, surfaces of metal implants can be modified either physically with roughned or patterned porous surfaces or layered with ceramic or composite for better new bone interaction at the interface.

Evaluation of biocompatibility of implants in new bone requires processing of bone with the implant-bone interface intact, to find out whether with time the tissue at the interface is bone or fibrous tissue. Hence, resin embedded sections which contain the bone with implant, thus preserving the bone-material interface are studied. They are stained with hematoxylin and eosin or Stevenel's blue stain and provide a good picture of this interface under transmitted light microscopy. In case of resorbable implants, it is also necessary to know whether new bone deposition is by conduction of the repair process from adjacent host bone otherwise known as osteoconduction or is it initiated by the material itself, otherwise known as osteoinduction. As it is difficult to determine where bone deposition began in a hematoxylin and eosin or Stevenel's blue stained section, this can be identified by labeling bone deposited with different colors of flurochromes. These dyes are injected into the animal at different time intervals following implantation till the end of the experiment. As the dye is deposited always in new bone matrix which is being deposited at that particular time, the representative color of each dye injected at a particular time can be seen in the sections, in areas of bone deposition. If yellow and green dyes were injected at one and six months respectively post implantation, and if the yellow dye is seen in the section in bone deposited inside the implant and the green colour is seen at a distance away, it is presumed that new bone deposition began by osteoinduction, i.e. was initiated by the material itself.

Tissue response at bone-implant interface can be seen in the following images.

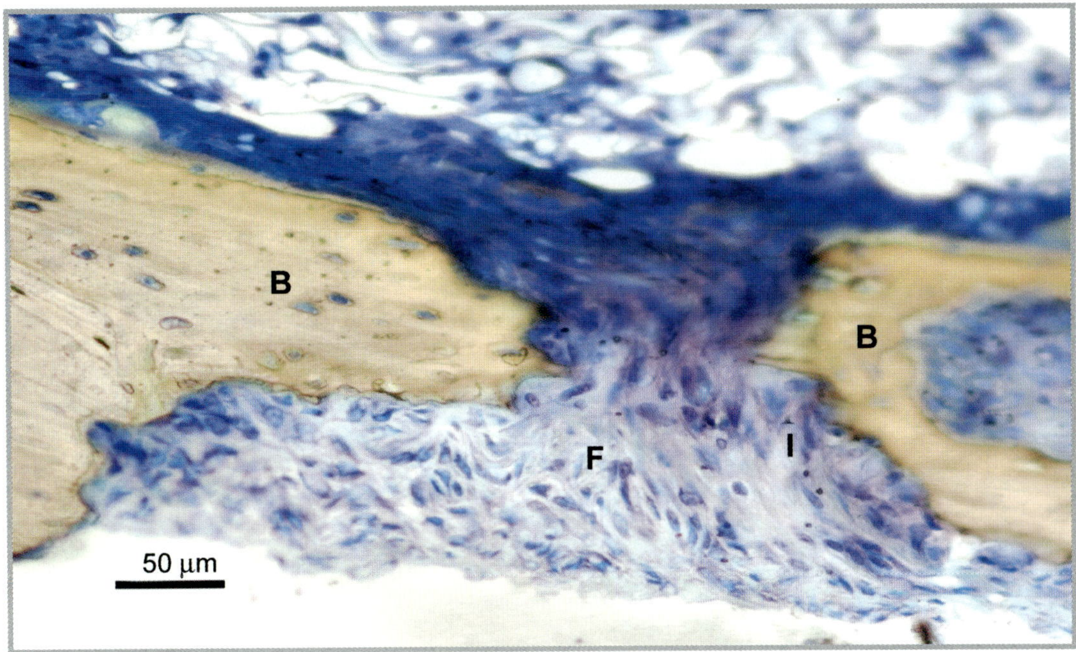

Figure 1 Tissue response to a fracture in bone. SVB x 20
The gap between the two edges of fractured long bone (B) is filled with inflammatory cells (I) and fibroblasts and fibrocytes (F)

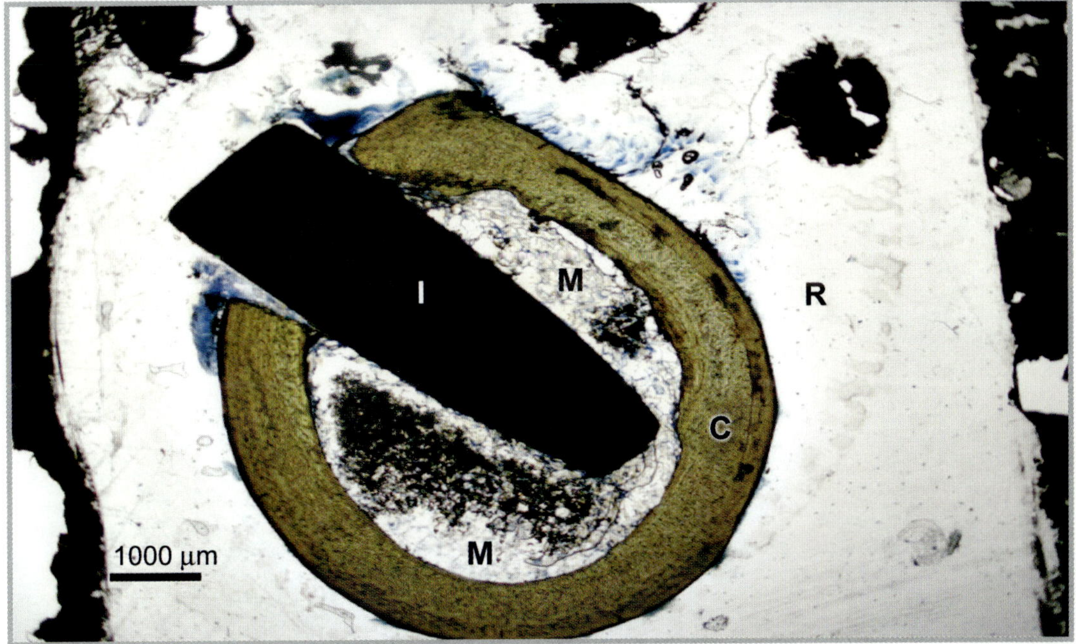

Figure 2 Tissue response to implant in bone. SVB x 1
Low magnification of a resin section (R) of titanium implant in bone. Cross-section of long bone cut perpendicularly to the long axis of the implant. Cortical bone (C) is seen all around with implant (I) in the implant site and marrow (M) in the center

Figure 3A Tissue response to implant in bone. Cross section of long bone cut perpendicularly to the long axis of the implant. SVB x 4
Implant (I) is seen in between both edges of the host bone. A space exists on either side of the implant. This space is initially filled with fibroblasts and fibrocytes stage in initial of healing. There is no new bone formation along both sides of host bone.

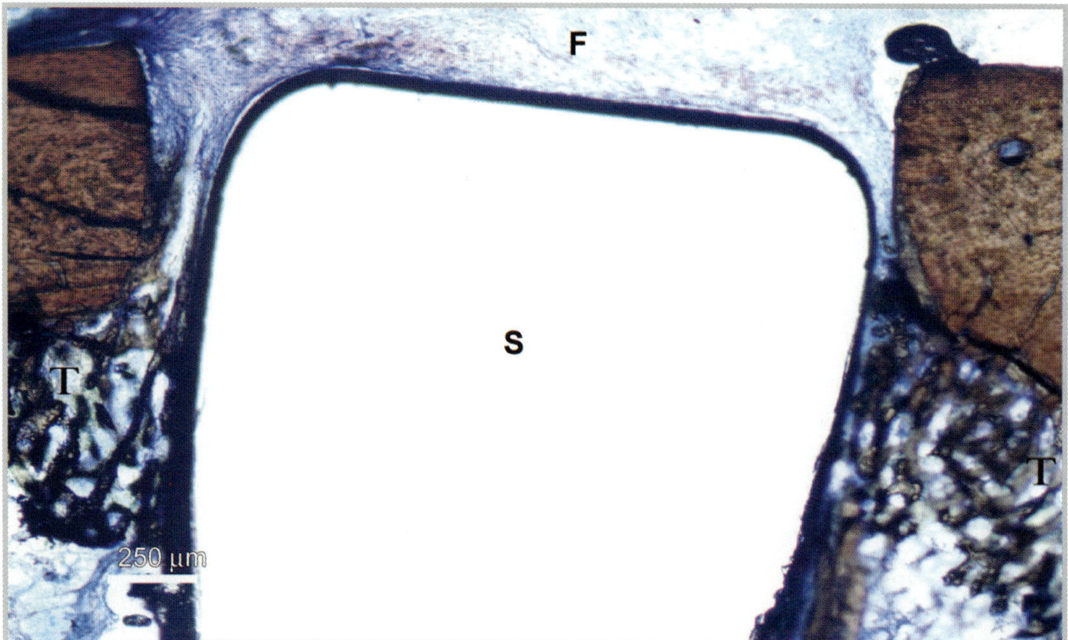

Figure 3B Cross, section of long bone cut perpendicularly to the long axis of the implant. SVB x 4
Implant site (S). Trabeculae of new bone (T) are seen at the inner edge of host bone otherwise known as the endosteal surface of the bone. Fibroblasts are seen on the outer surface known as periosteal surface. Implant positioning in evaluation of biocompatibility is very important

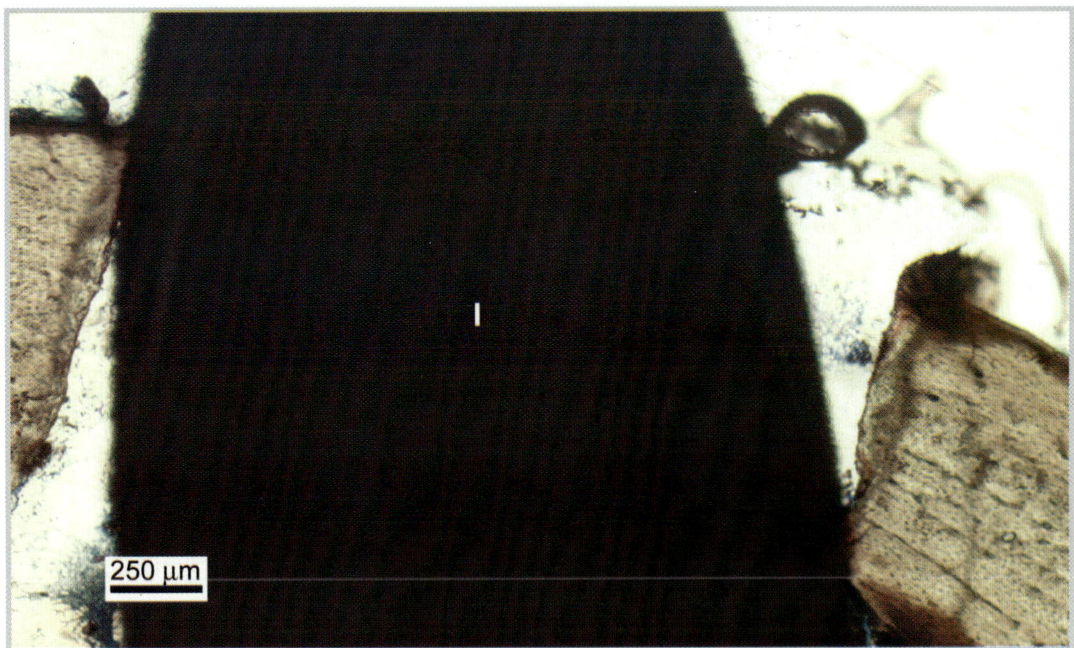

Figure 3C Cross-section of long bone cut perpendicularly to the long axis of the implant. SVB x 4 Oblique placement of implant results in larger interfacial space with long time persistence of fibrous tissue and delayed healing

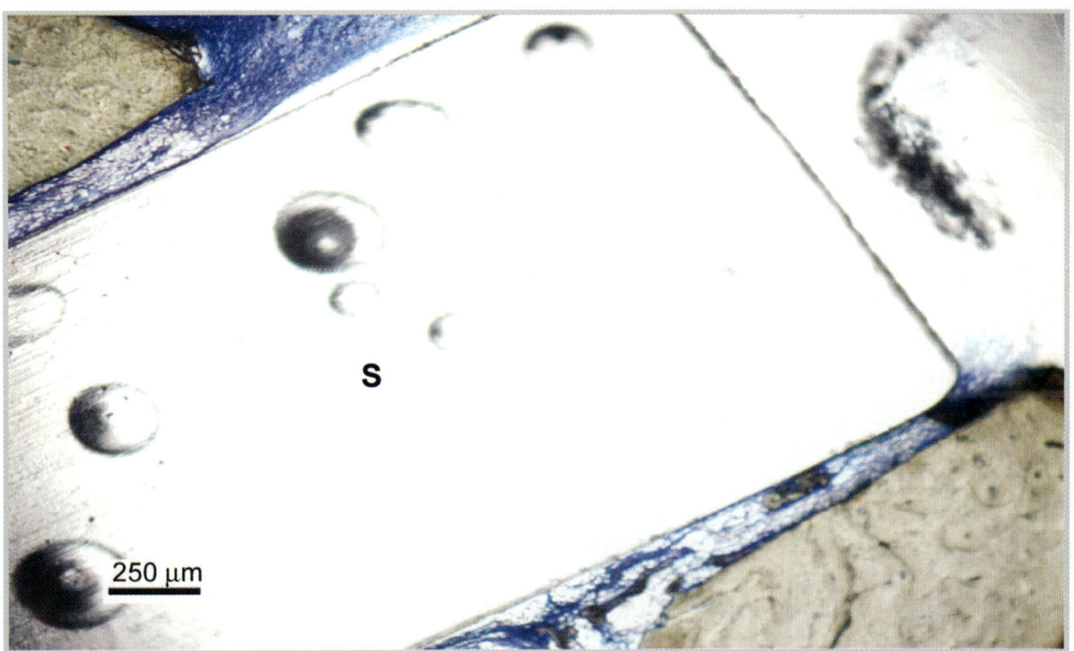

Figure 3D Cross-section of long bone cut perpendicularly to the long axis of the implant. SVB x 4 Perpendicular placement ideally press fit with scant interfacial space is ideal

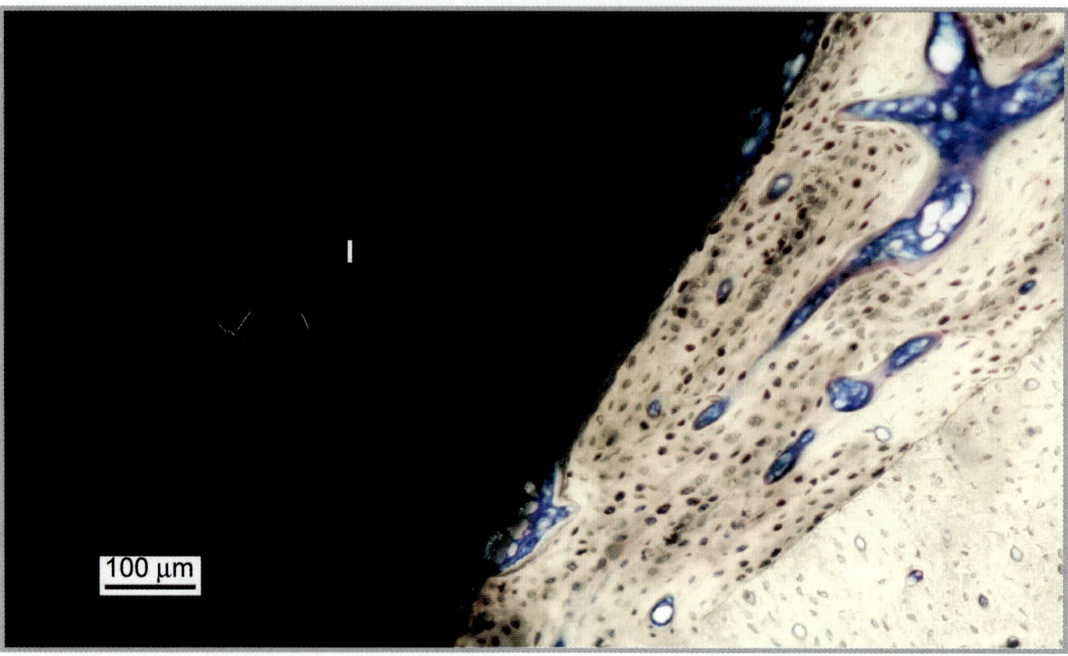

Figure 3E Cross-section of long bone cut perpendicularly to the long axis of the implant. SVB x 10 Press fit results in good and early mature bone deposition at the interface

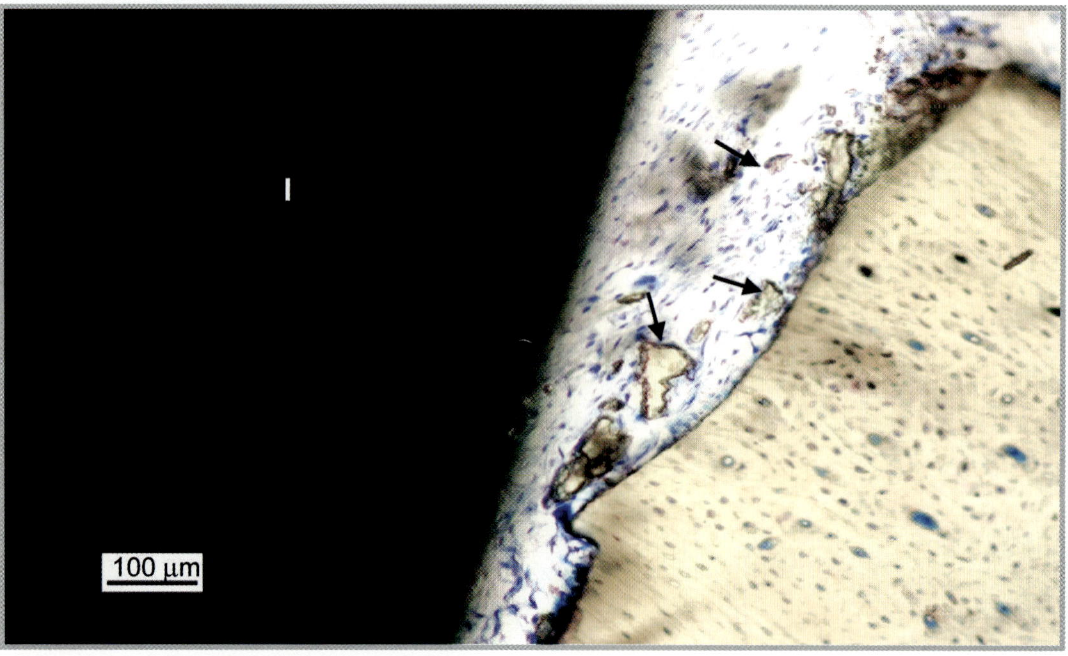

Figure 4A Tissue response to implant in bone. SVB x 10
Fragments of dead bone (↑) at the interface following implantation procedure. Bone fragments during drilling, should be removed prior to implantation

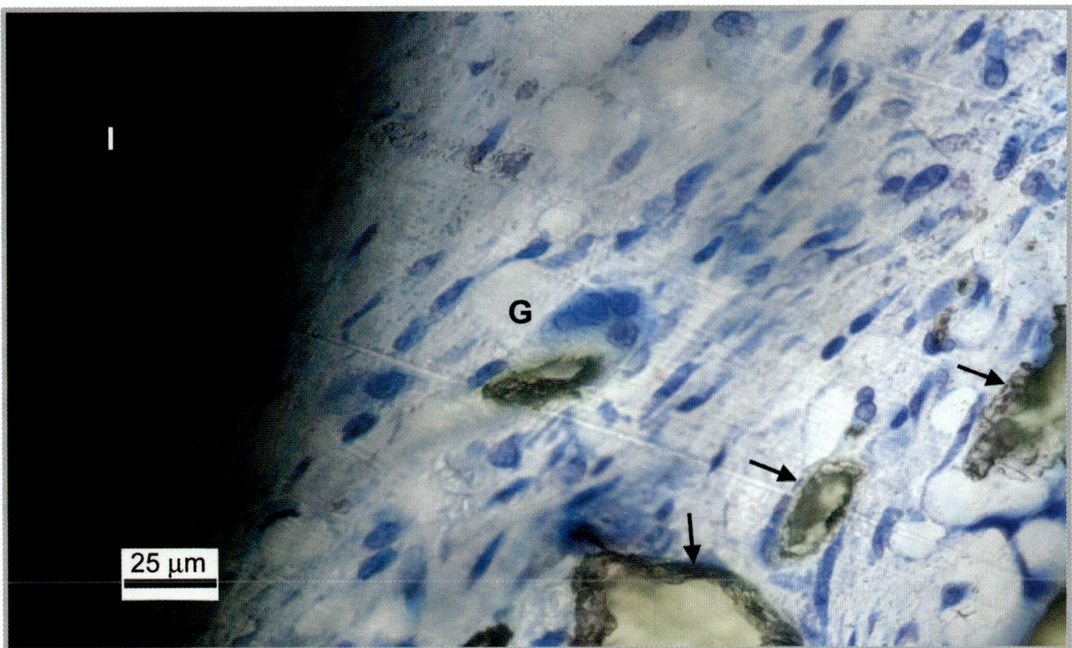

Figure 4B Tissue response to implant in bone. SVB x 40
Fragments of dead bone (↑) at the interface initiate an inflammatory reaction with macrophages and foreign body giant cell formation (G)

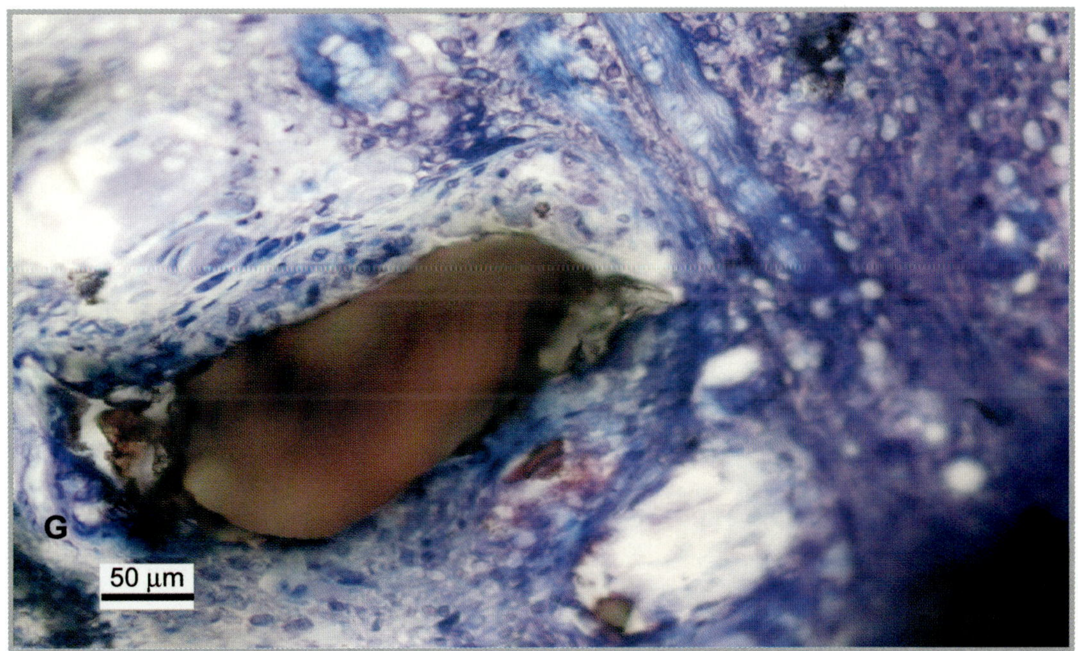

Figure 4C Tissue response to implant in bone. SVB x 20
Macrophages and foreign body giant cell (G) formation around fragment of dead bone

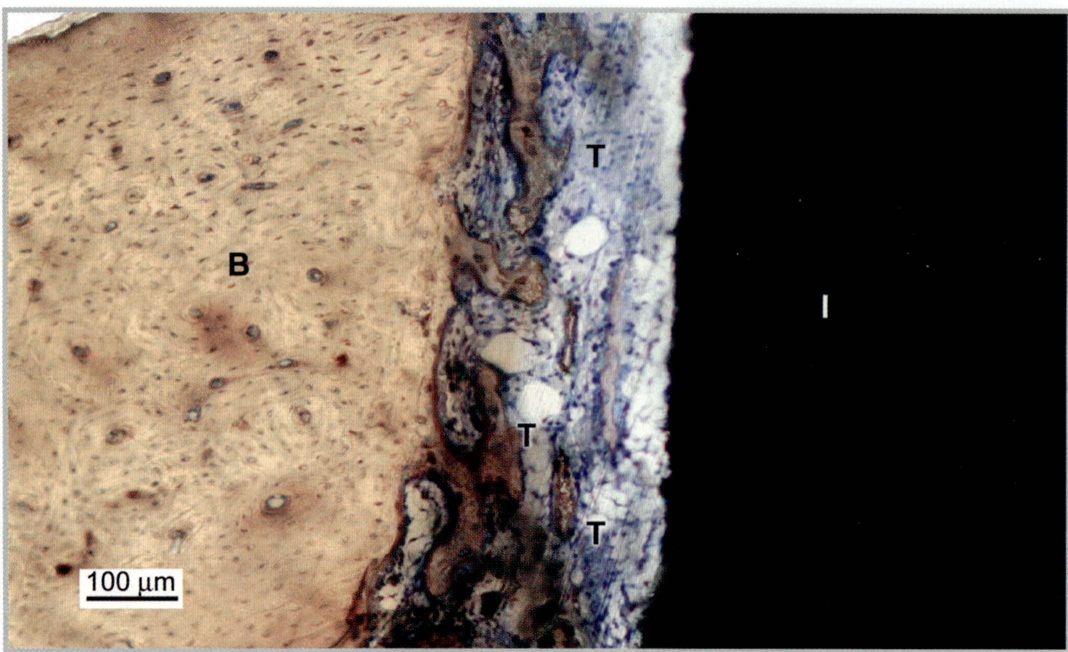

Figure 5A Tissue response to implant in bone. SVB x 10
New bone trabeculae (T) seen along the host bone growing into the space between host bone (B) and implant (I)

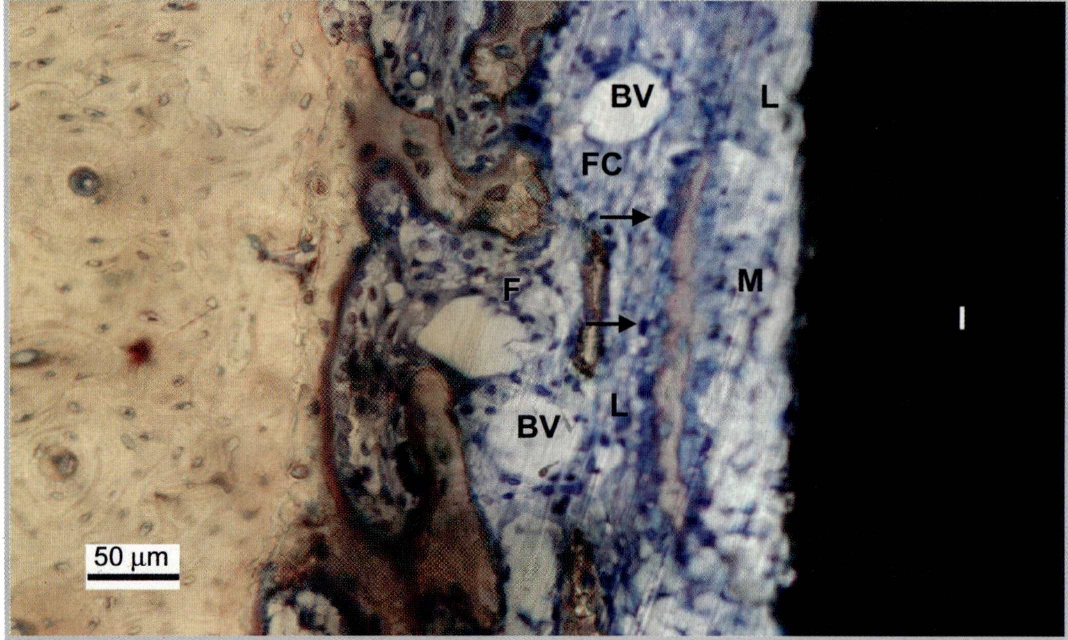

Figure 5B Tissue response to implant in bone. SVB x 20
Higher magnification with macrophages (M), lymphocytes (L), fibroblasts (F) and fibrocytes (FC) and new blood vessels (BV) indicating angiogenesis are seen. Occasional osteoblasts (↑) lining the new bone are observed

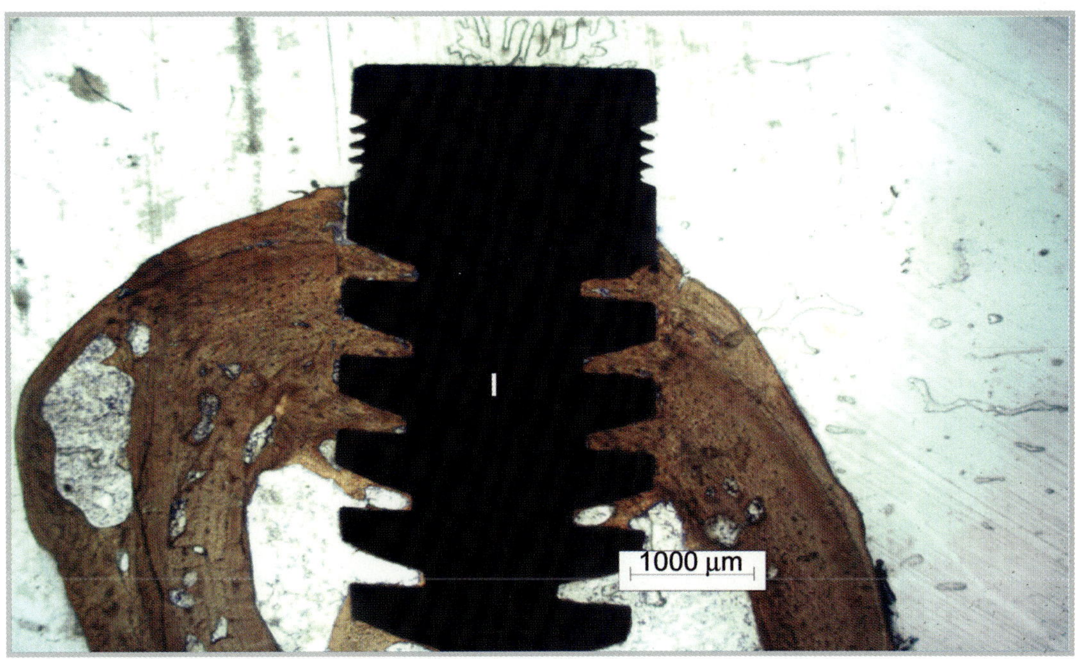

Figure 6A Tissue response to implant in bone. SVB x 1
Metal implant (I) surface modified physically with grooves

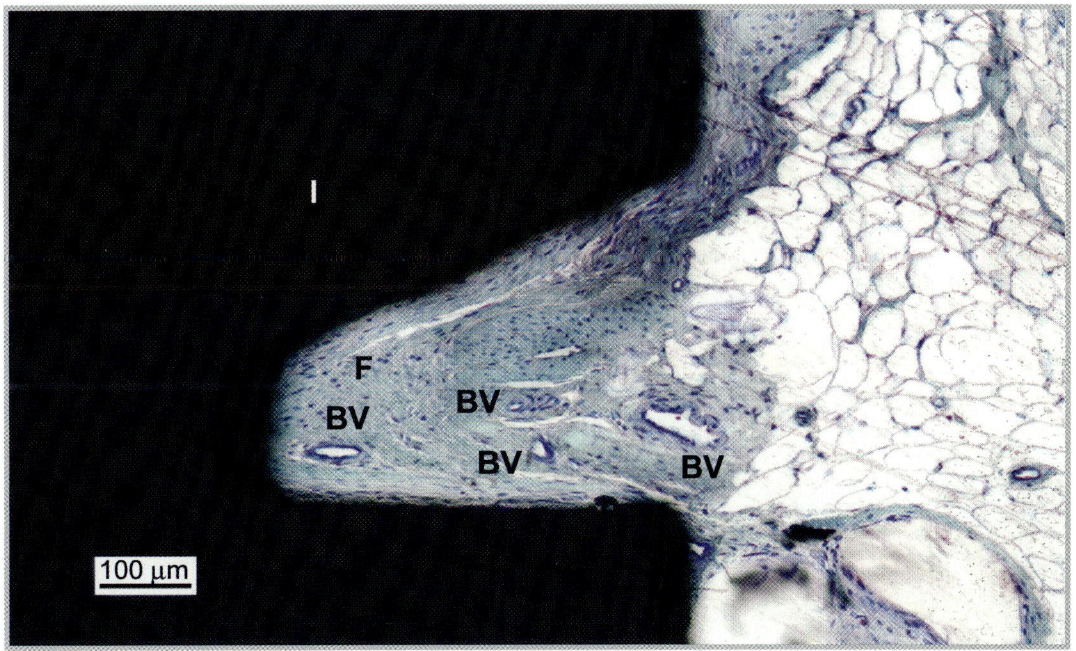

Figure 6B Tissue response to implant in bone. SVB x 10
Fibrous tissue (F) growing into the groove. New blood vessels (BV) are seen

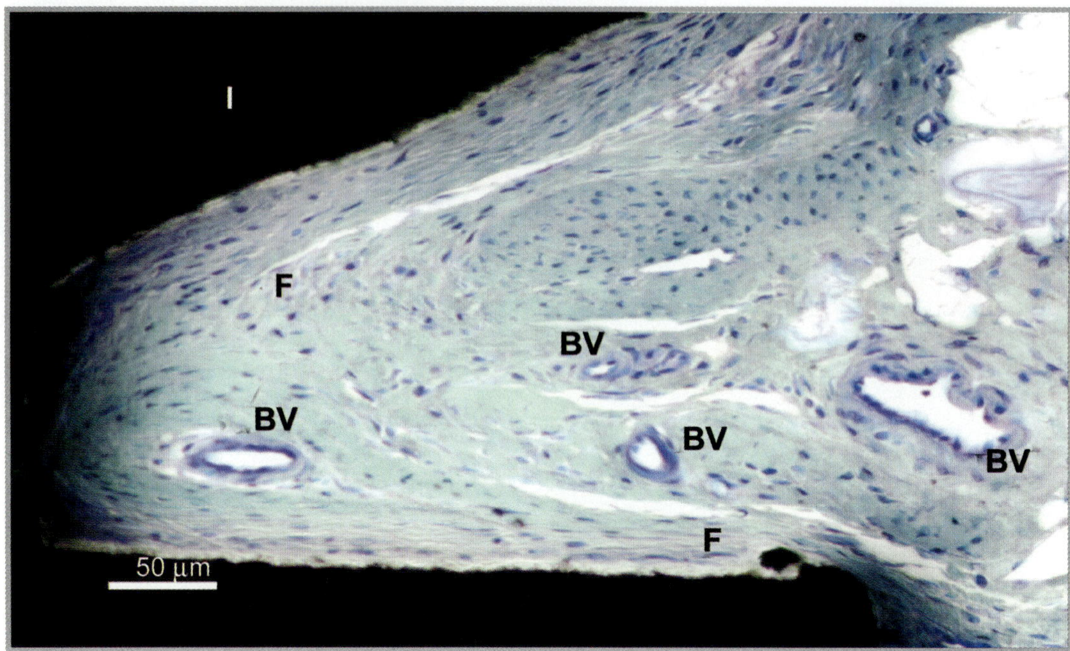

Figure 6C Tissue response to implant in bone. SVB x 20
Higher magnification of the fibrous tissue (F) with numerous new blood vessels (BV)

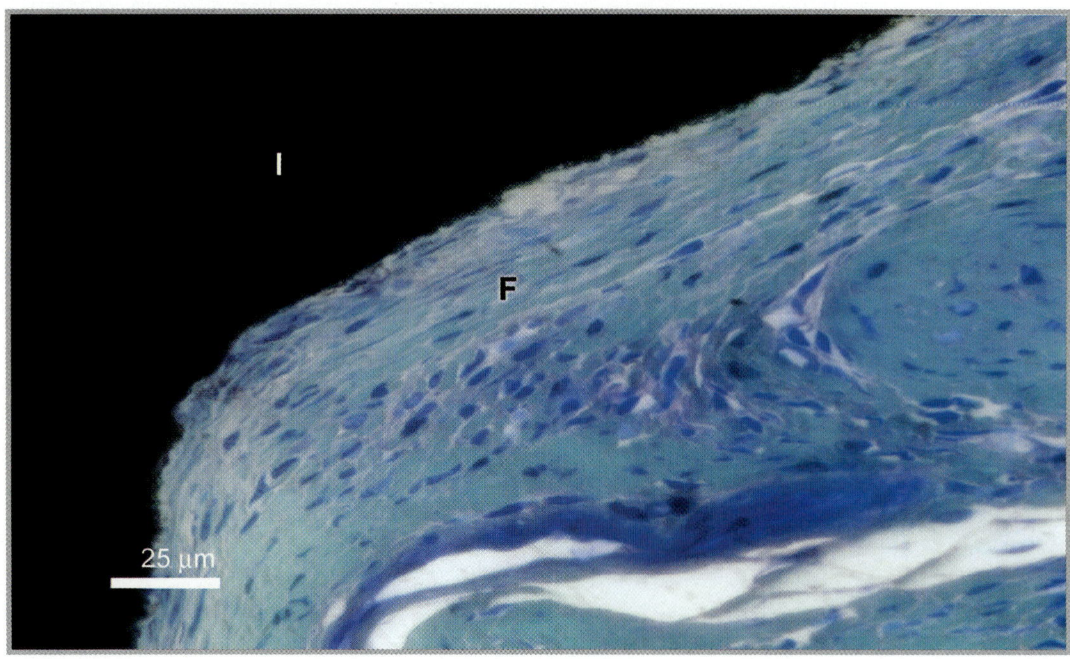

Figure 6D Tissue response to implant in bone. SVB x 40
Numerous fibroblasts (F) at the implant interface

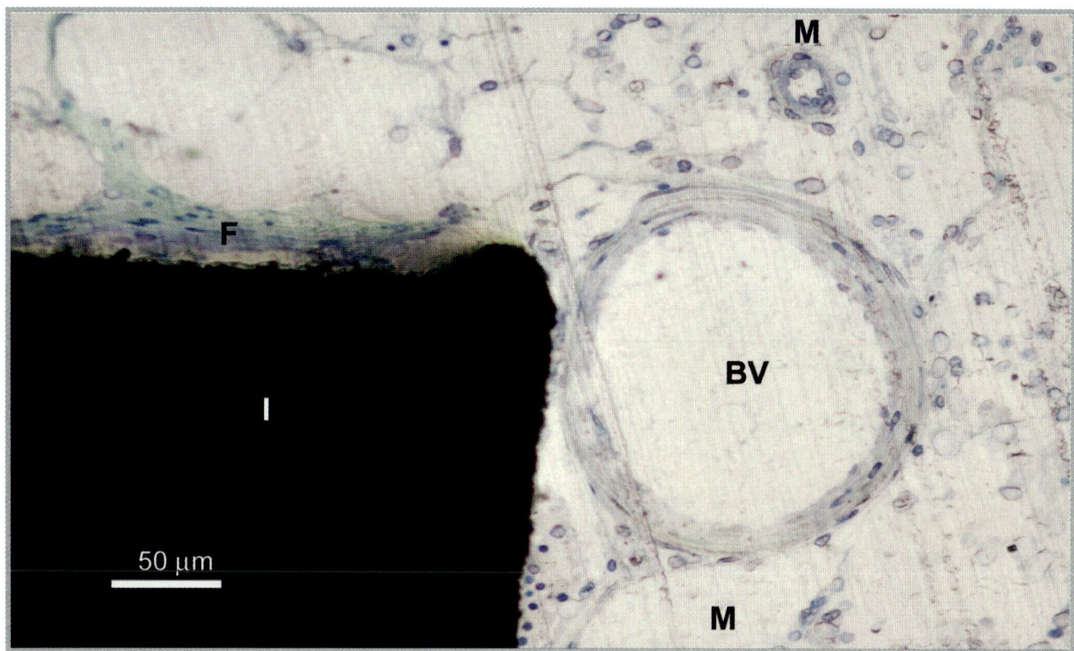

Figure 7 Tissue response to implant in bone. SVB x 20
Distal end of implant in marrow (M). Marrow cells, fibrocytes (F) and a large blood vessel (BV) are seen

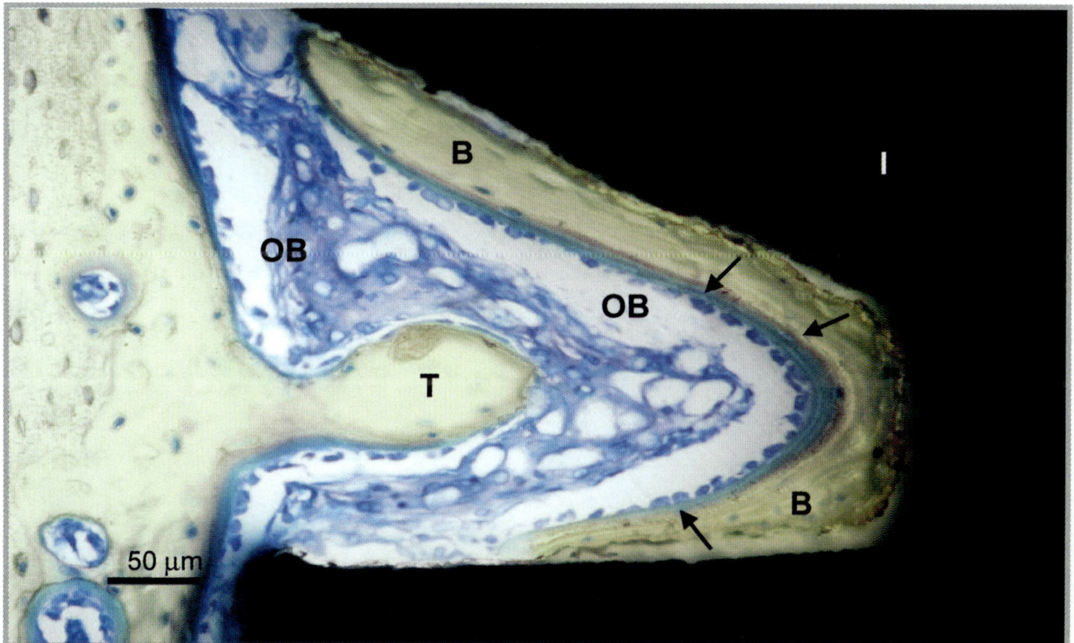

Figure 8 Tissue response to implant in bone. SVB x 20
New woven bone (B) being laid down at the implant surface. Osteoblasts (OB) line the osteoid (↑) layer adjacent to the new bone. The osteoblasts lay down the bone matrix known as osteoid which is calcified to form mature bone. New bone trabeculae (T) are also observed from host bone at left

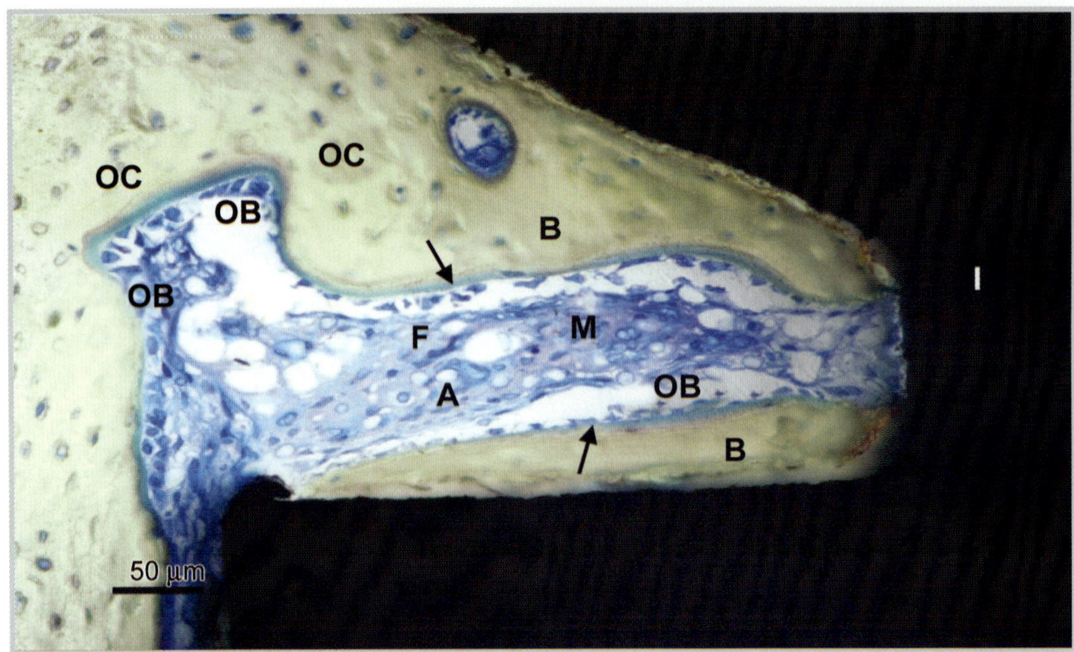

Figure 9 Tissue response to implant in bone. SVB x 20
Fibrous tissue (F) being replaced by new woven bone (B) at the interface. Osteoblasts (OB) line the osteoid (↑) layer adjacent to the new bone. Osteoblasts embedded in the new bone matrix, otherwise known as osteocytes (OC) are noted. Fibrous tissue (A) with fibrocytes and occasional macrophages (M) also persist

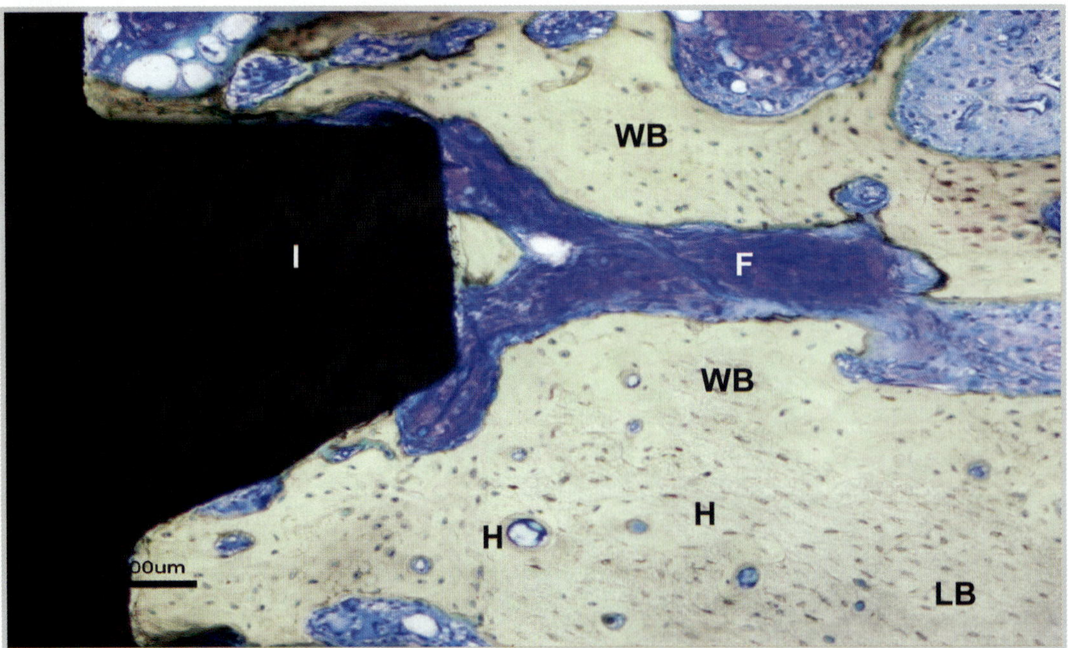

Figure 10 Tissue response to implant in bone. SVB x 10
Islands of fibrous tissue (F) with new woven bone (WB) and lamellar bone (LB) at implant interface. Numerous small Haversian canals (H) are present in the new bone

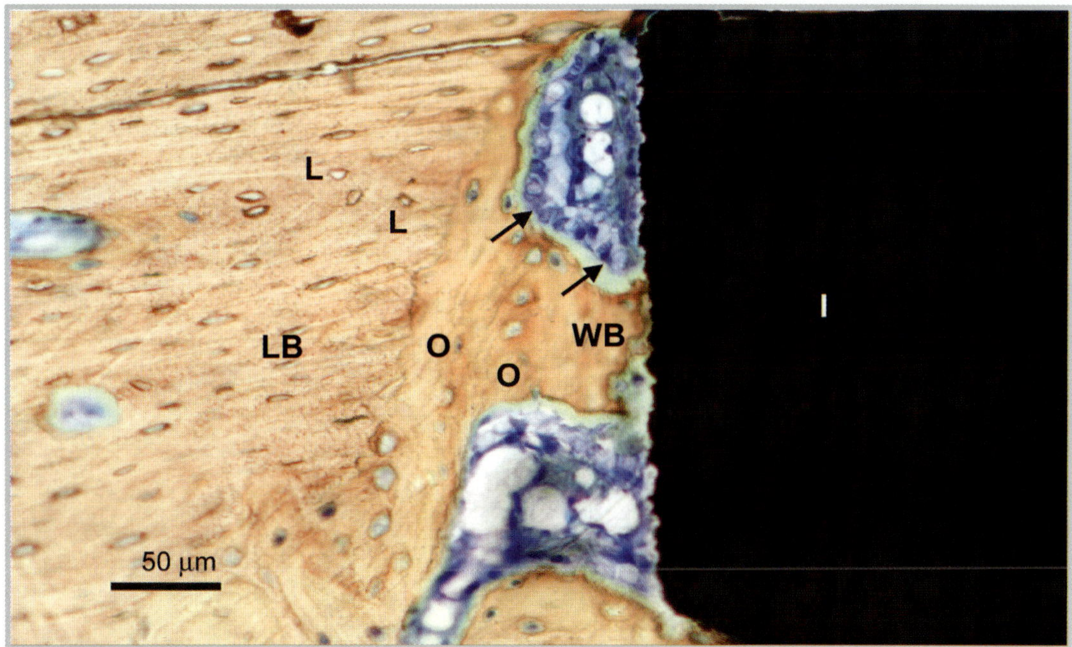

Figure 11 Tissue response to implant in bone. SVB x 20
Mature lamellar host bone (LB) is well-demarcated from new woven bone (WB) adjacent to implant surface. Osteoblasts (↑) and osteocytes (O) in new bone and empty lacunae (L) in host bone are seen

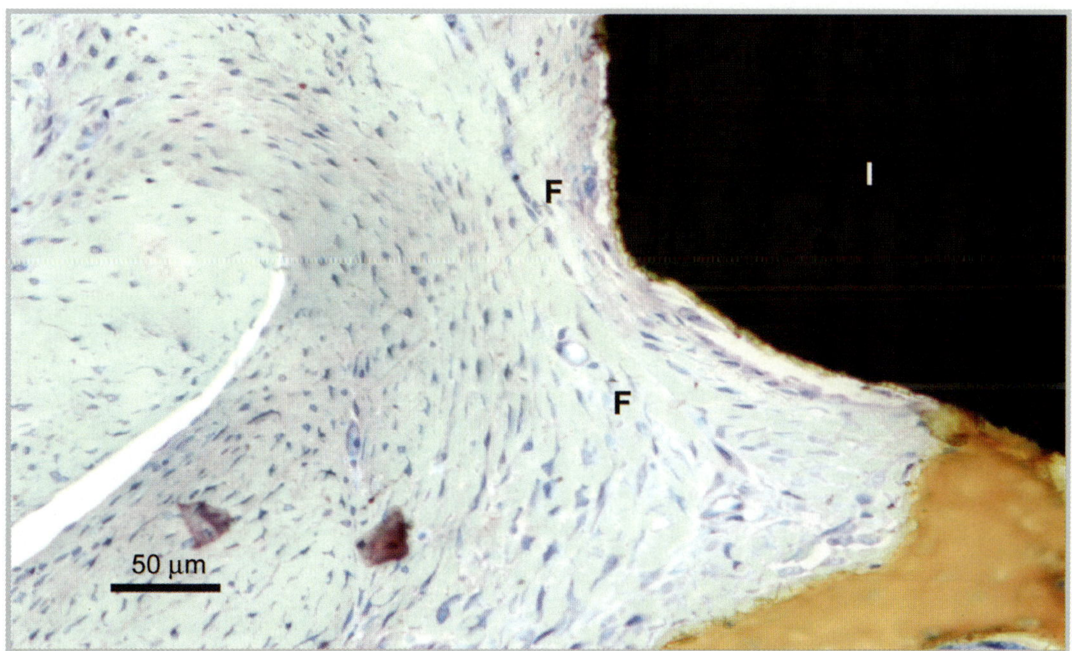

Figure 12 Tissue response to implant in bone. SVB x 20
Fibrous tissue (F) at implant interface

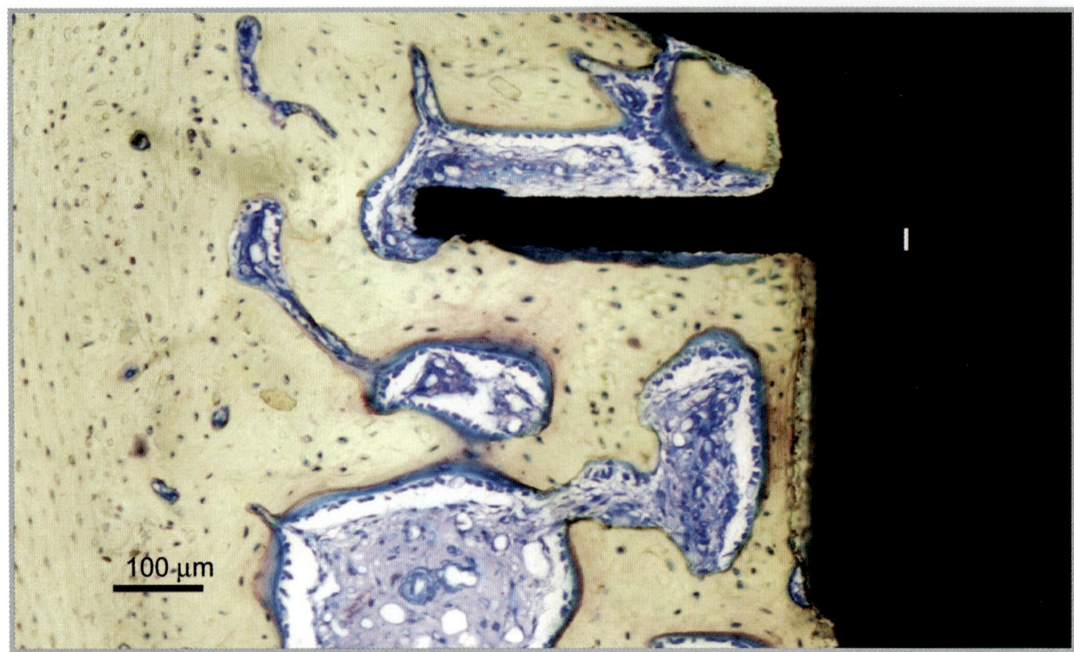

Figure 13 Tissue response to implant in bone. SVB x 10
Bone deposition at implant interface along the bulk implant as well around pegs on the modified surface

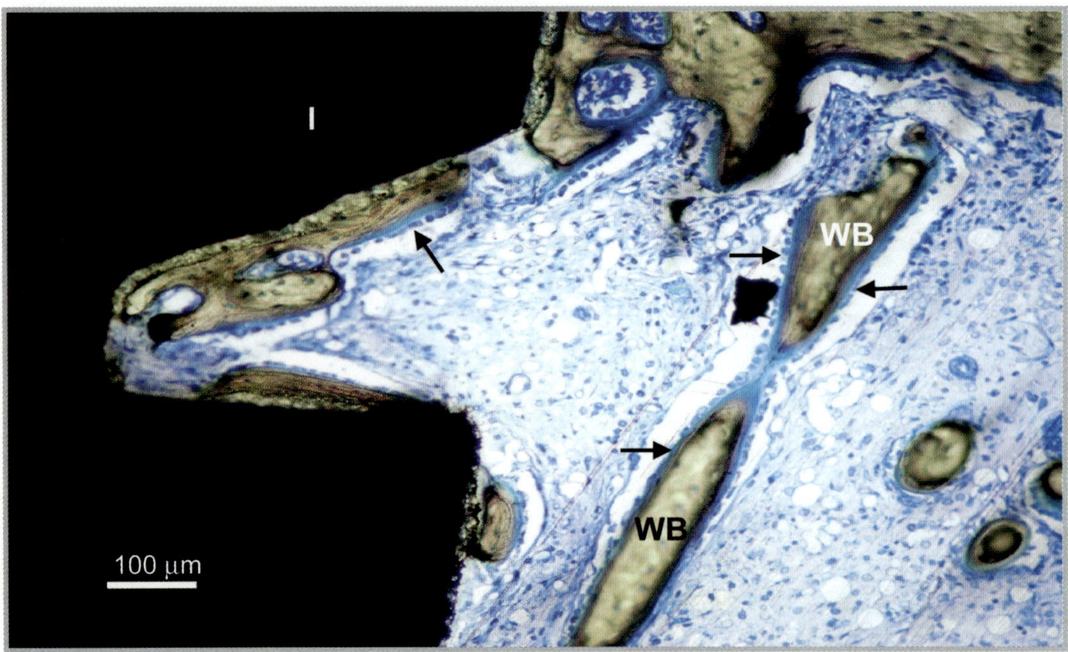

Figure 14 Tissue response to implant in bone. SVB x 10
Fragments of new bone with numerous osteoblasts (↑)

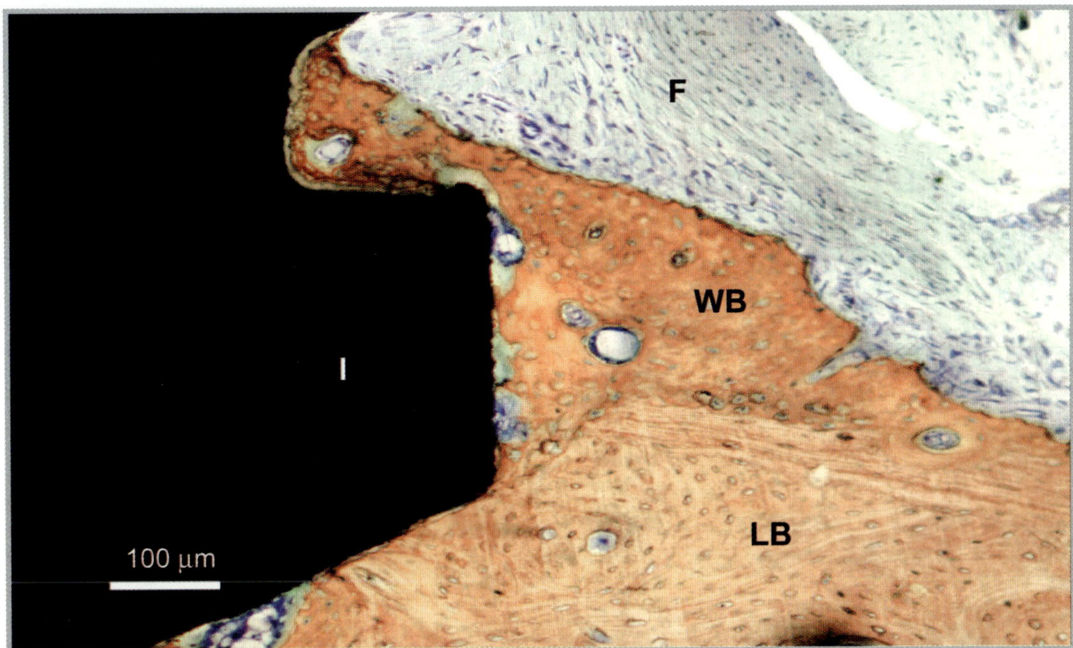

Figure 15 Tissue response to implant in bone. SVB x 10
Lamellar (LB) and woven bone (WB) and fibrous tissue (F) with fibrocytes and fibroblasts at implant interface

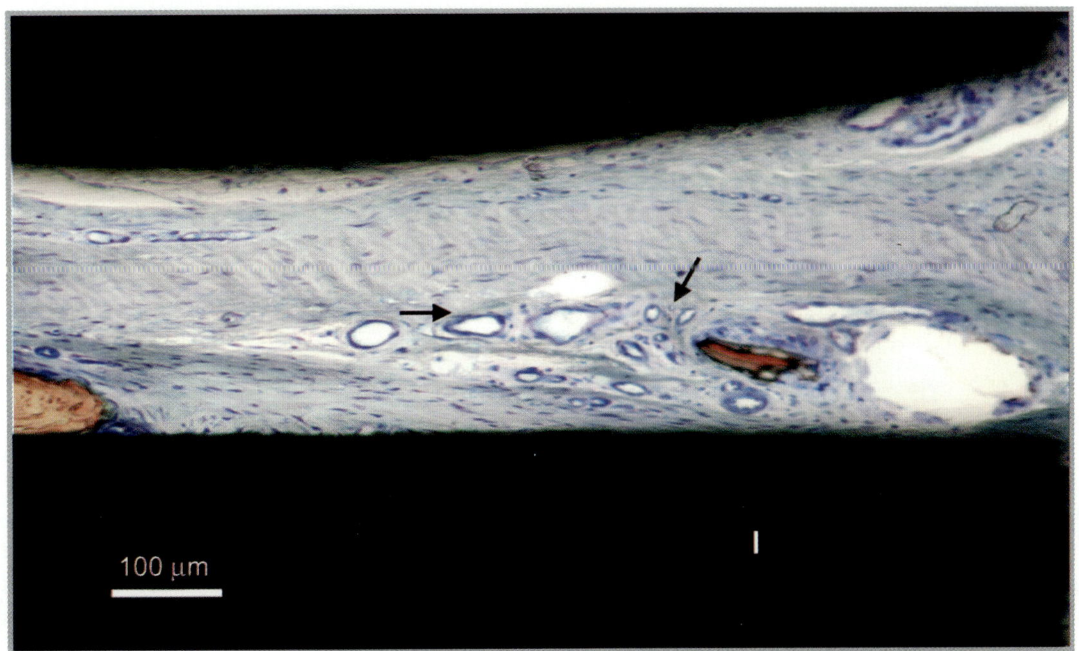

Figure 16 Tissue response to implant in bone. SVB x 10
Fibrous tissue in the grooves of a metal implant with angiogenesis (↑)

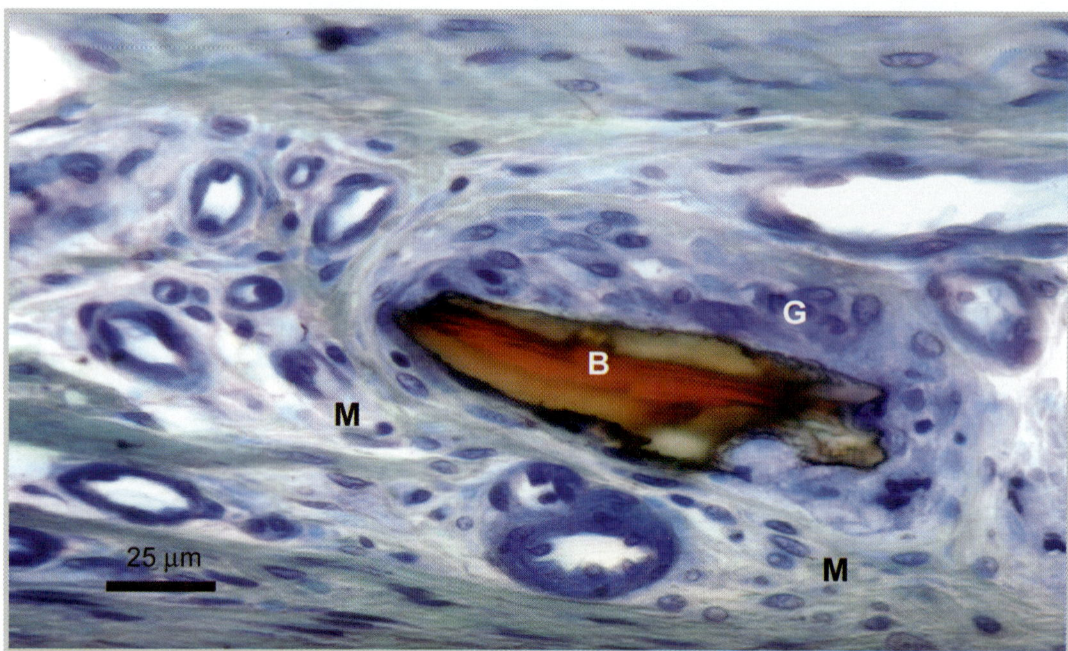

Figure 17 Tissue response to implant in bone. SVB x 40
Fragment of dead bone (B). There are no lacunae and no osteoblasts. Numerous macrophages (M) and a foreign body type of giant cell (G) are seen

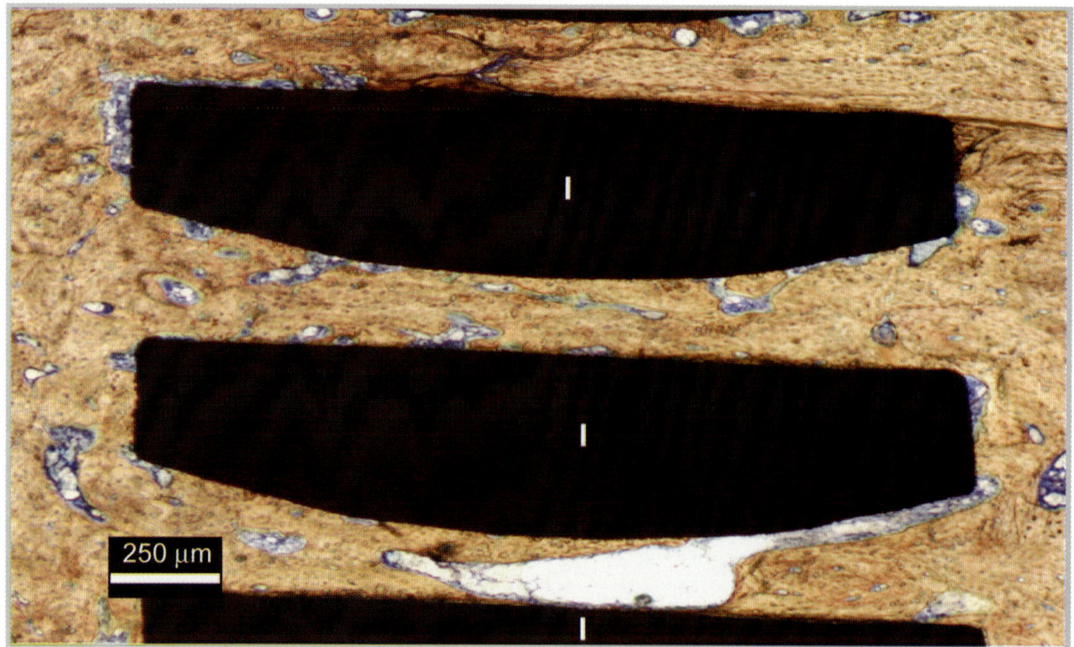

Figure 18A Tissue response to implant in bone. SVB x 4
Good woven bone deposition in the grooves of a metal implant with close apposition of bone on to metal surface

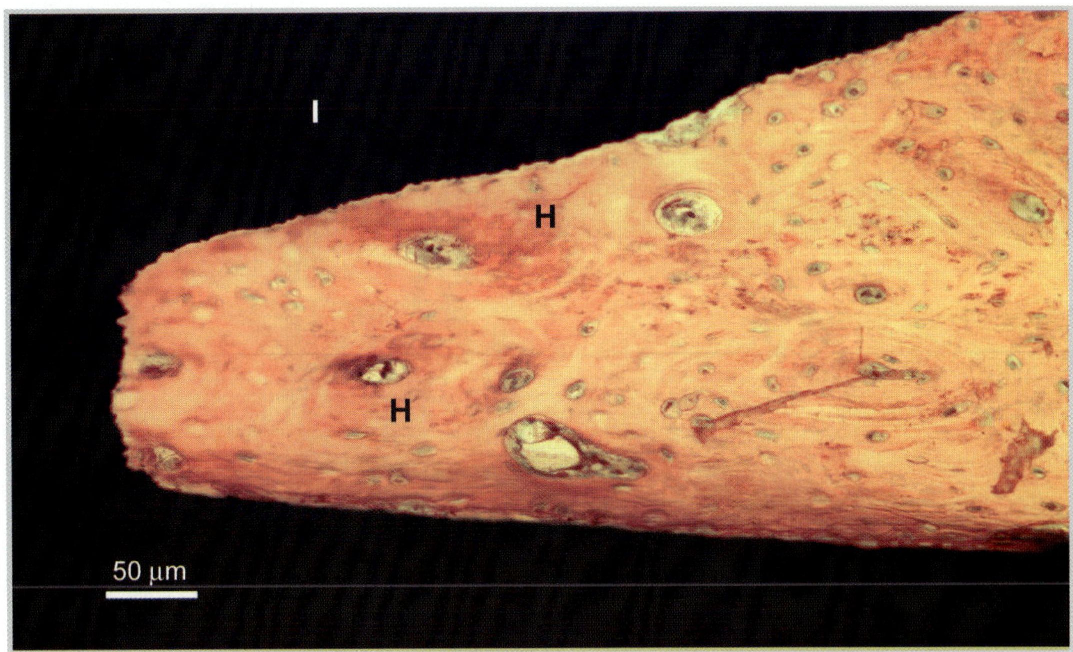

Figure 18B Tissue response to implant in bone. SVB x 20
Close apposition of bone on to metal surface. Well-formed Haversian systems (H) are seen

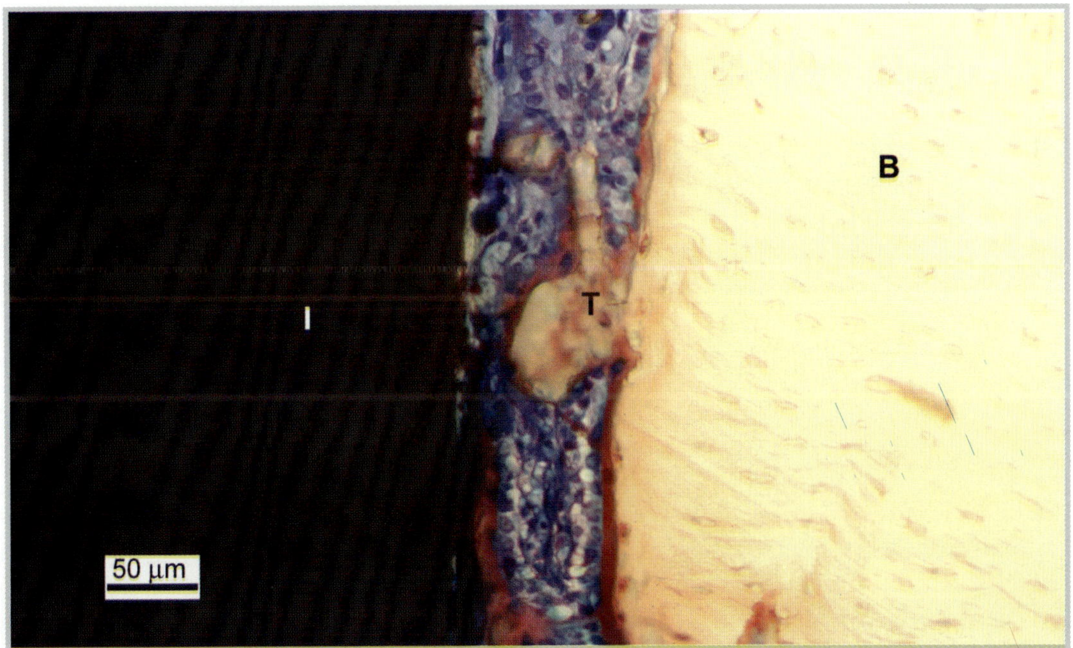

Figure 19A Tissue response to implant in bone. SVB x 20
Evaluation of biocompatibility of a metal rod in long bone at one week. Macrophages and fibroblasts are seen at the implant (I)—bone (B) interface, as well as trabeculae (T) of new woven bone from the host bone

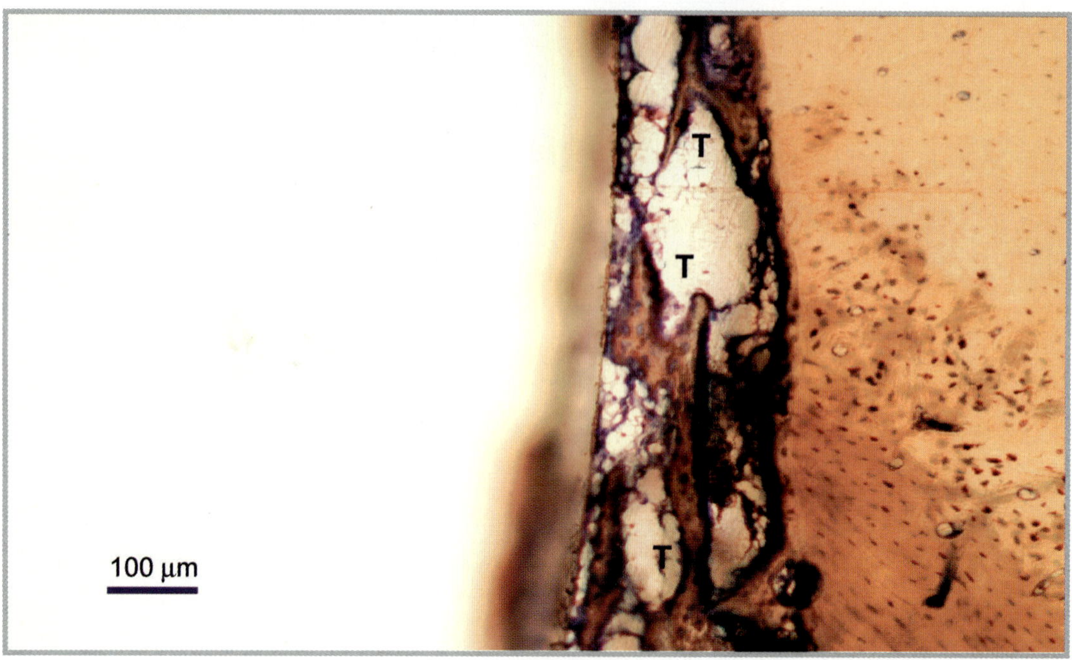

Figure 19B Tissue response to implant in bone. SVB x 10
Lower magnification of new bone trabeculae (T) at the interface

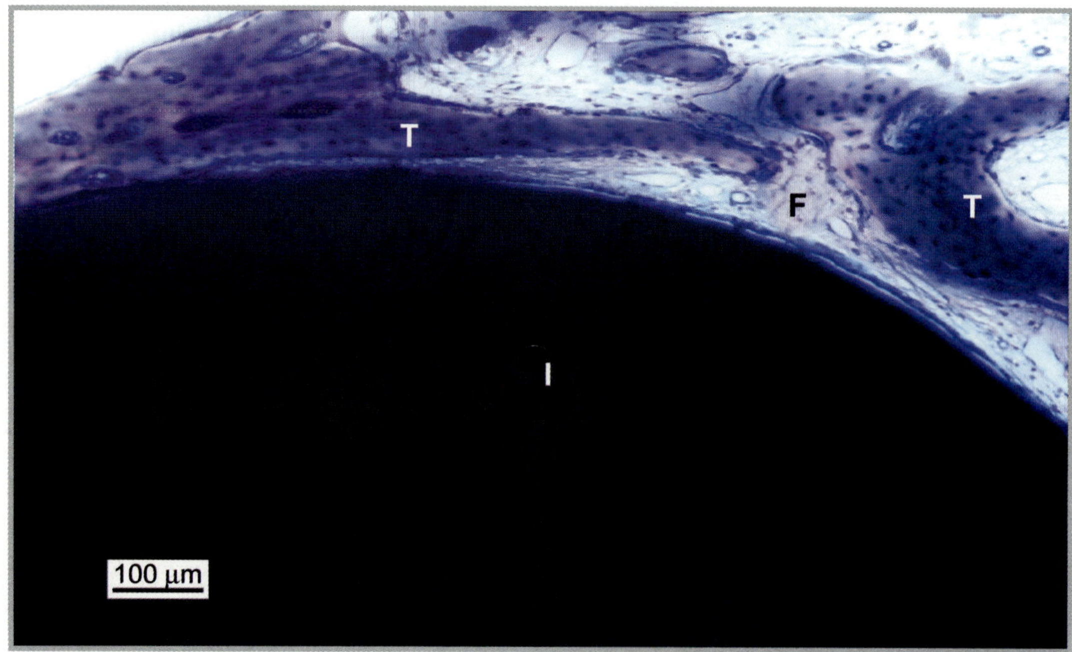

Figure 19C Tissue response to implant in bone. SVB x 10
Evaluation of biocompatibility of a metal rod in long bone at four weeks. Bone trabeculae (T) as well as fibrous tissue (F) around proximal end of implant

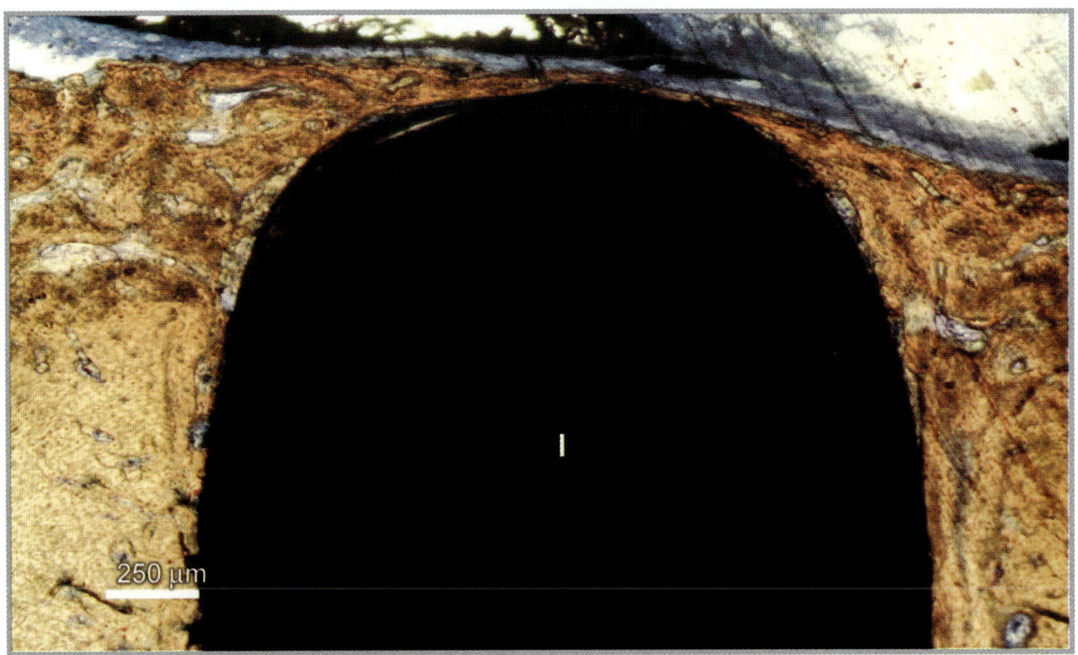

Figure 19D Tissue response to implant in bone. SVB x 4
Mature bone around proximal end and sides of implant

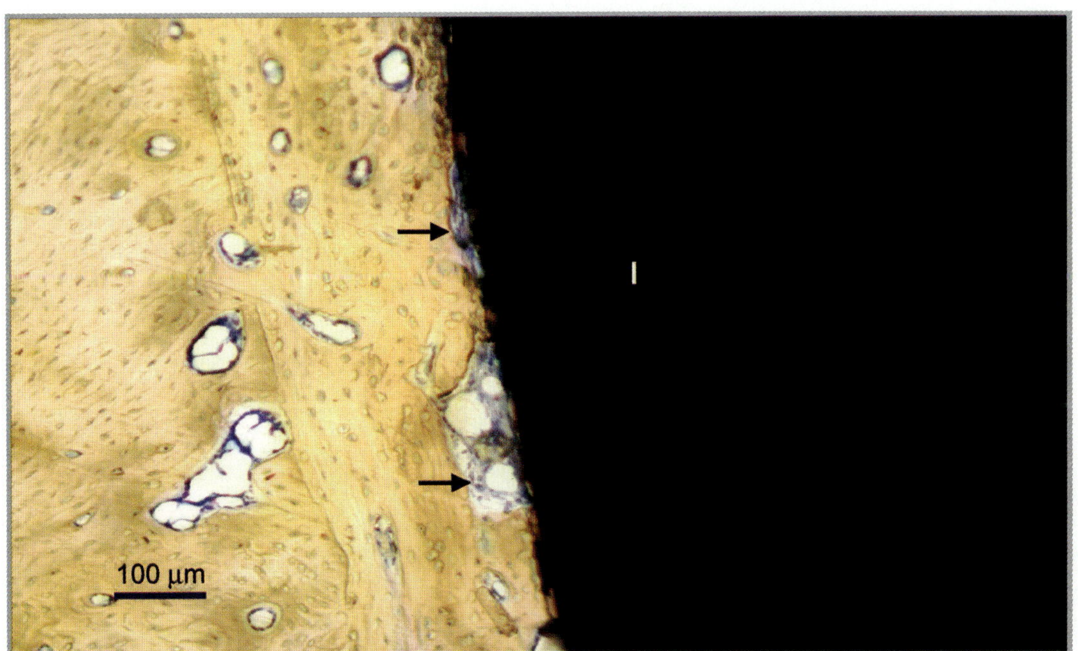

Figure 19E Tissue response to implant in bone. SVB x 10
Occasional cellular areas (↑) noted at the interface

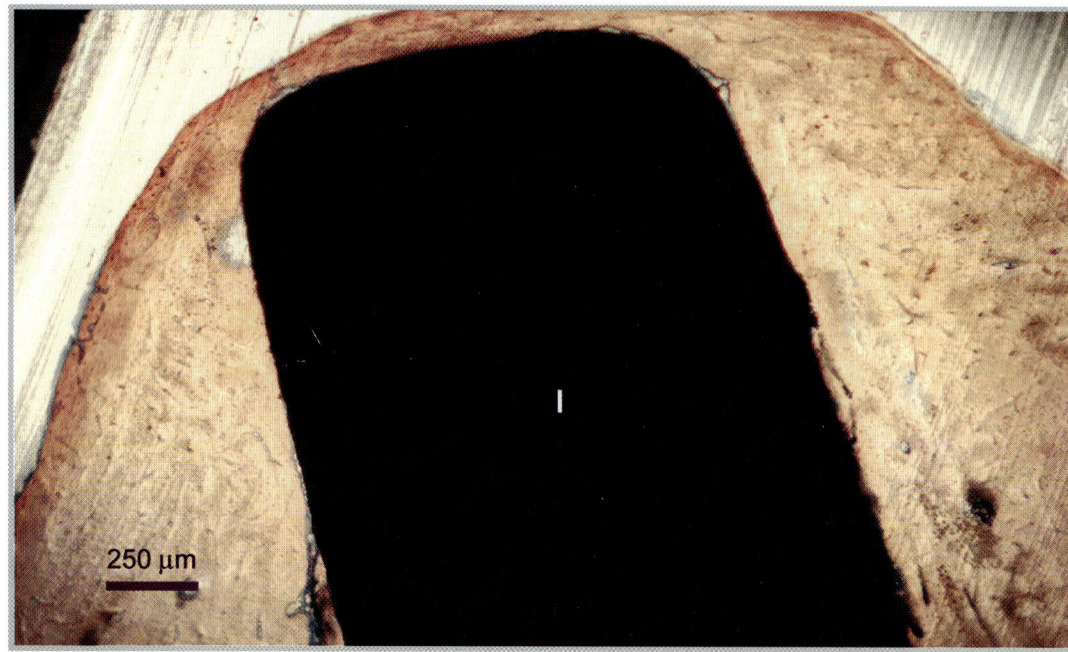

Figure 19F Tissue response to implant in bone. SVB x 4
Evaluation of biocompatibility of a metal rod in long bone at twelve weeks. Good biocompatibility of implant with bone as evidenced by mature bone at the interface

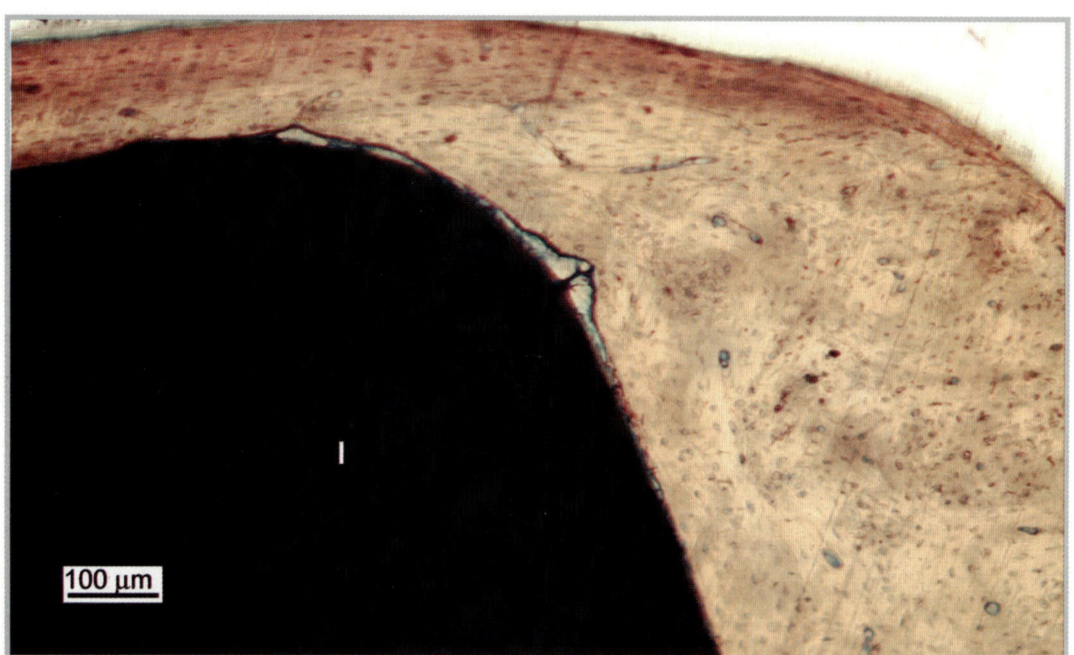

Figure 19G Tissue response to implant in bone. SVB x 10
Mature bone at the interface

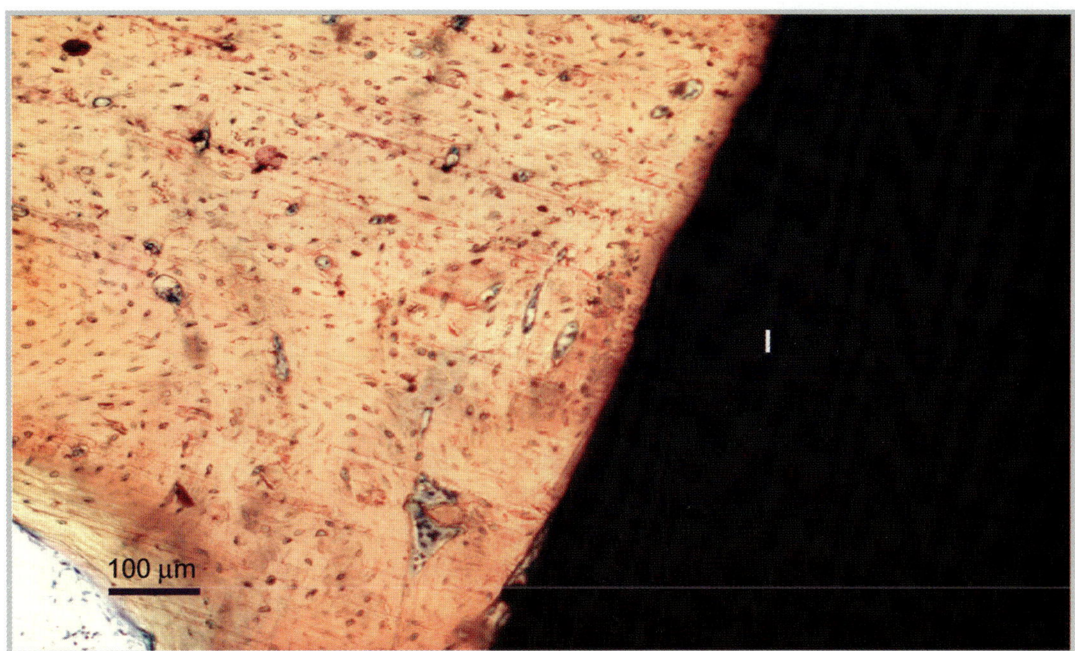

Figure 19H Tissue response to implant in bone. SVB x 10
Mature bone at the interface. There is absence of inflammation and fibrosis

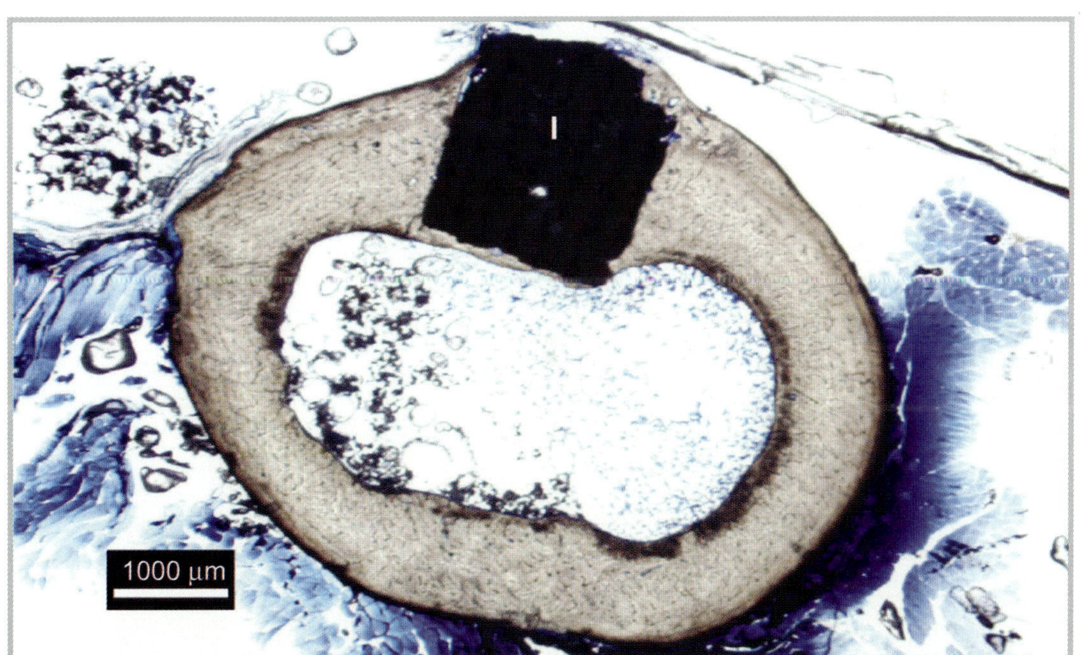

Figure 20 Tissue response to implant in bone. SVB x 1
Resin cross-section of a porous rod shaped ceramic polymer composite implant (I) in long bone

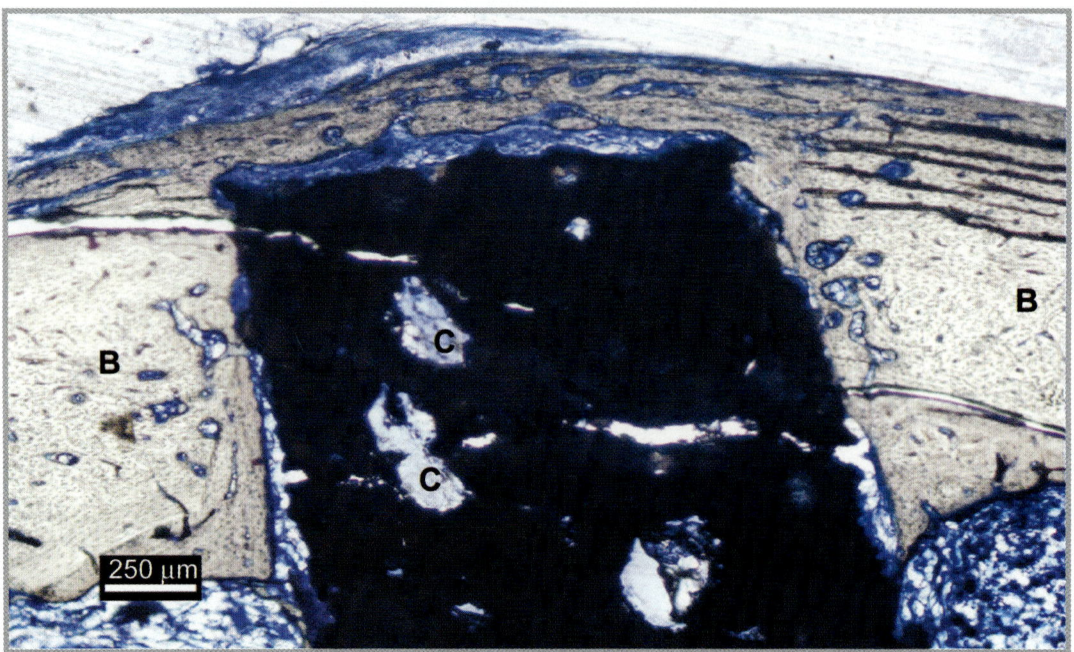

Figure 21A Tissue response to implant in bone. SVB x 4
Evaluation of biocompatibility of a rod shaped ceramic polymer composite implant in long bone (B) at four weeks. Islands of cellular tissue (C) noted in the implant

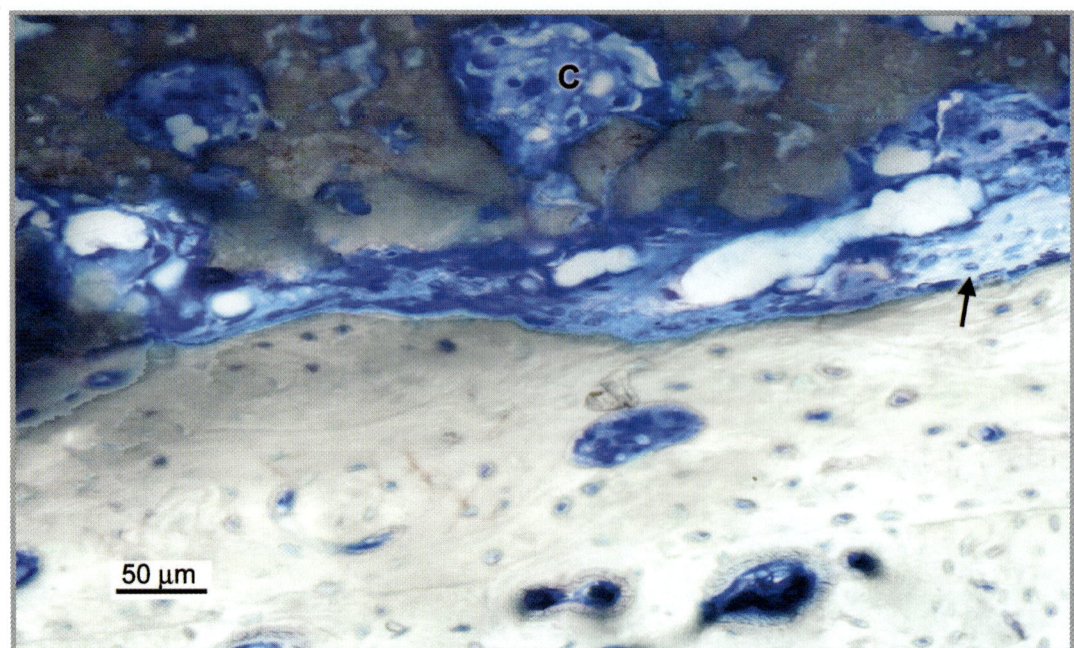

Figure 21B Tissue response to implant in bone. SVB x 20
Macrophages and fibroblasts (↑) at the interface as well as in the material (C)

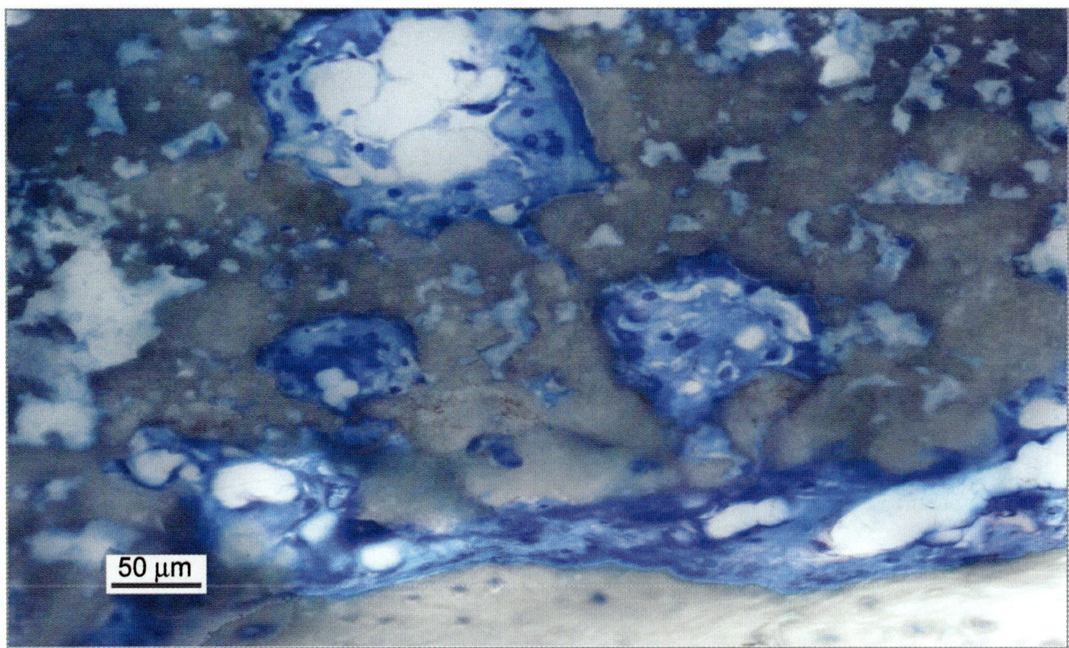

Figure 21C Tissue response to implant in bone. SVB x 20
Higher magnification of macrophages and fibroblasts at the interface as well as in the material

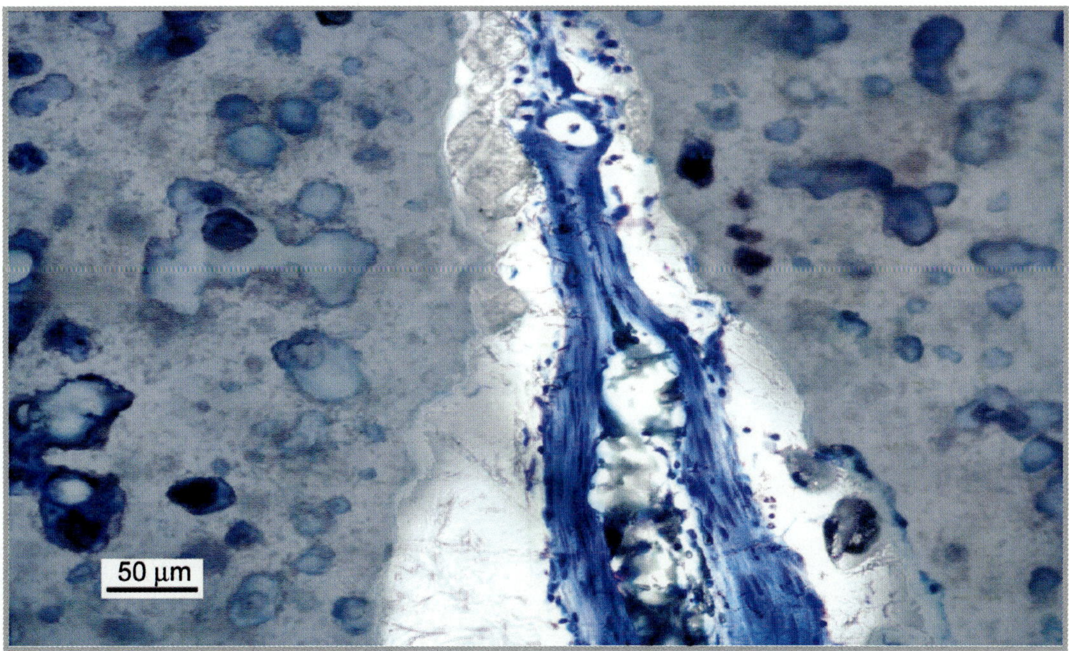

Figure 21D Tissue response to implant in bone. SVB x 20
Fibrocytes in crevices of material

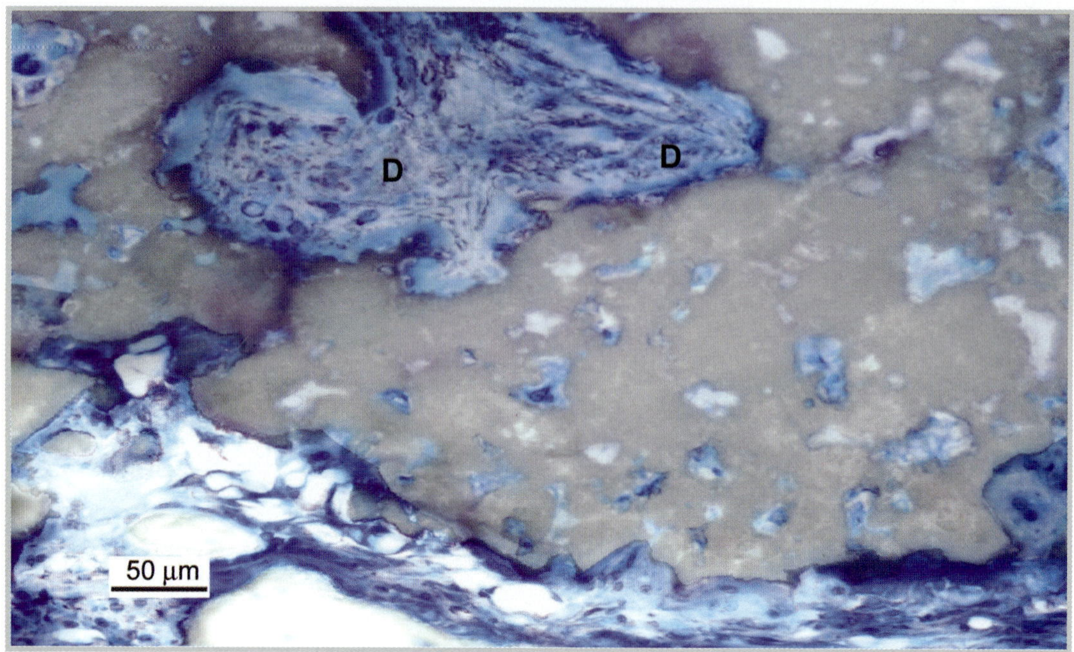

Figure 21E Tissue response to implant in bone. SVB x 20
Fibrocytes and material debri (D) in crevices of the material

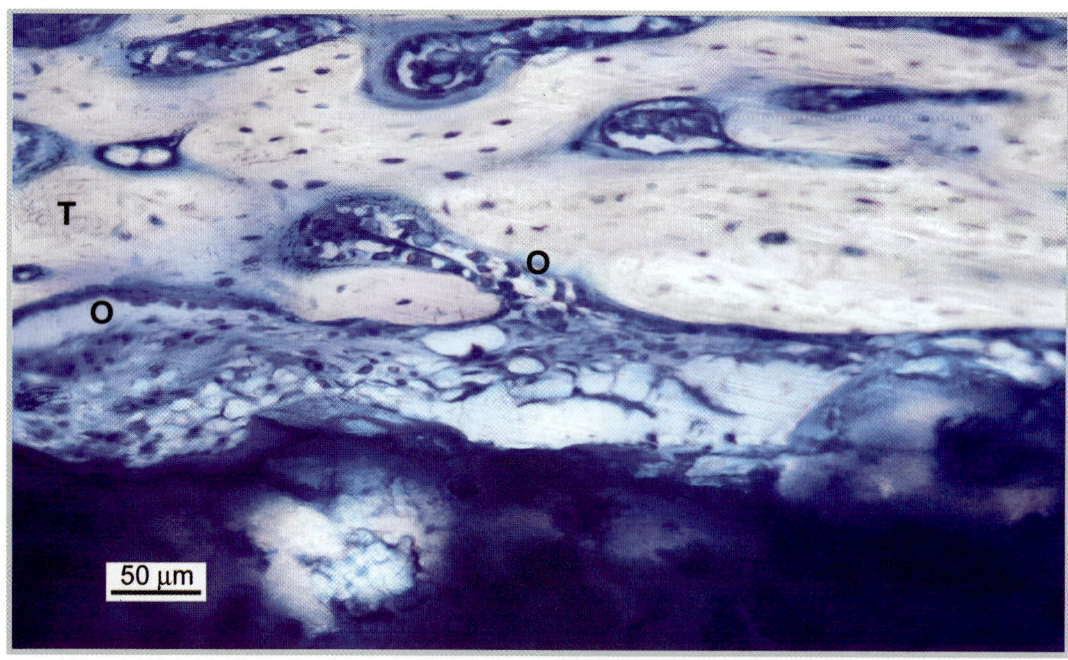

Figure 21F Tissue response to implant in bone. SVB x 20
New bone trabeculae (T) at the implant interface with osteoblasts (O)

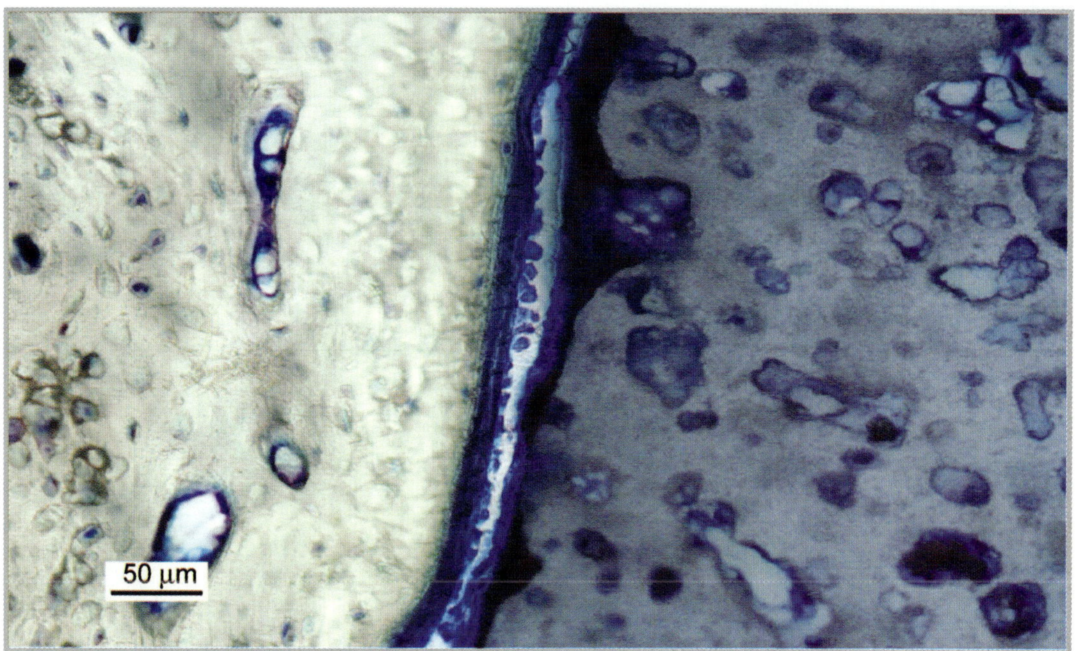

Figure 21G Tissue response to implant in bone. SVB x 20
New woven bone at the implant interface with osteoblasts

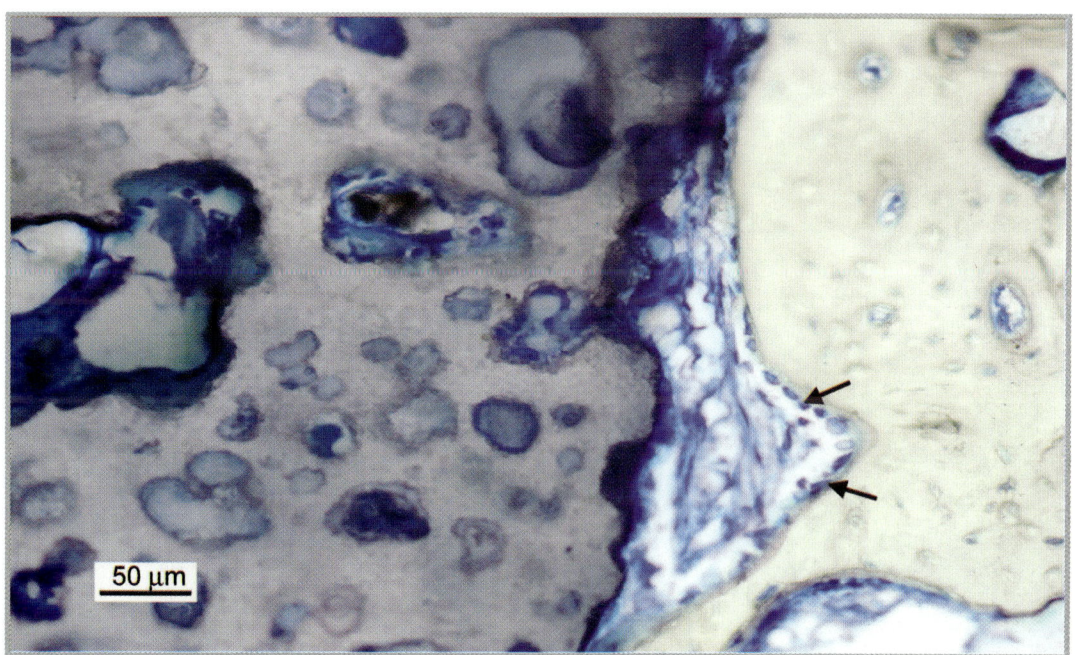

Figure 21H Tissue response to implant in bone. SVB x 20
New bone trabeculae at the implant interface with osteoblasts (↑)

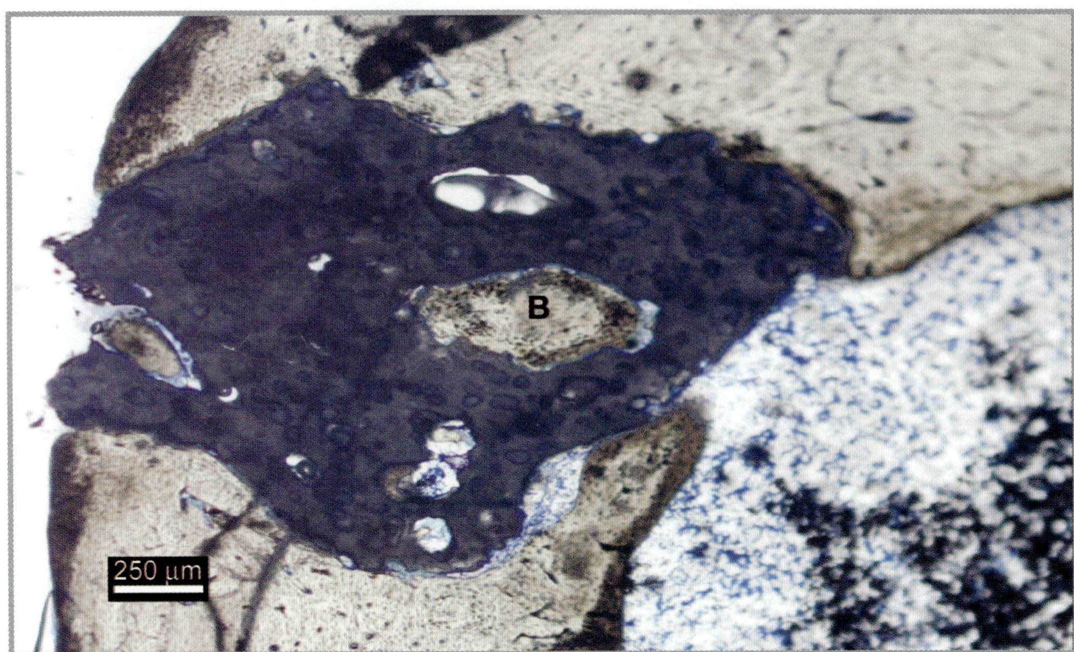

Figure 21I Tissue response to implant in bone. SVB x 4
Islands of mature bone (B) formation in the implant at twelve weeks post-implantation

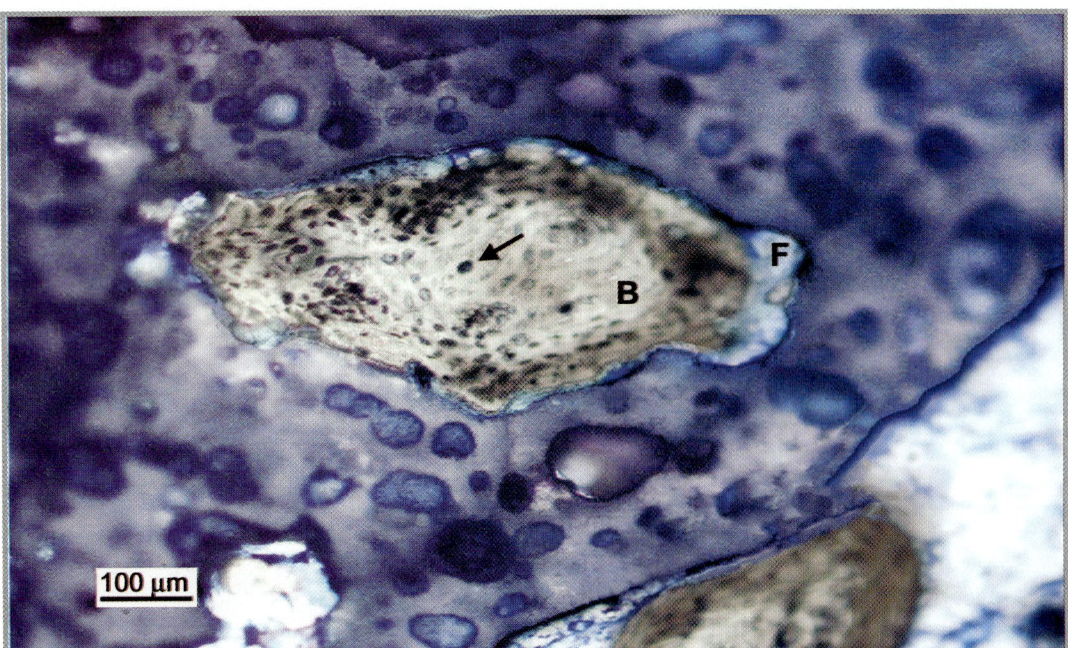

Figure 21J Tissue response to implant in bone. SVB x 10
Higher magnification of islands of mature bone (B) formation in the implant with formation of Haversian canals (↑). Occasional fibrocytes (F) persist at the periphery

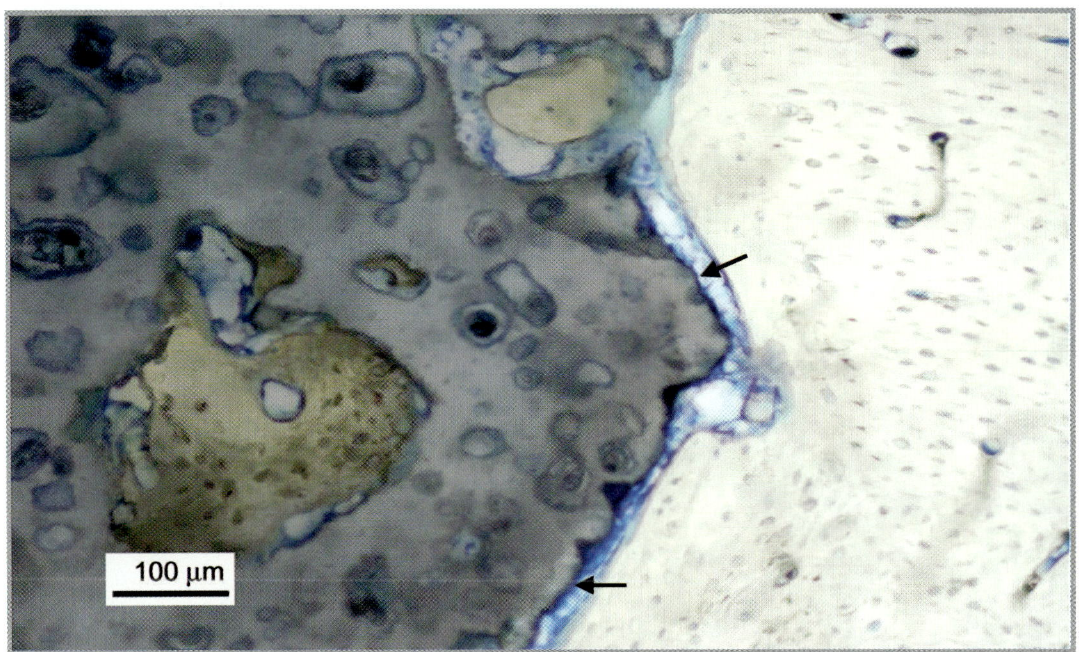

Figure 21K Tissue response to implant in bone. SVB x 10
Thin layer of fibrocytes (↑) at the bone material interface

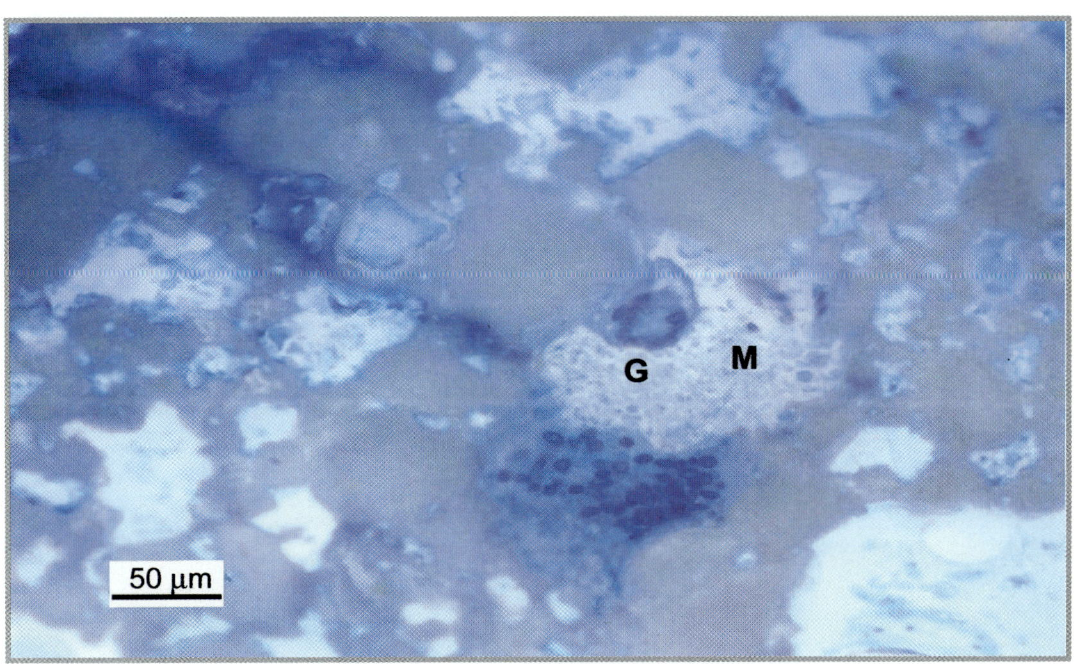

Figure 21L Tissue response to implant in bone. SVB x 20
Persistence of macrophages (M) and giant cells (G) in the material

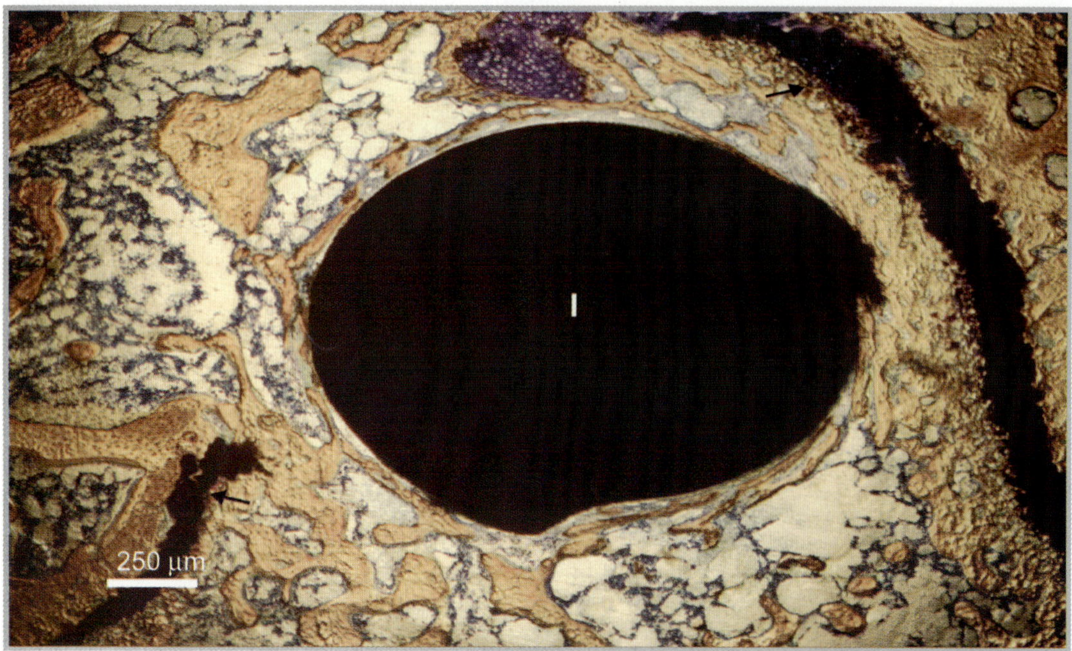

Figure 22A Tissue response to implant in bone. SVB x 4
Evaluation of biocompatibility of a rod shaped metal implant with a modified surface with nanoparticles in lateral condyle of long bone at four weeks. Cross-section of implant in the cancellous bone

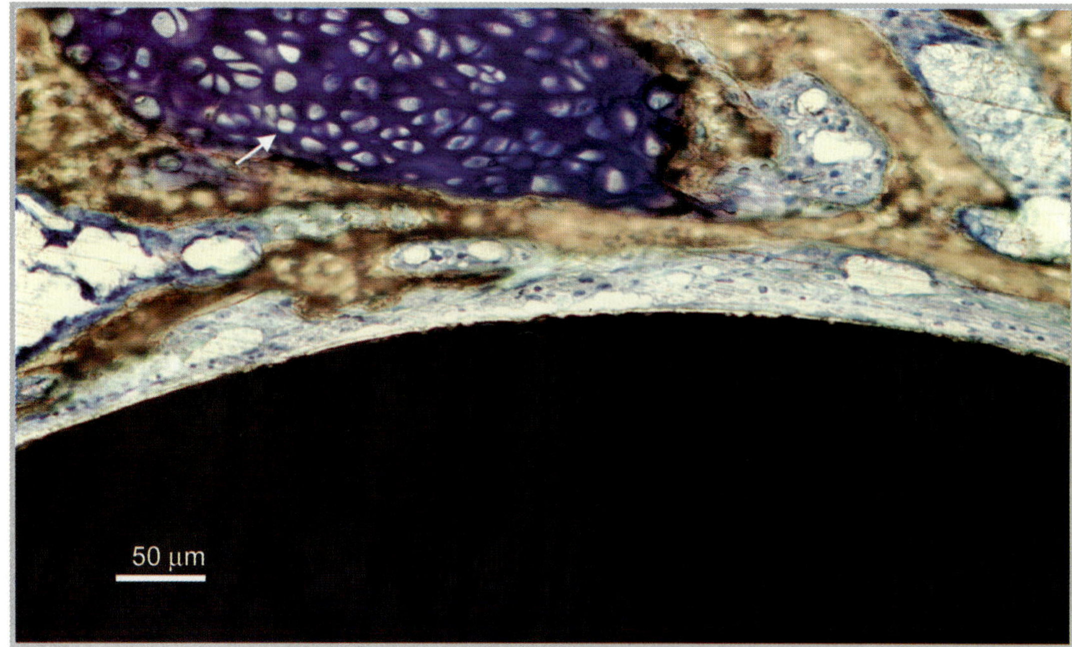

Figure 22B Tissue response to implant in bone. SVB x 10
Higher magnification showing cartilage plate made up of cartilage cells known as chondrocytes (↑)

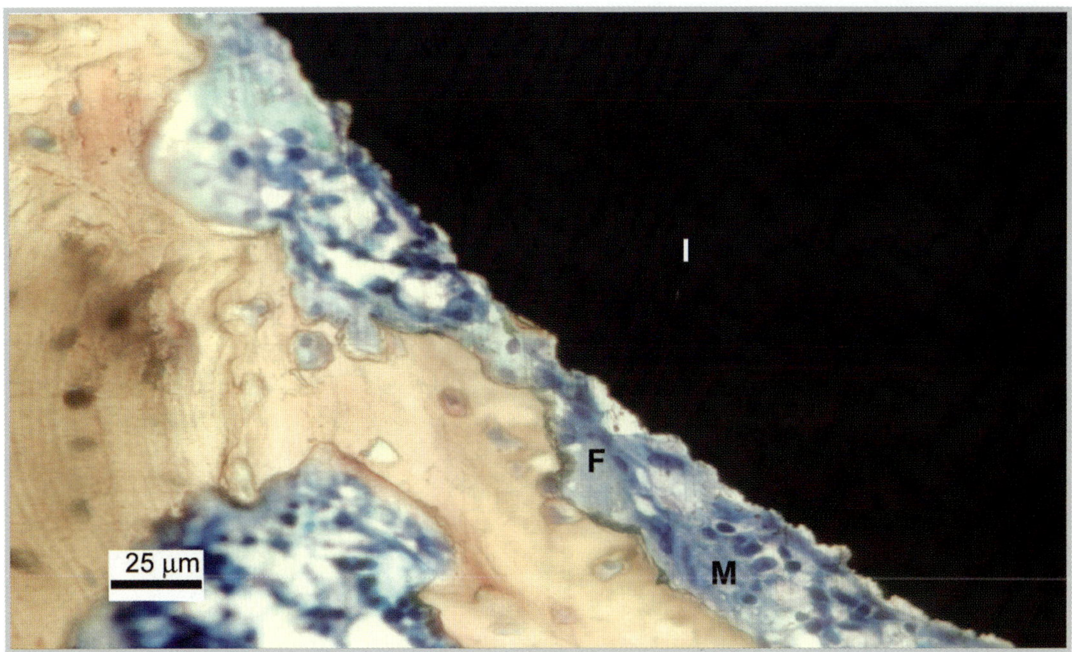

Figure 22C Tissue response to implant in bone. SVB x 40
Higher magnification with macrophages (M) and fibroblasts (F) at implant interface

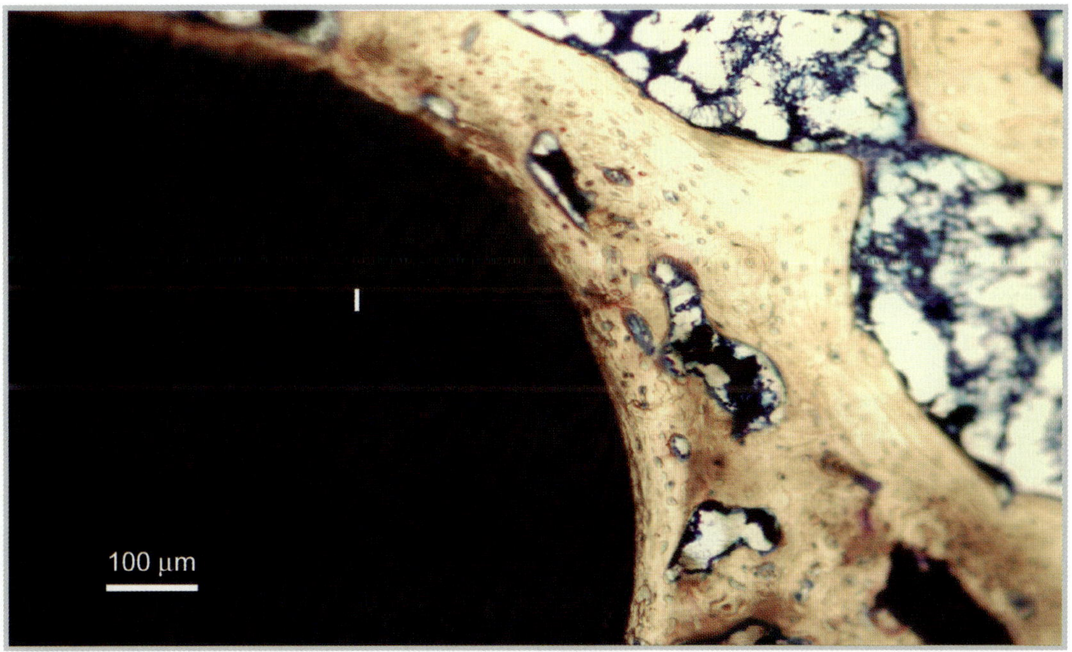

Figure 22D Tissue response to implant in bone. SVB x 10
Higher magnification with mature bone formation at another area of the implant interface

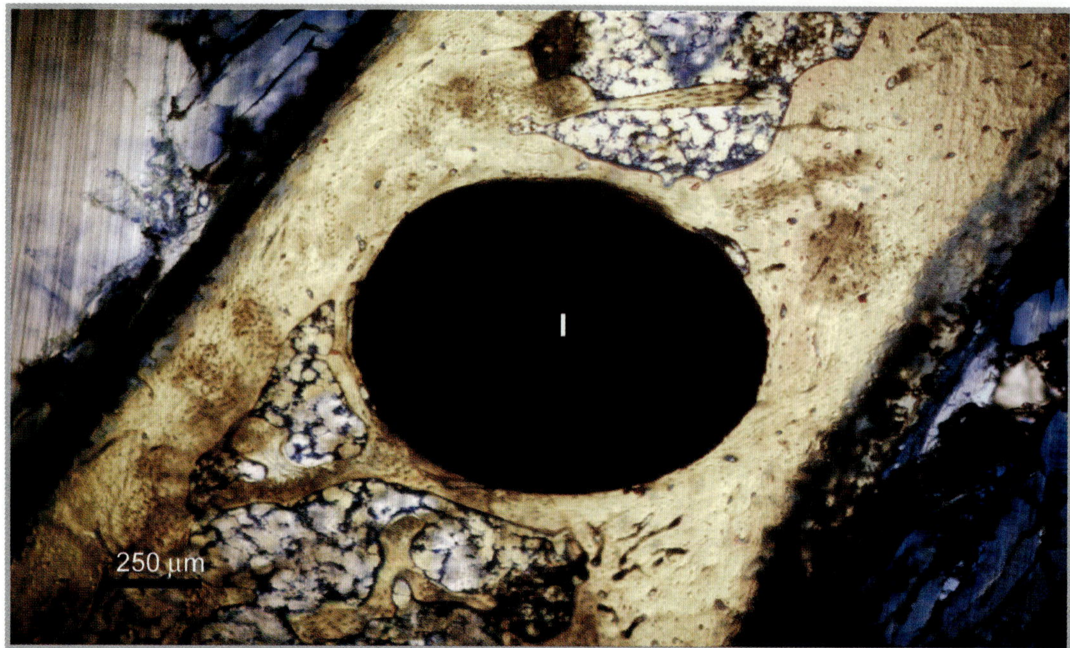

Figure 22E Tissue response to implant in bone. SVB x 4
Evaluation of biocompatibility of a rod shaped metal implant with a modified surface with nanoparticles in lateral condyle of long bone at eight weeks. Dense new bone from adjoining host bone surround the implant

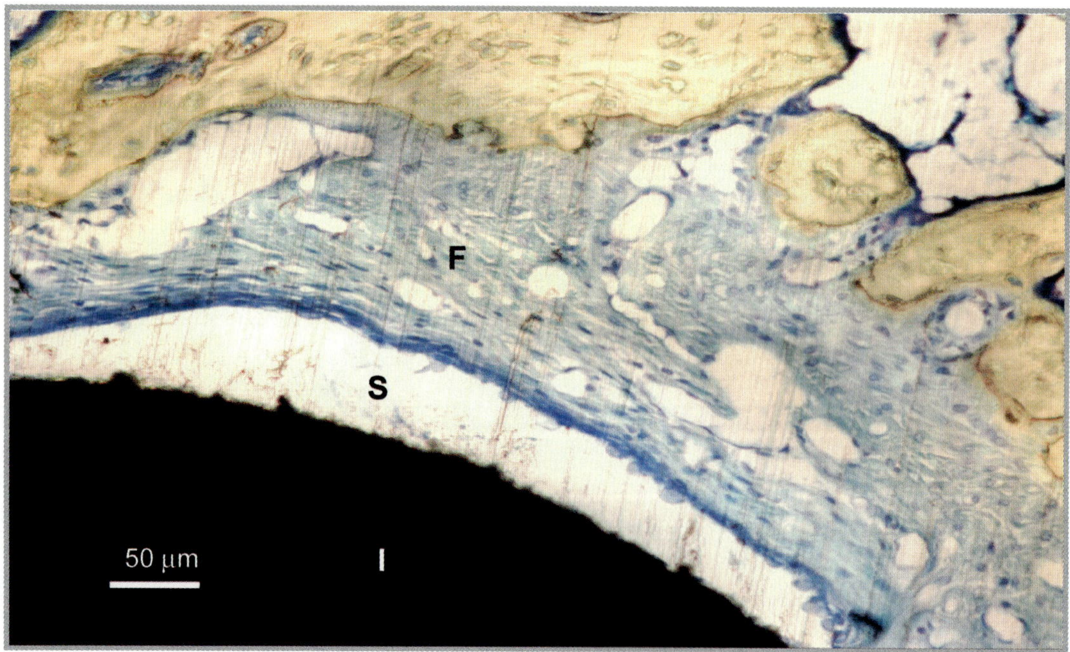

Figure 22F Tissue response to implant in bone. SVB x 20
Higher magnification showing persisting fibrosis at some areas at interface. Artifactural space (S) seen

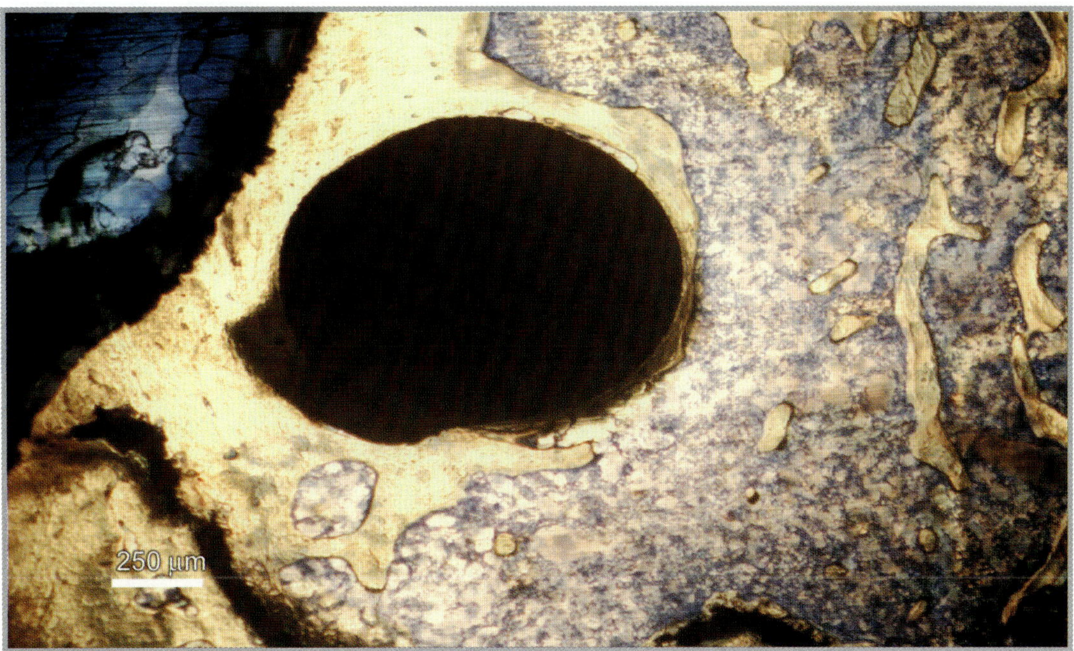

Figure 22G Tissue response to implant in bone. SVB x 4
Mature bone and marrow around implant

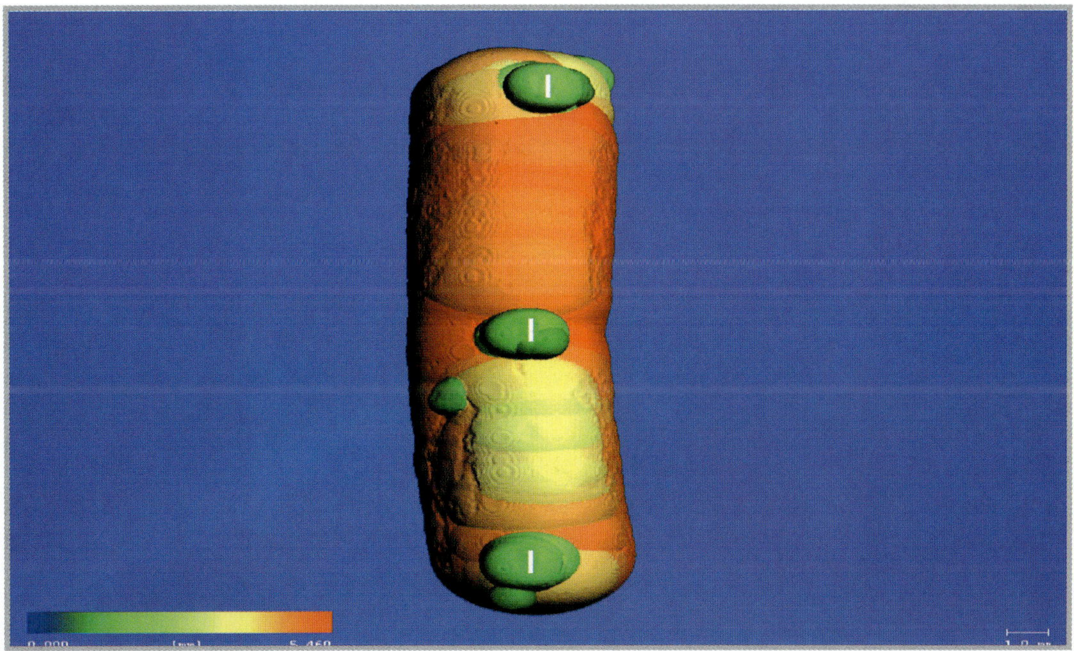

Figure 23A Tissue response to implant in bone. Gross non-identification of implants in bone. When identification of resorbable implants is not possible, micro-computerized tomography helps in locating the implants (I) in the bone

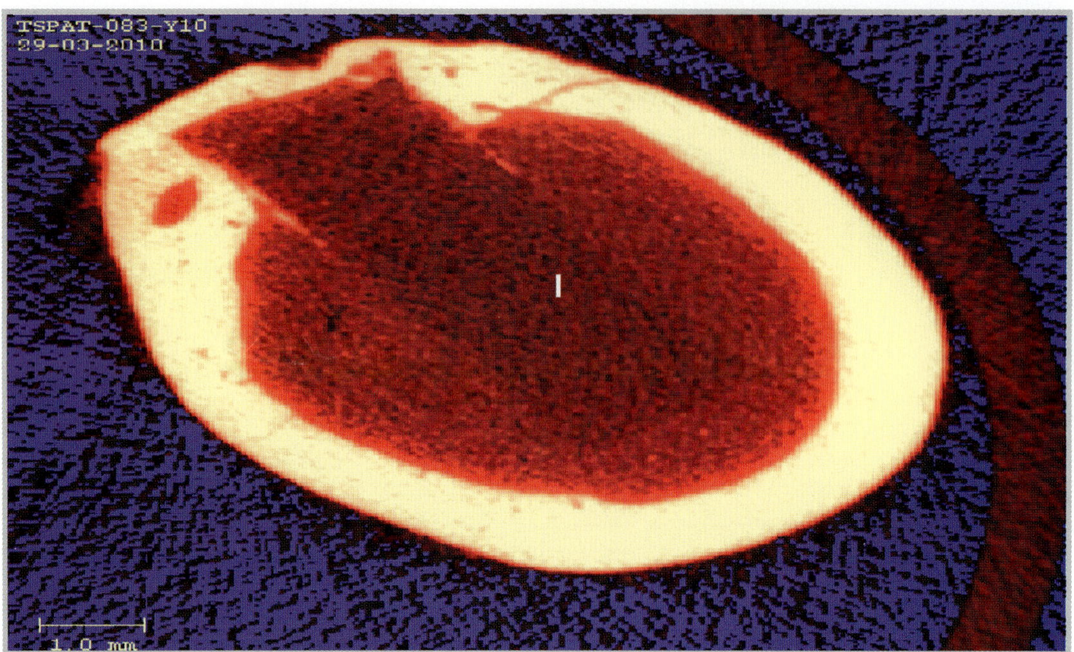

Figure 23B Tissue response to implant in bone. Gross non-identification of implant. Micro-computerized tomography of cross-section of bone with implant

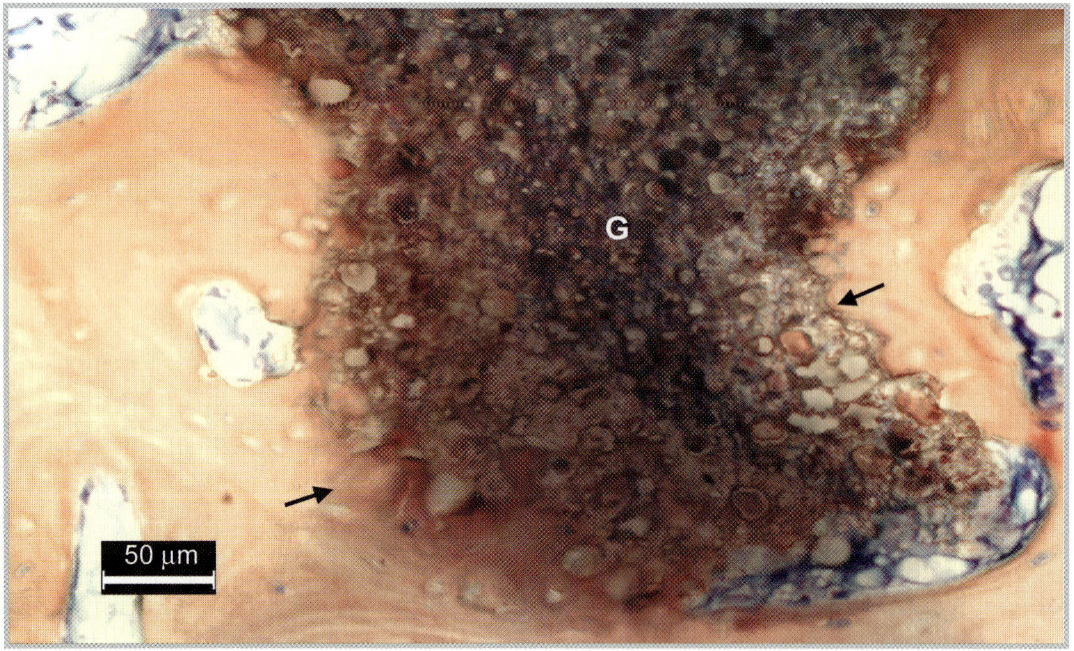

Figure 24A Tissue response to implant in bone. SVB x 20
Implantation of resorbable granules in bone
Resorbable granules (G) being replaced by areas of new bone (↑) as granules resorb

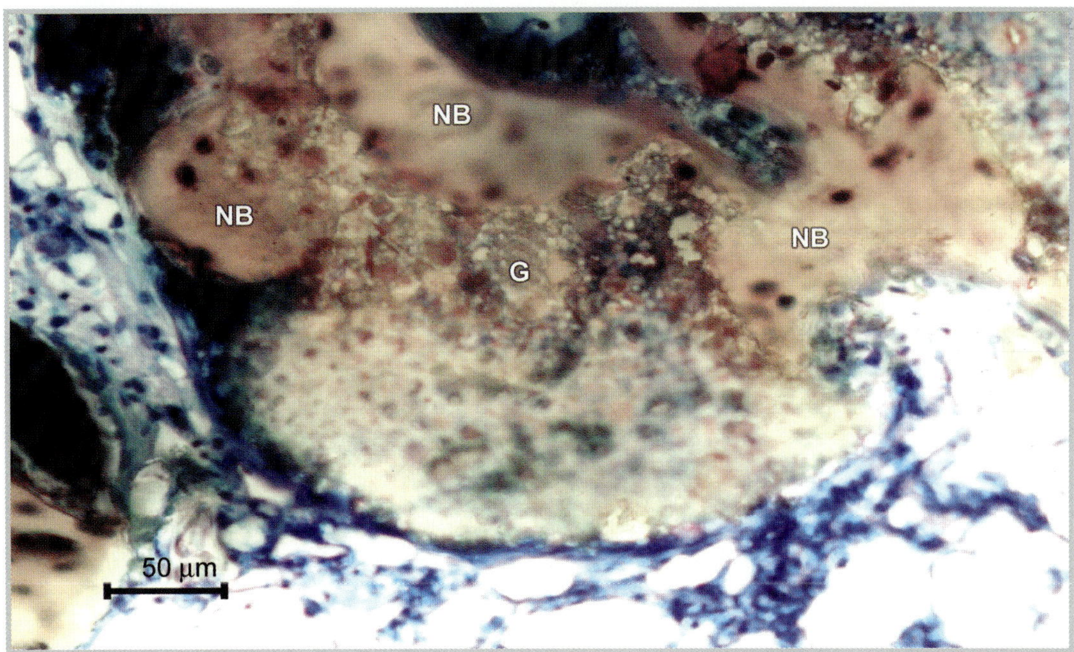

Figure 24B Tissue response to implant in bone. SVB x 20
Implantation of resorbable granules in bone
New woven bone (NB) with osteocytes, and adjacent granules (G)

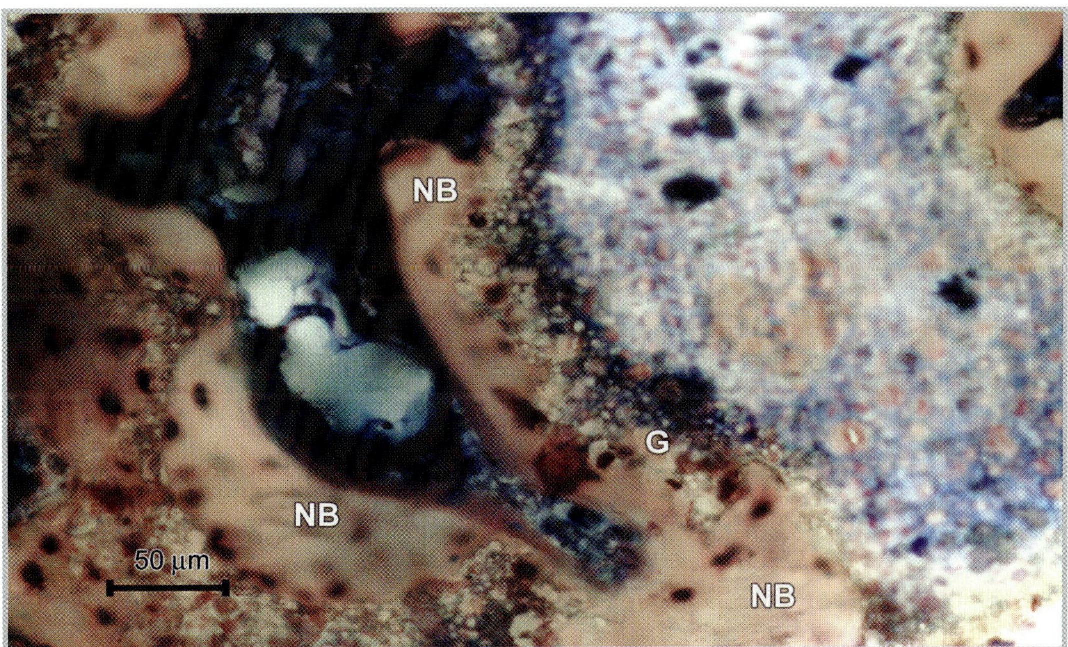

Figure 24C Tissue response to implant in bone. SVB x 20
Implantation of resorbable granules in bone
Higher magnification with resorbable granules (G) embedded in new bone (NB) as they resorb

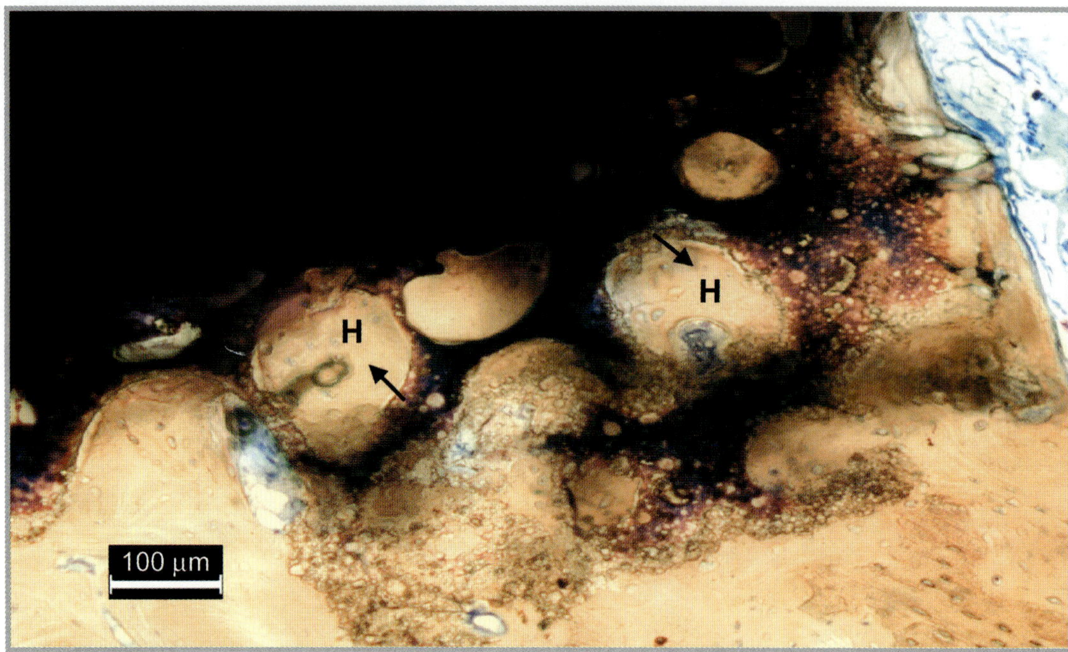

Figure 25 Tissue response to implant in bone. SVB x 10
Lamellar bone (↑) with formation of Haversian canals (H) seen in resorbable implant at twelve weeks post-implantation

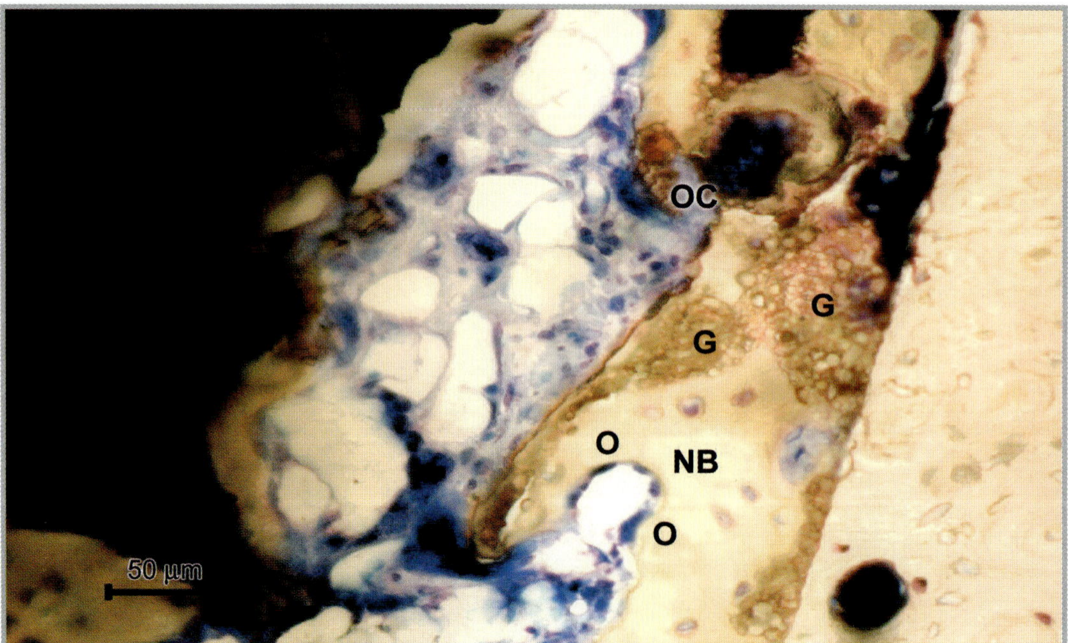

Figure 26A Tissue response to implant in bone. SVB x 20
Resorbable implant in bone
Osteoblasts (O) line new bone (NB) deposited as granules (G) resorb. Osteoclasts (OC) are also seen

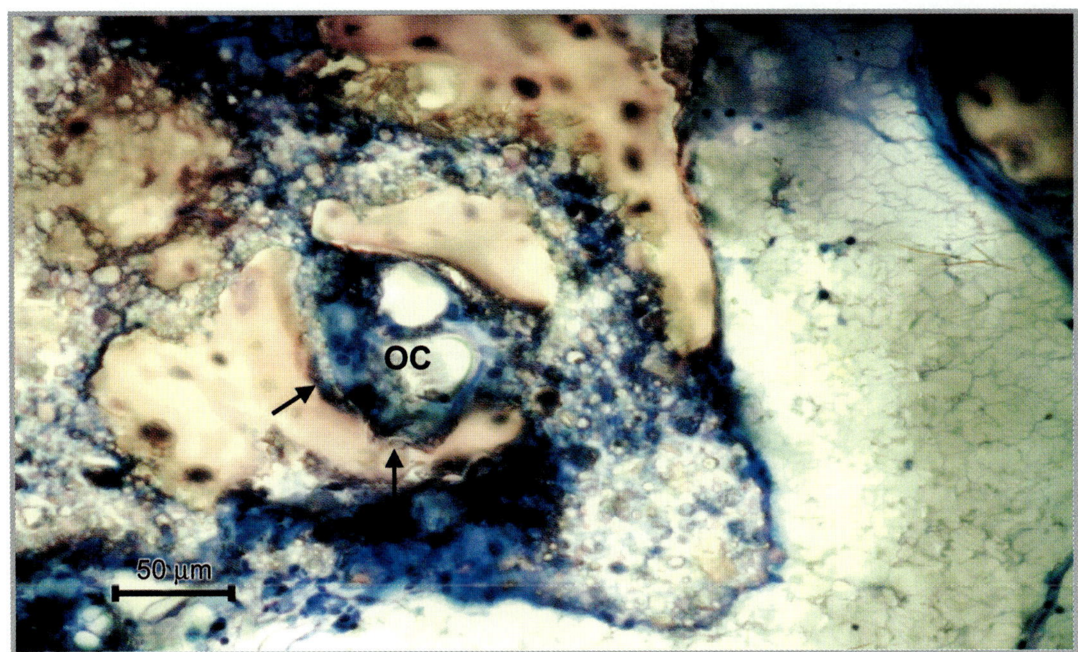

Figure 26B Tissue response to implant in bone. SVB x 20
Resorbable implant in bone
Osteoclasts (OC) with resorption bay (↑)

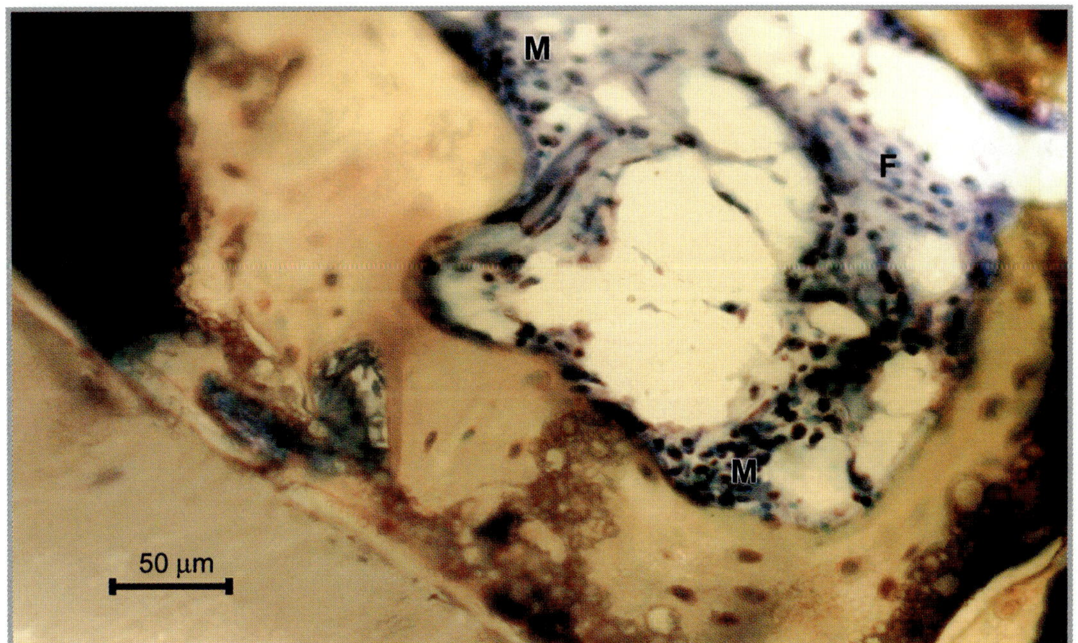

Figure 26C Tissue response to implant in bone. SVB x 20
Resorbable implant in bone
Fibroblasts (F) and macrophages (M) persist

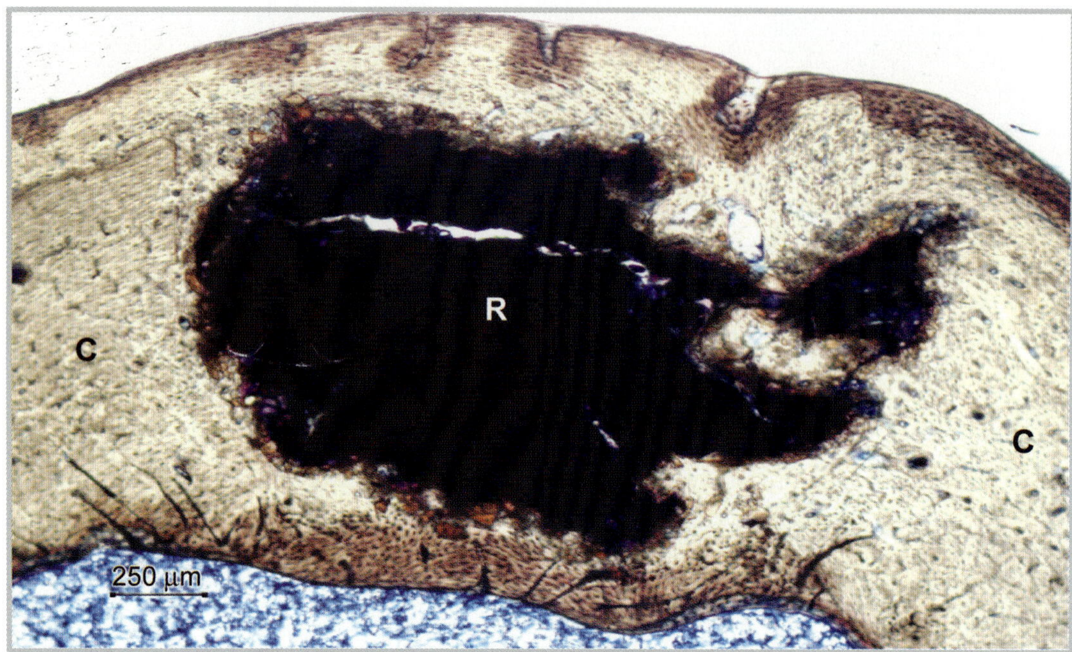

Figure 27A Tissue response to implant in bone. SVB x 4
Well-defined resorbable implant (R) in cortical bone (C)

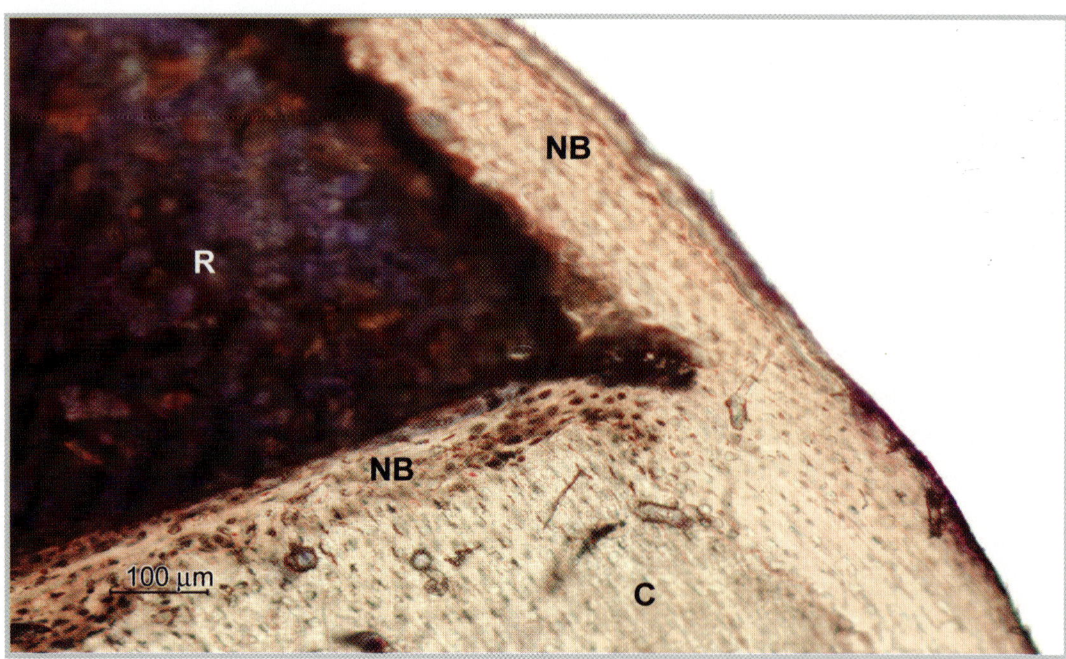

Figure 27B Tissue response to implant in bone. SVB x 10
New lamellar bone (NB) deposited at implant (R)-host bone (C) interface as well as across proximal end of implant

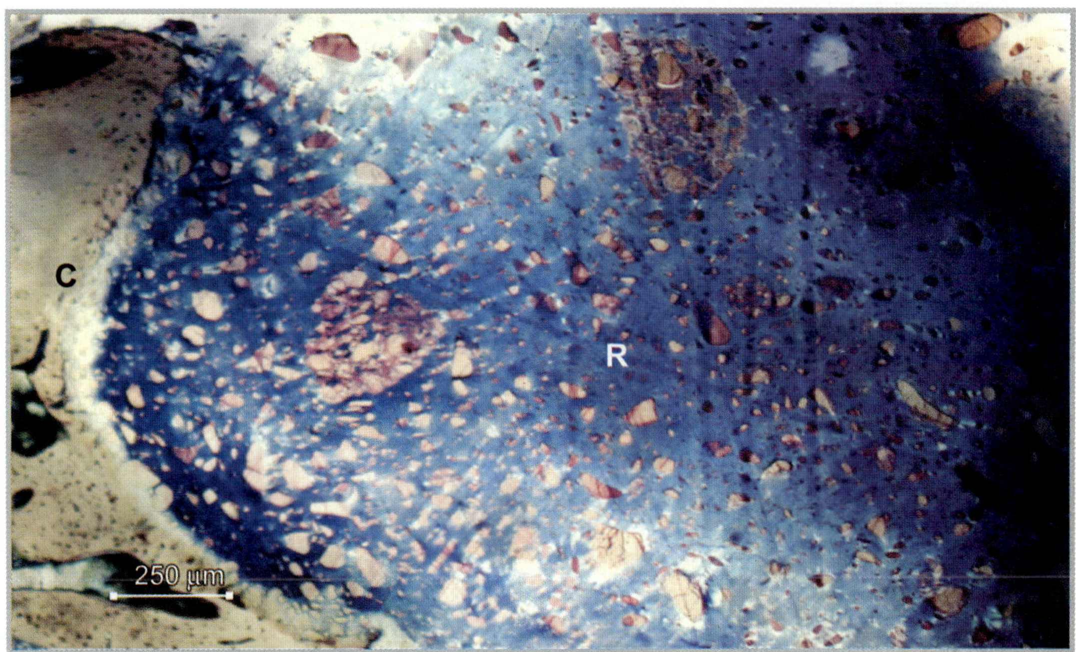

Figure 28 Tissue response to implant in bone. SVB x 4
Cortical bone (C) at interface with resorbable implant (R)

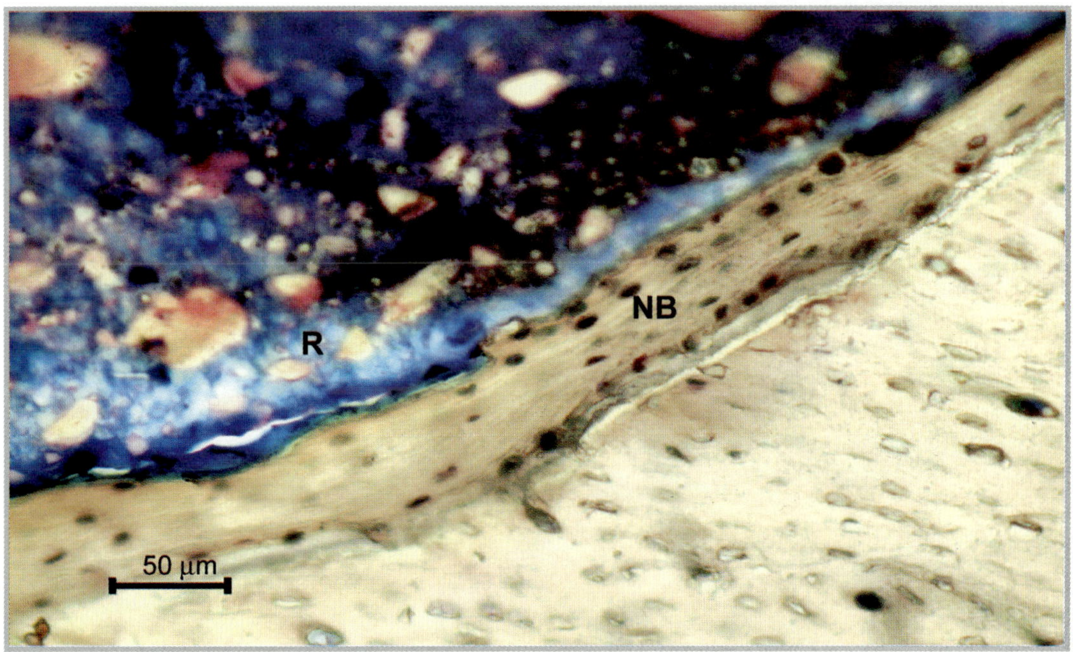

Figure 29 Tissue response to implant in bone. SVB x 20
Layer of new bone (NB) at interface with resorbable implant (R)

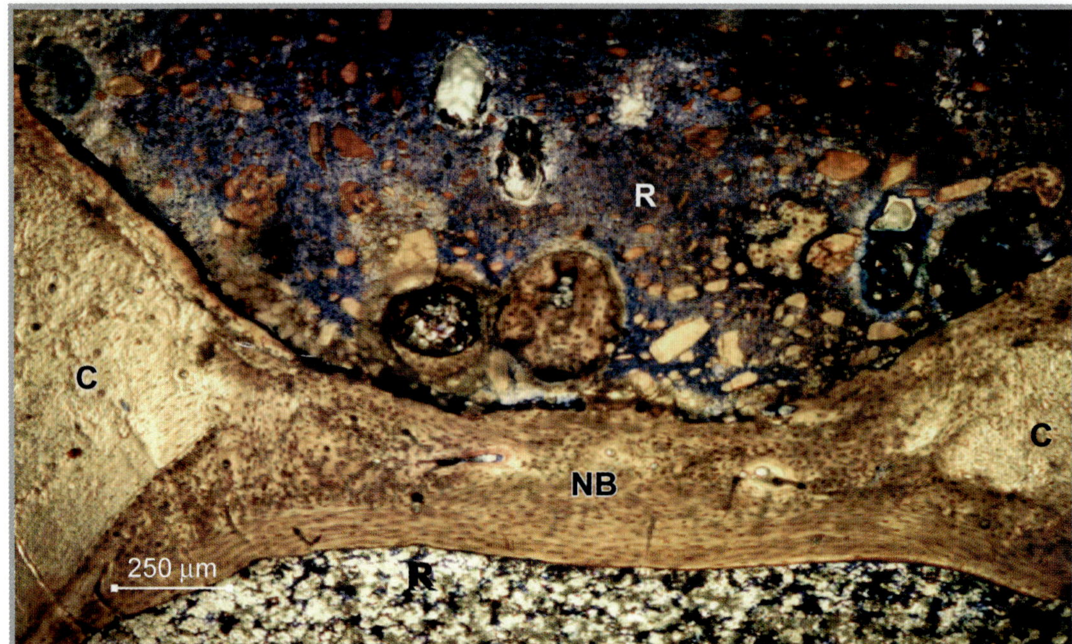

Figure 30 Tissue response to implant in bone. SVB x 4
New bone (NB) forms a bridge with host cortical bone (C) on both sides, beneath the resorbable implant (R)

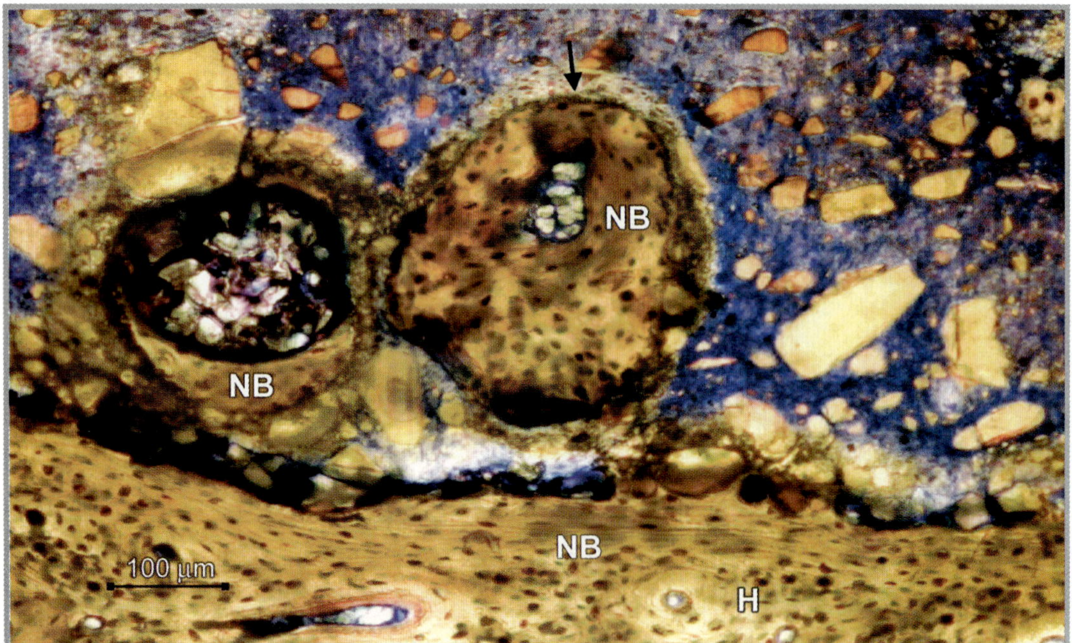

Figure 31A Tissue response to implant in bone. SVB x 10
Lamellar bone (NB) with Haversian canals (H) at the resorbable implant interface. Bone with osteocytes adjacent to granules (↑)

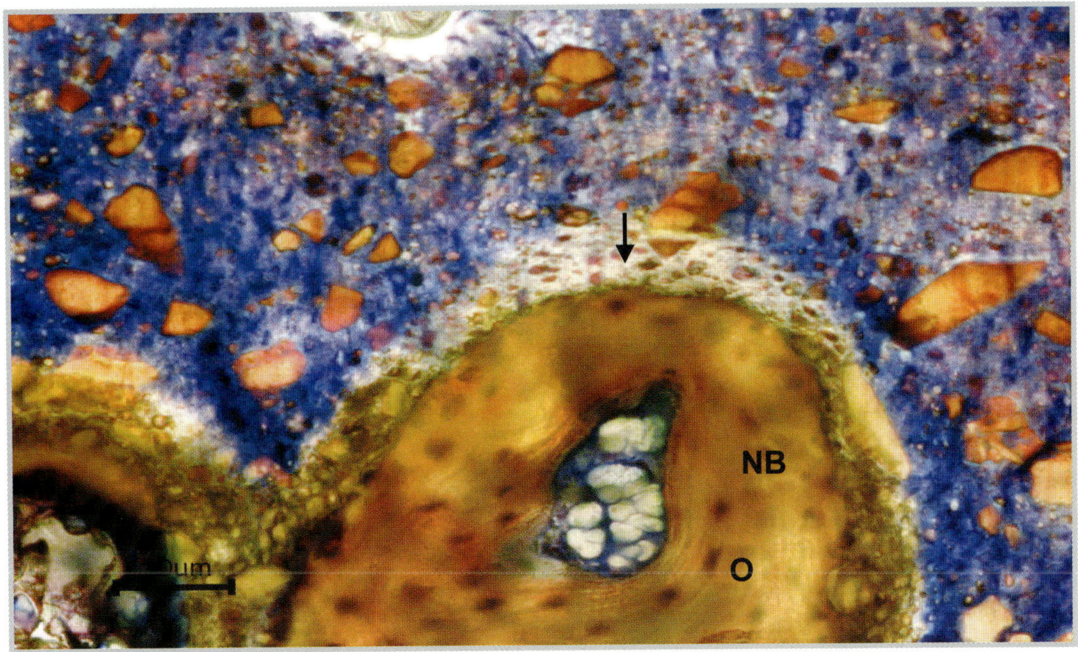

Figure 31B Tissue response to implant in bone. SVB x 20
Lamellar bone formation (NB) with osteocytes (O). Resorbing granules (↑) seen at interface

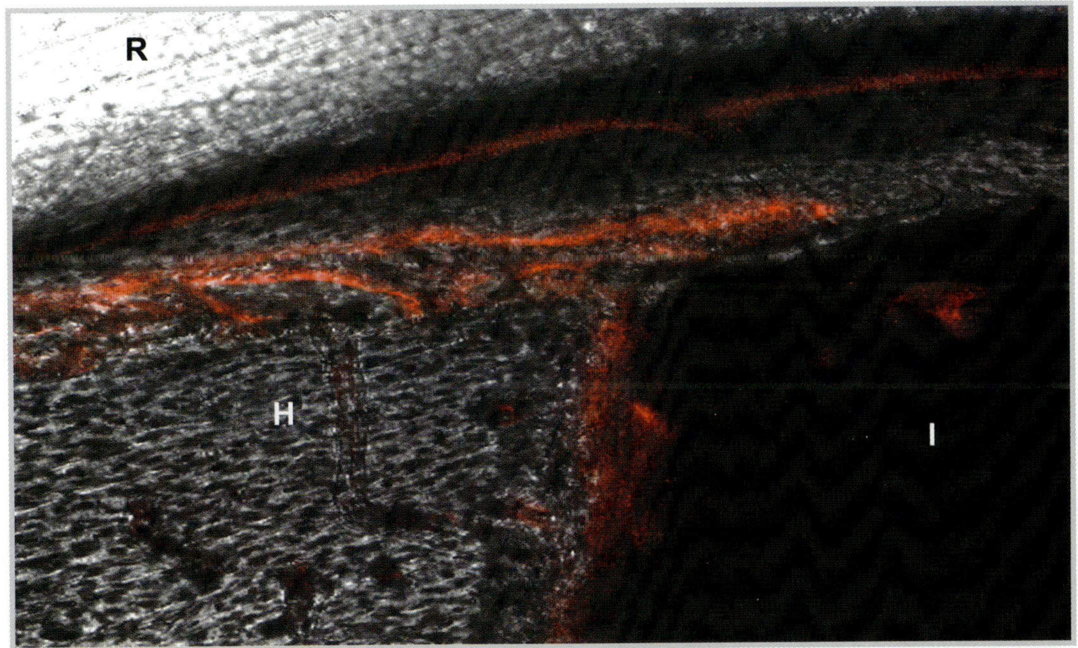

Figure 32 Injected flurochrome stains new bone deposited at time of injection. Resin (R) section of bone showing flurochrome stained (red) areas of new bone formation between host bone (H) and implant (I) and also in the implant

4

Preclinical Evaluation of Biomaterials and Medical Devices

When a material is found biocompatible in tissue, it is used as such to replace diseased tissue, e.g. as a wound dressing or a cardiac patch. It is also used in the fabrication of a medical device either singly or as multiple different components of a medical device. Prior to use in humans, these materials or devices are evaluated for the performance in their final end use application sites in animal models. Assessment is carried out by elective necropsy at specific time periods and gross examination and microscopy of tissue response. The pictures in this chapter are of materials and devices received in the laboratory for preclinical evaluation.

Valve replacement of the mitral, tricuspid, aortic or pulmonary valves of the heart are either artificial or natural. Artificial or mechanical prosthesis generally consist of a sewing ring and leaflets. The sewing ring is usually of metal covered with a fabric which facilitates the anchorage of the valve to the surrounding heart muscle or myocardium. The circumferential measurement of the sewing ring is very important and must be suitable for the diseased valve being removed as well as the age of the patient. These features are also adhered to when the valves are tested in preclinical studies. Surgical suturing of the sewing ring is important to prevent gaps being left resulting in a leakage of blood from outflow chamber into inflow chamber, otherwise known as paravalvular leaks. These leaks can be identified during gross examination of the valve. Formation of thrombi on valve leaflets cause blood flow obstruction. One of the histological features examined during preclinical studies is the extent of tissue overgrowth on the inner margin of the sewing ring, otherwise known as pannus. This ledge or shelf of tissue is responsible for narrowing the lumen of the valve as well as is a cause of obstruction of valve leaflets. Slowing of blood flow through the valve can cause deposition of thrombi on the valve struts. Bioprosthetic valves are made of decellularized tissue like pericardium or natural valve cusps and have a metal cage, sewing ring and struts. The decellularized tissue for the valve cusps is placed on the metal struts. Evaluation includes assessment of calcification in the cusps over long periods of implantation which leads to stiffness and valve dysfunction. Grafts used to replace segments of diseased blood vessels are evaluated preclinically in animal models for their patency over long periods, ingrowth of tissue externally and formation of neointima and endothelization. Vascular stents are placed in coronary blood vessels and assessed for patency as well as restenosis due to neointimal proliferation. Natural decellularized tissues are assessed for their immunogenecity and survival with good healing and replacement with normal host tissue. Initiation of calcification with extension is assessed microscopically. Embolizing agents for aneurysms are evaluated for their capability to cause obstruction to blood flow without causing any complication.

Scaffolds seeded with cells are tested by placing the scaffold in the end application site and assessed for gradual host tissue formation along with slow degradation of scaffold without any adverse tissue response.

Dental filling materials are assessed for their effect on pulp cells by making a cavity in the tooth, filling it with the material and then examining the underlying dentine, odontoblasts and other pulp cells. However, a cautionary measure is the minimum dentine thickness which should be ascertained when making the cavity.

These are a few examples of features of assessment in preclinical evaluation of devices. The important point for all devices is the selection of an appropriate animal model, the site of implantation and the surgical technique to ensure proper functional, gross and histological assessment.

Gross and histological features are seen in the following images.

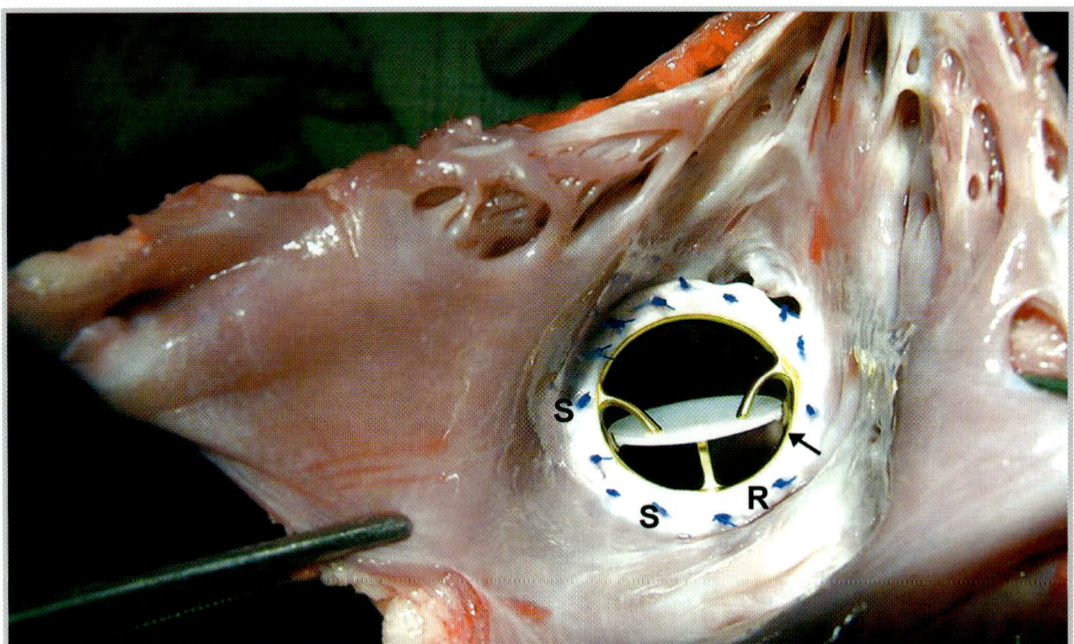

Figure 1 Mechanical heart valve. Gross image. Mechanical heart valve in situ in the heart. The metal cage (↑) with sewing ring (R) made of fabric is sewed on to the adjoining heart muscle with sutures (S)

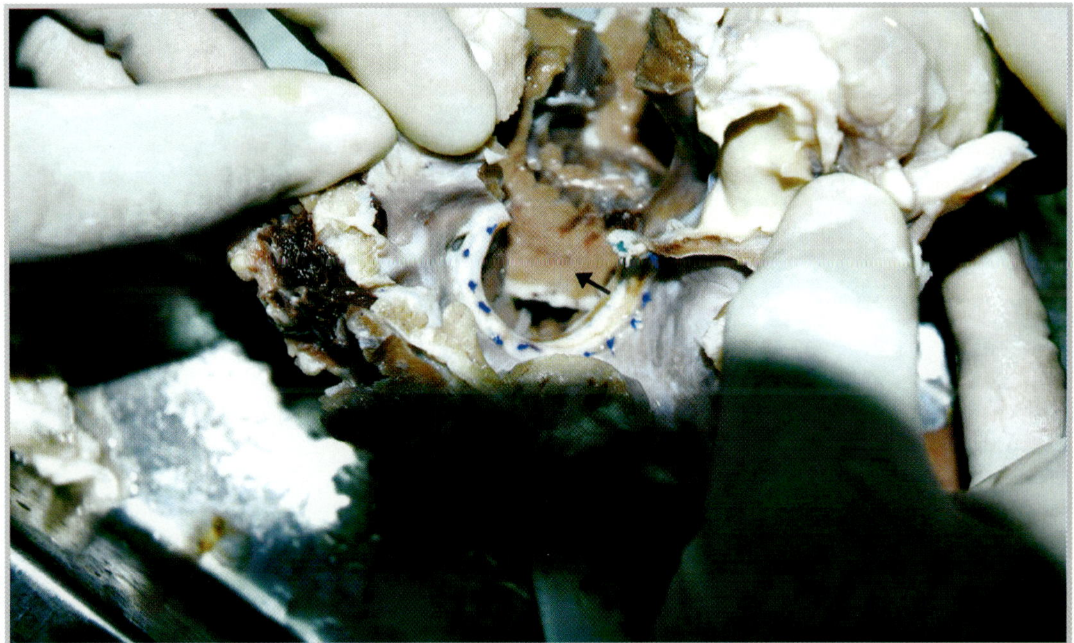

Figure 2 Mechanical heart valve. Gross image. The valve is removed from the sewing ring. A section (↑) perpendicular to the sewing ring is taken and processed for histological evaluation. The plane of embedding is very important to enable examination of the pannus formation and tissue ingrowth

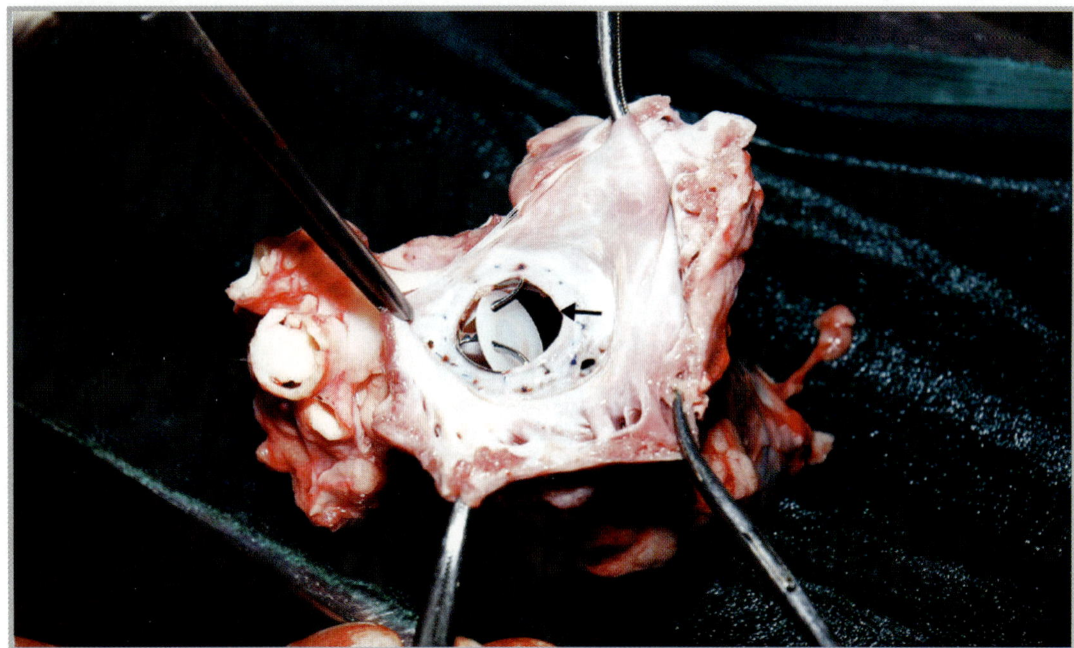

Figure 3A Mechanical heart valve. Gross image
Pannus formation (↑) along one edge of sewing ring

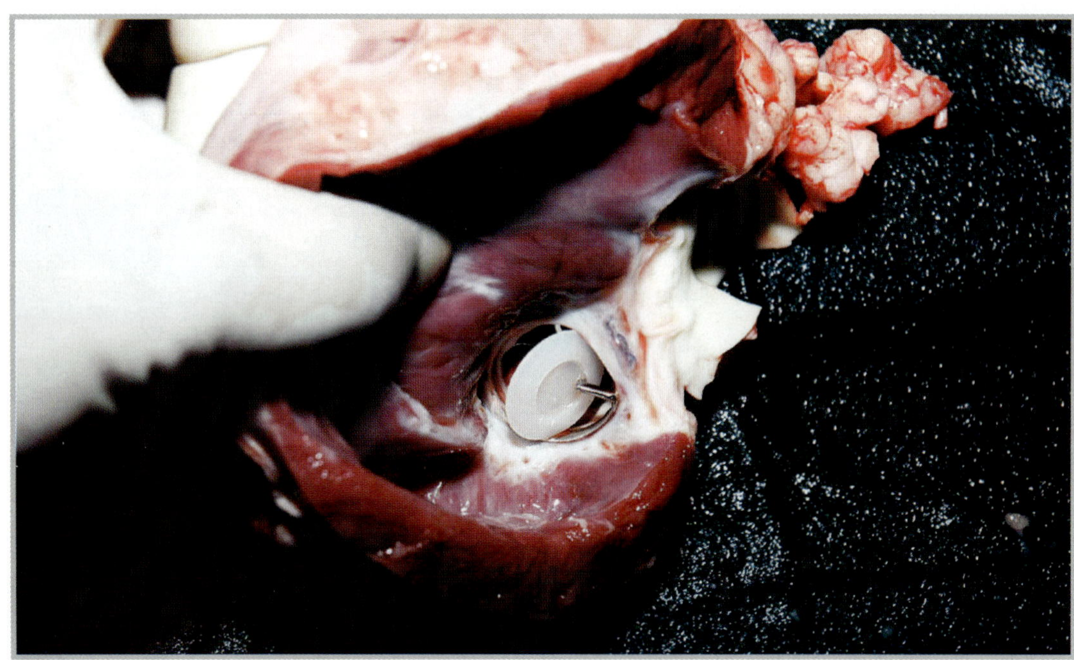

Figure 3B Mechanical heart valve. Gross image
Obstruction of disk movement due to pannus formation

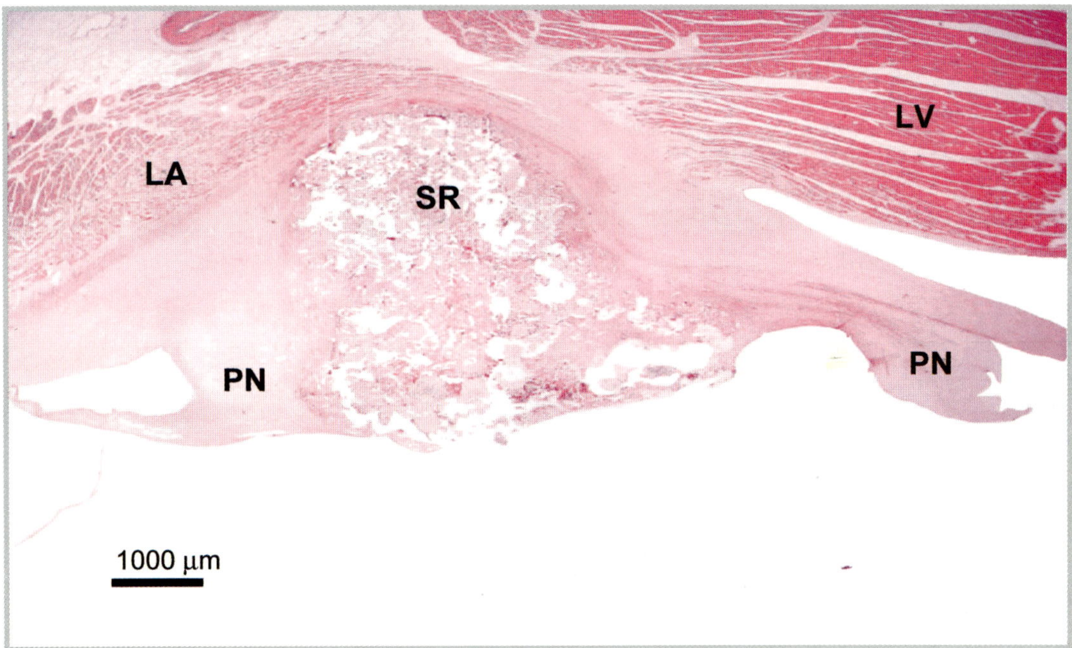

Figure 4 Mechanical heart valve. H & E x 1
Cross-section of sewing ring (SR) which is removed off the metal cage to identify tissue ingrowth into the fabric and the extent of pannus formation (PN). Left atrial (LA) and left ventricular (LV) host tissue is seen

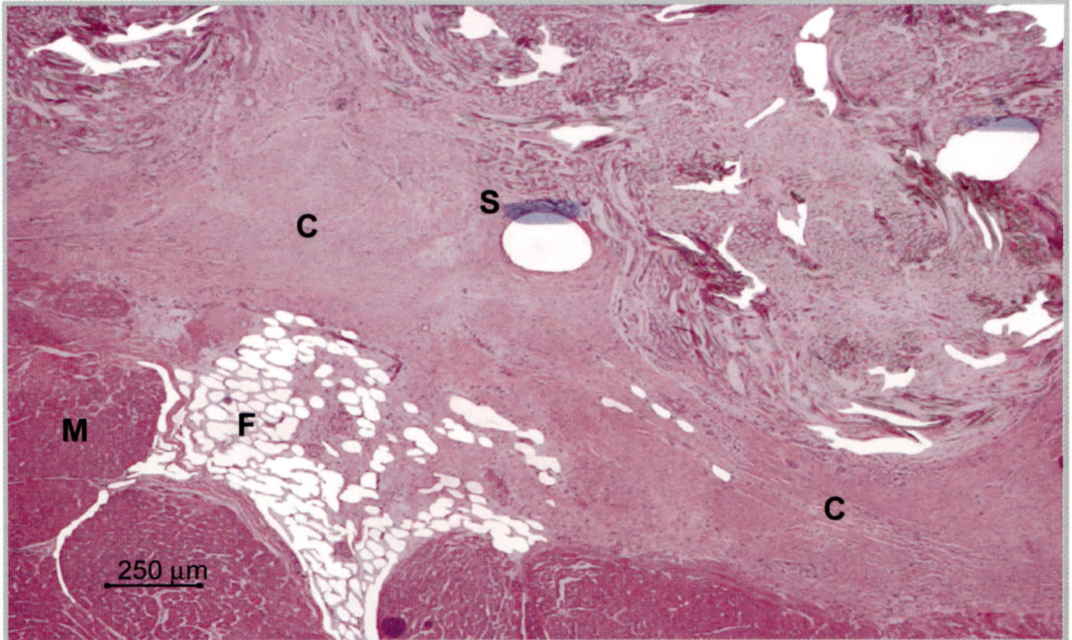

Figure 5A Mechanical heart valve. H & E x 4
Cross-section of the sewing ring and adjoining myocardium (M). Dense collagen (C) is seen at the sewing ring-myocardium interface and around suture (S). Fragments of sutures (blue) and fat (F) is seen

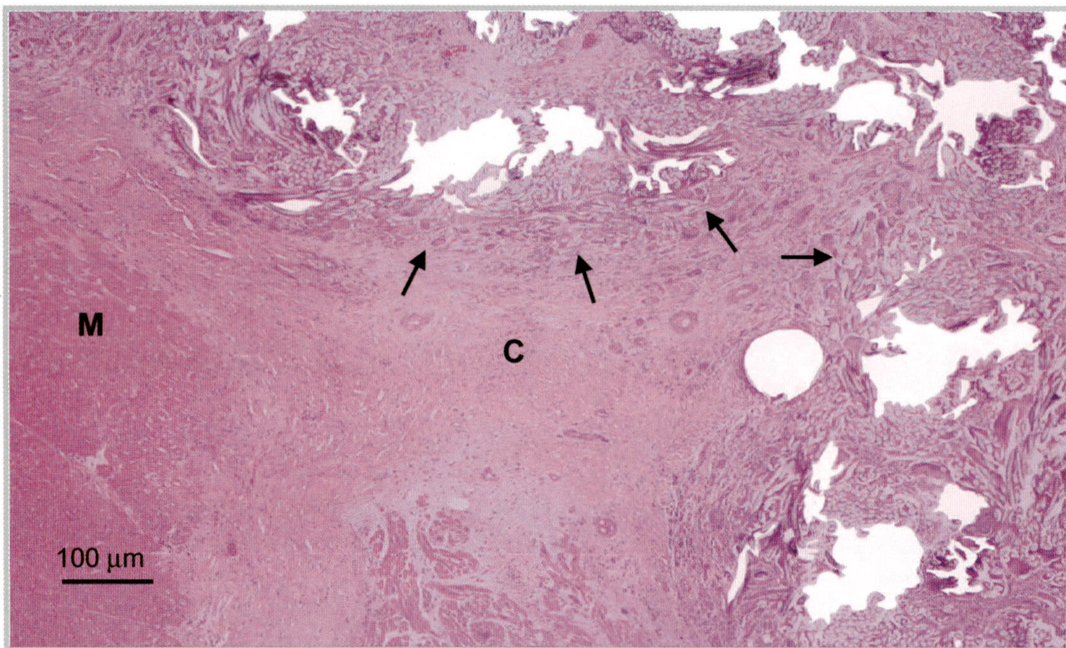

Figure 5B Mechanical heart valve. H & E x 10
Foreign body type of giant cells (↑) surround the sewing ring as well as present in the intercises of the sewing ring

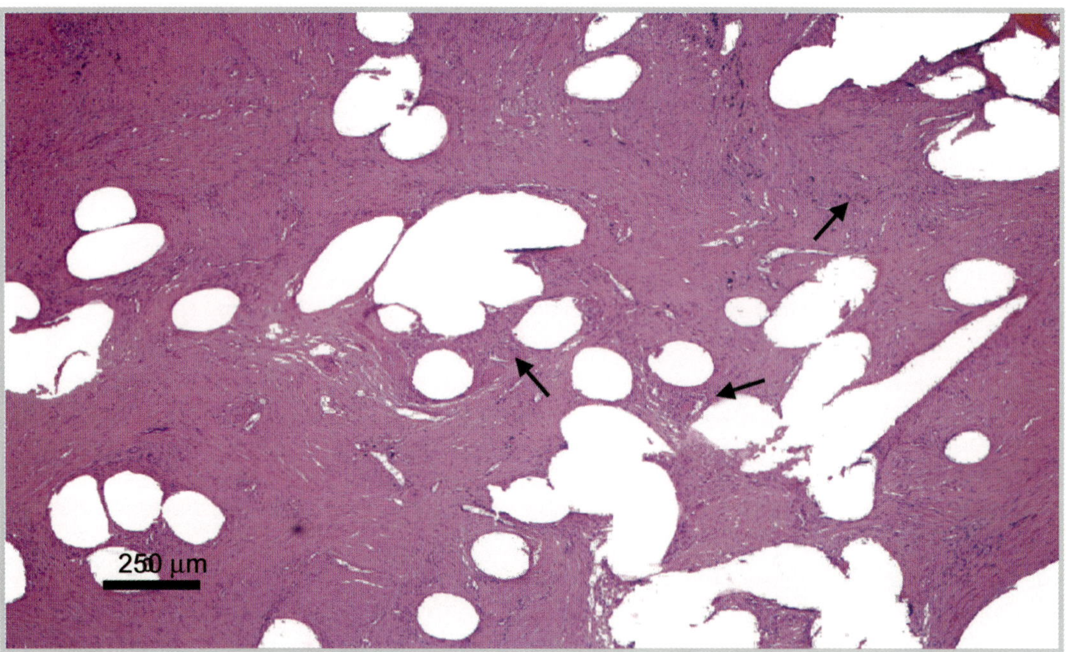

Figure 6A Mechanical heart valve. H & E x 4
Cross-section of the sewing ring. Clear spaces indicate the areas of fabric fibers with infiltrating inflammatory cells (↑)

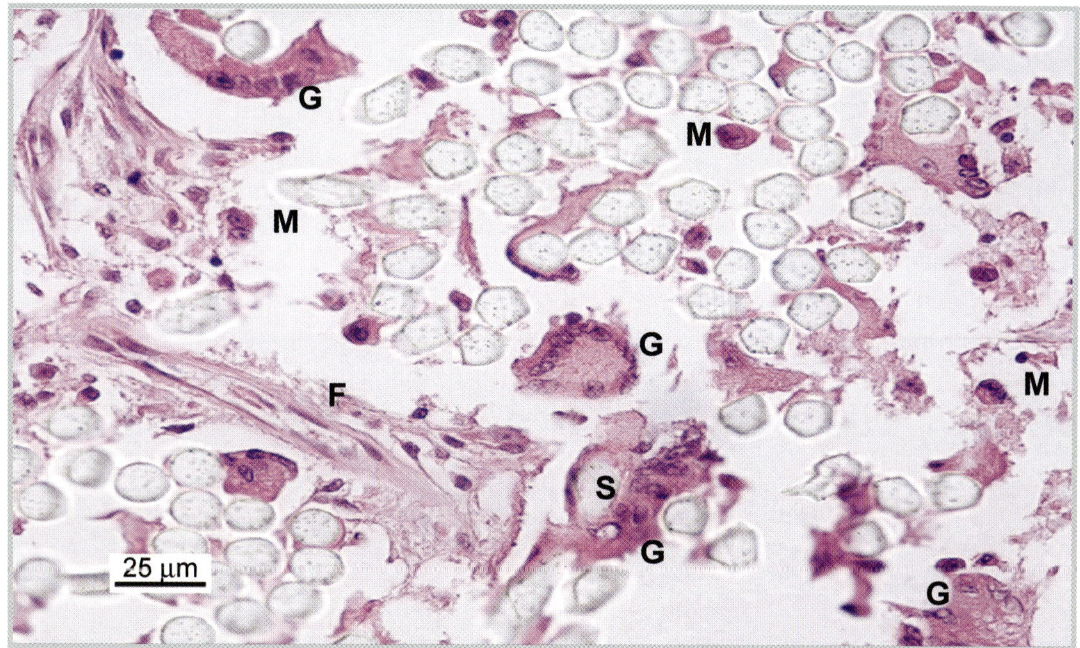

Figure 6B Mechanical heart valve. H & E x 40
Cross-section of the sewing ring. Macrophages (M), fibrocytes (F) and numerous foreign body type of giant cells (G) persisting for long periods post implantation

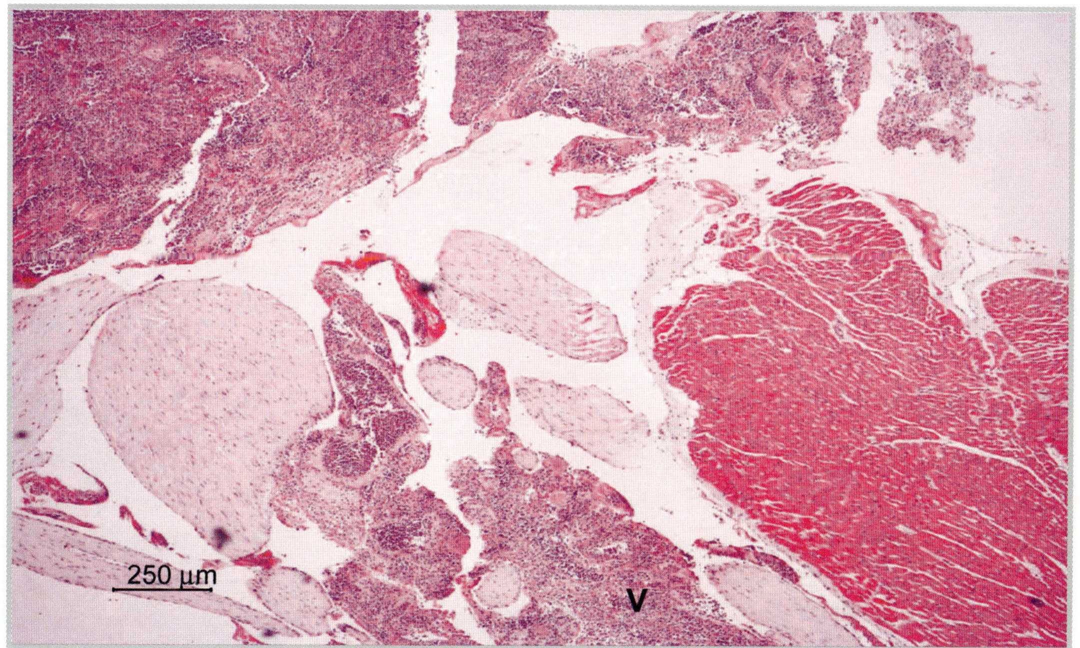

Figure 7 Mechanical heart valve. H & E x 4
Fragments of vegetation (V) in ventricle

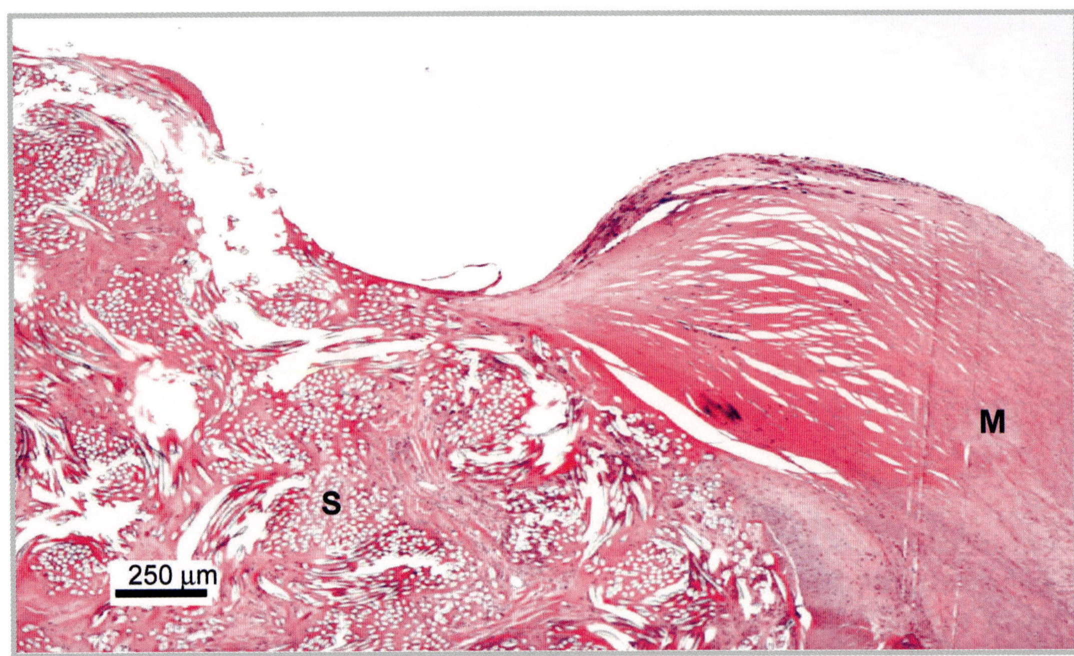

Figure 8 Mechanical heart valve. H & E x 4
Cross-section of the sewing ring (S) with adjacent myocardium (M)

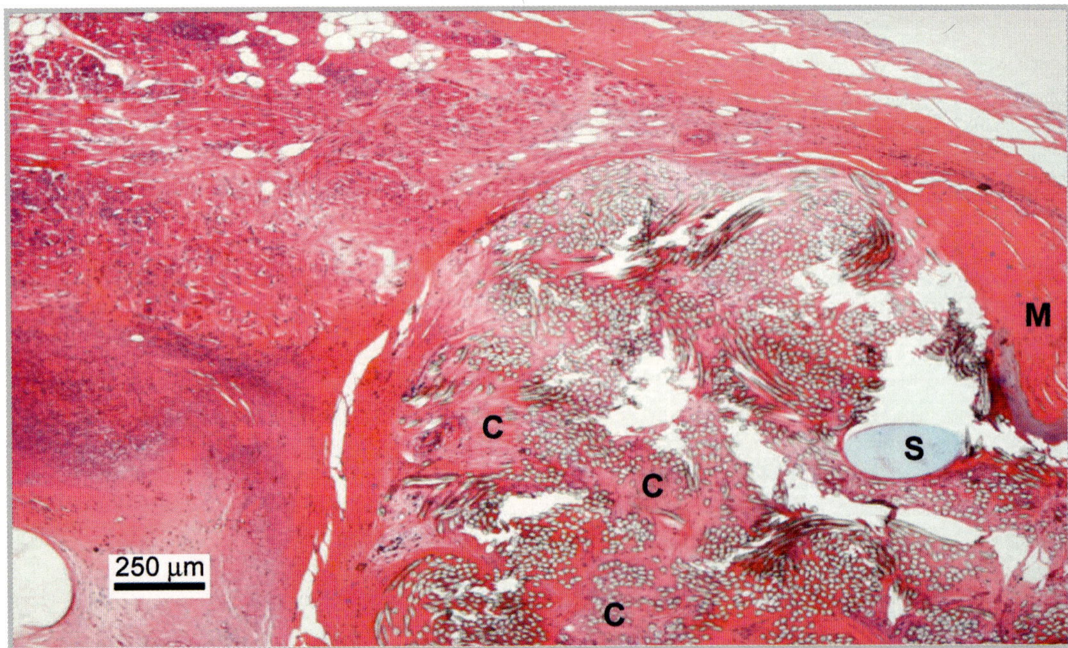

Figure 9A Mechanical heart valve. H & E x 4
Cross-section of the sewing ring, cross and longitudinal sections of individual fibers of the fabric with fibrocytes and collagen (C) in between. Cross-section of suture (S) is present at interface with myocardium (M)

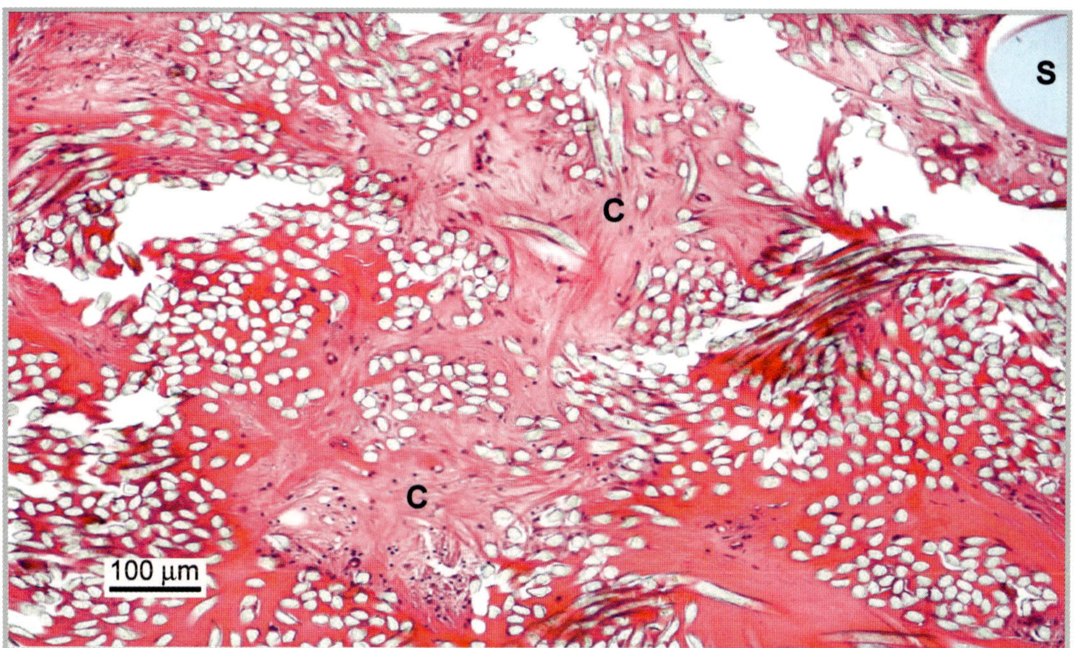

Figure 9B Mechanical heart valve. H & E x 10
Higher magnification with strands of collagen (C) in between the sewing ring fibers

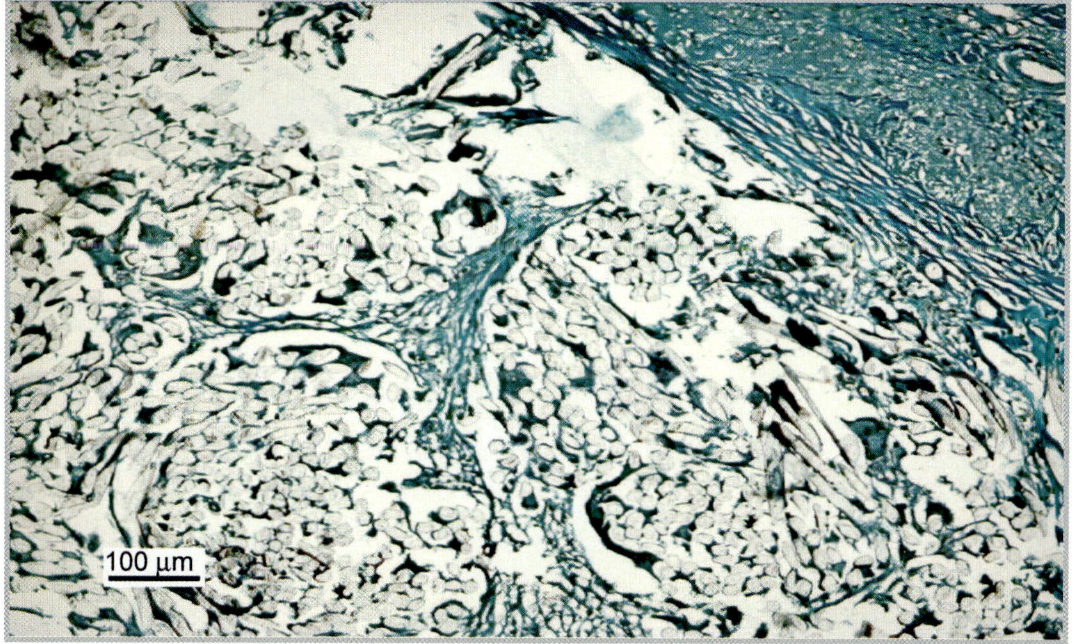

Figure 10 Mechanical heart valve Masson's Trichrome stain x 10
Cross-section of the sewing ring showing greenish blue collagen in between the fibers

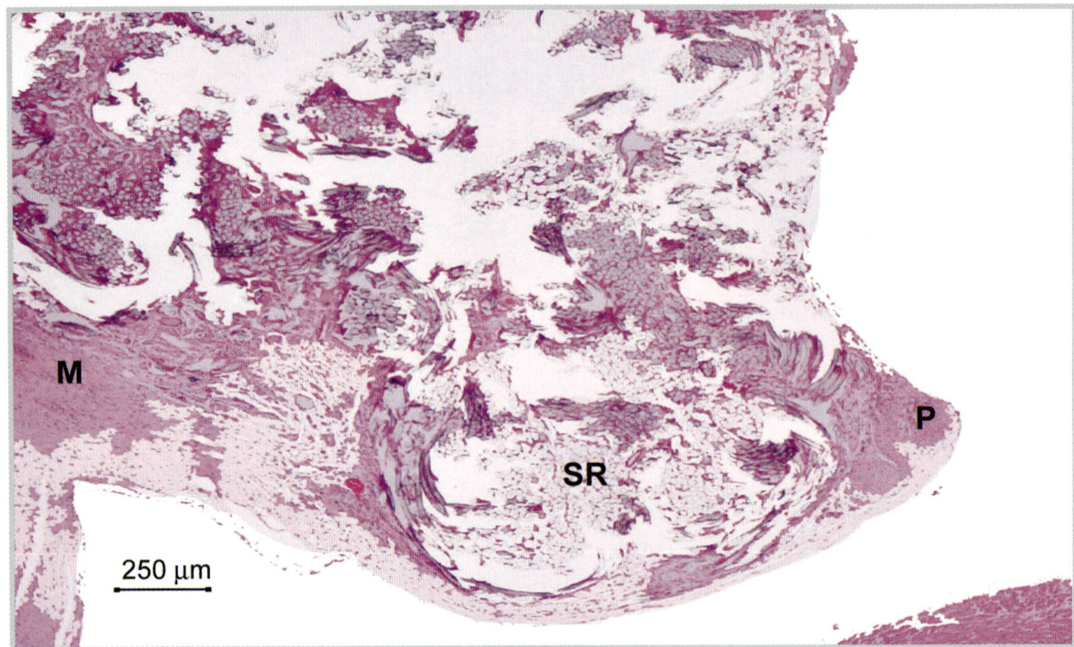

Figure 11A Mechanical heart valve. H & E x 4
Cross-section of sewing ring (SR) which is sewed on to the myocardium (M). Early pannus (P) formation over sewing ring

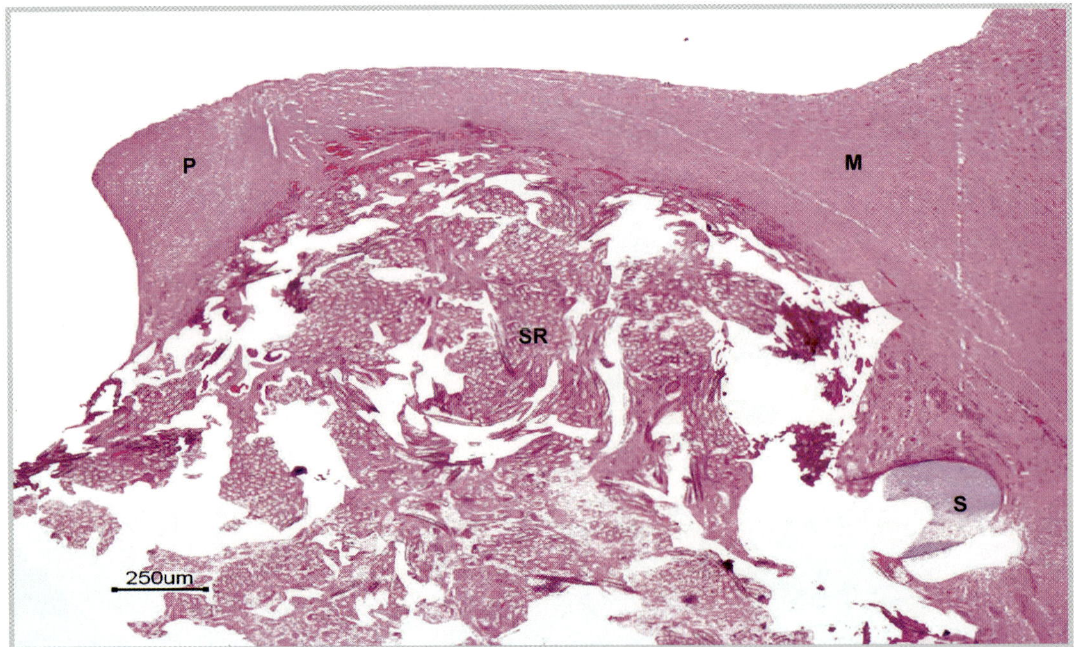

Figure 11B Mechanical heart valve. H & E x 4
Cross-section of sewing ring (SR) which is sewed on to the myocardium (M) with suture site (S). Moderate pannus (P) formation over sewing ring

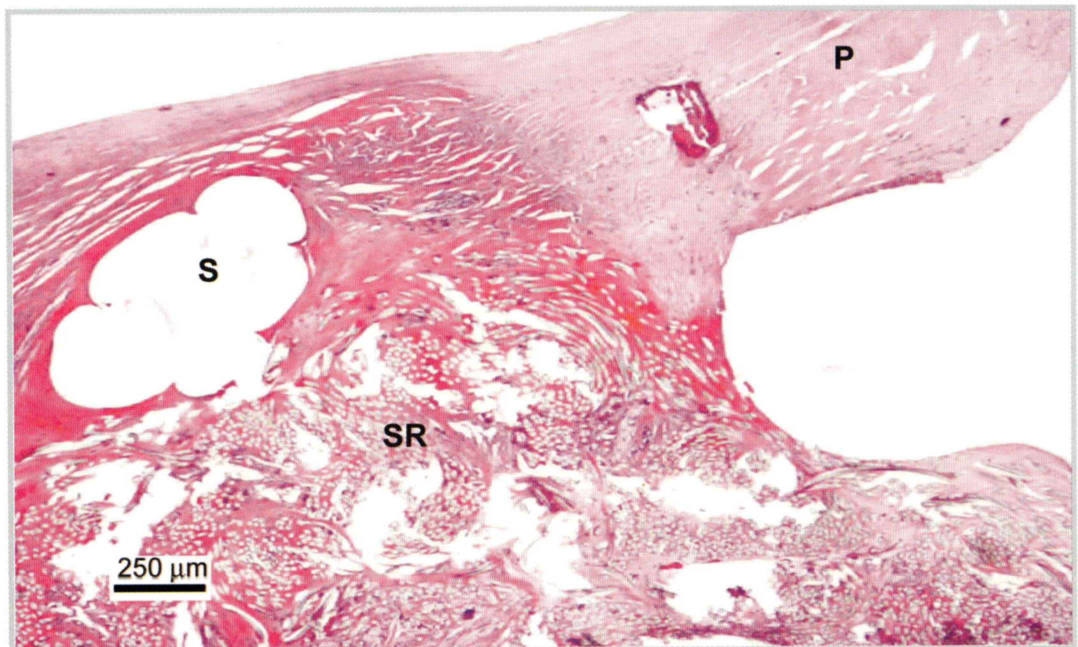

Figure 11C Mechanical heart valve. H & E x 4
Cross-section of sewing ring (SR) which is sewed on to the myocardium (M) with suture site (S). Thick pannus (P) formation over sewing ring

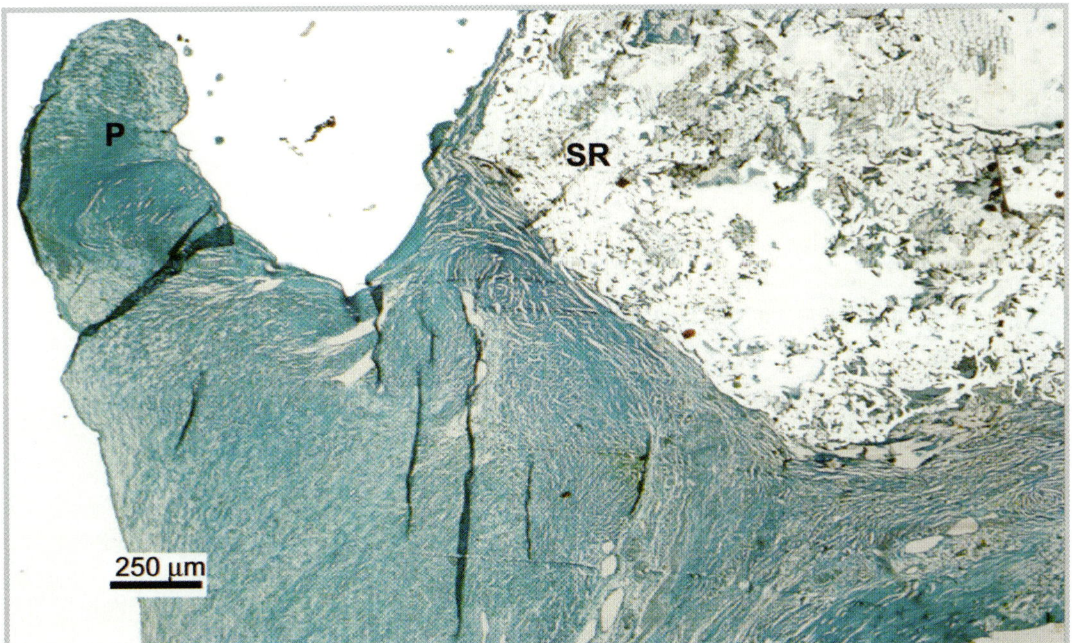

Figure 12 Mechanical heart valve. Masson's Trichrome stain x 4
Cross-section of the sewing ring (SR) showing pannus (P) with greenish blue collagen extending from the sewing ring

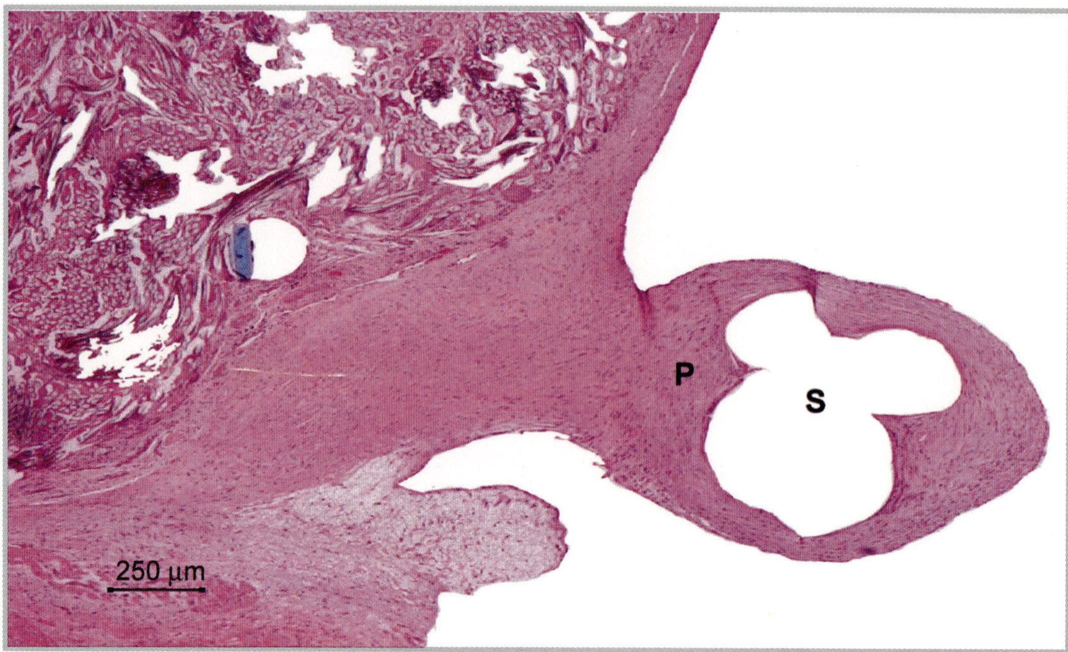

Figure 13 Mechanical heart valve. H & E x 4
Pannus growth (P) involving extending end of suture (S). The length of suture stub was too long

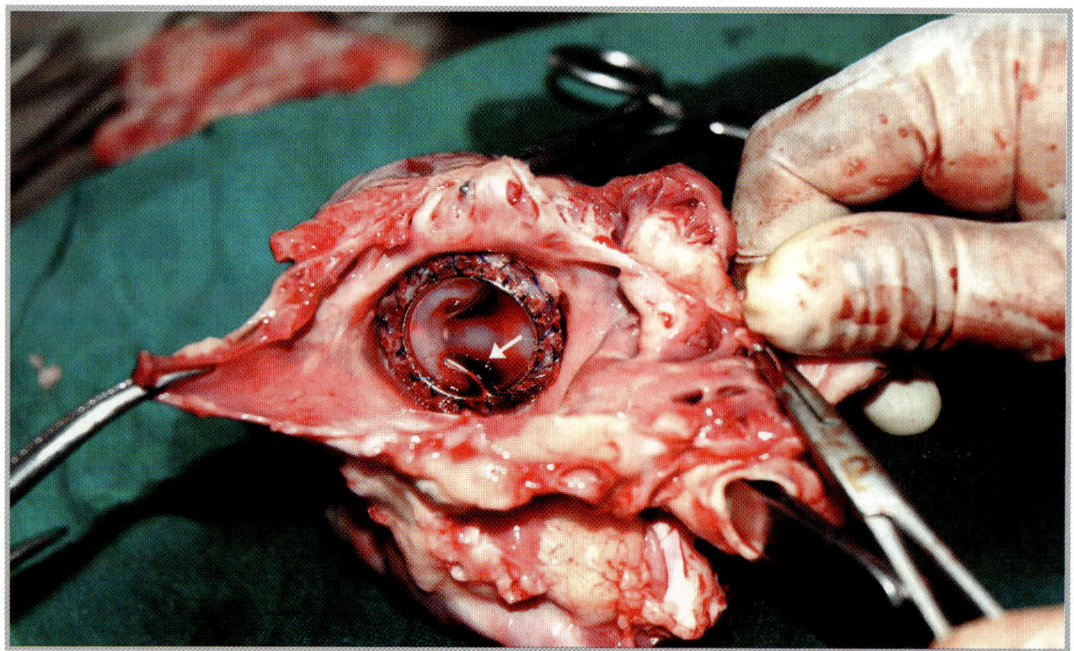

Figure 14 Mechanical heart valve. Gross image
Fresh blood clot (↑) on disk of the valve. The clot is soft and bright red

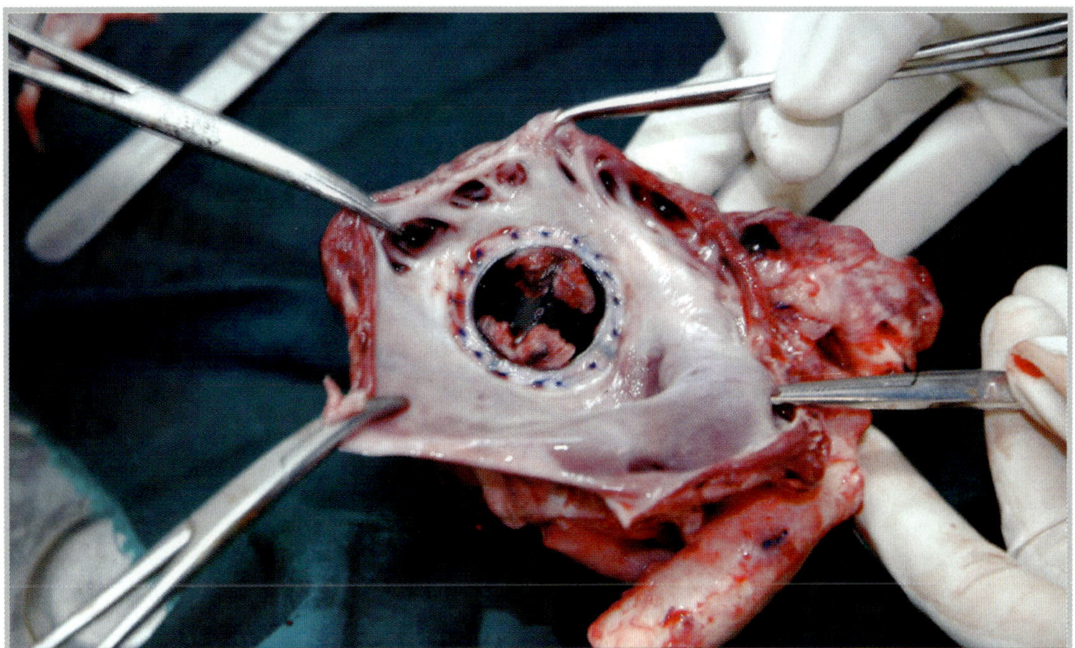

Figure 15A Mechanical heart valve. Gross image. Thrombus formation Thrombi on valve leaflets

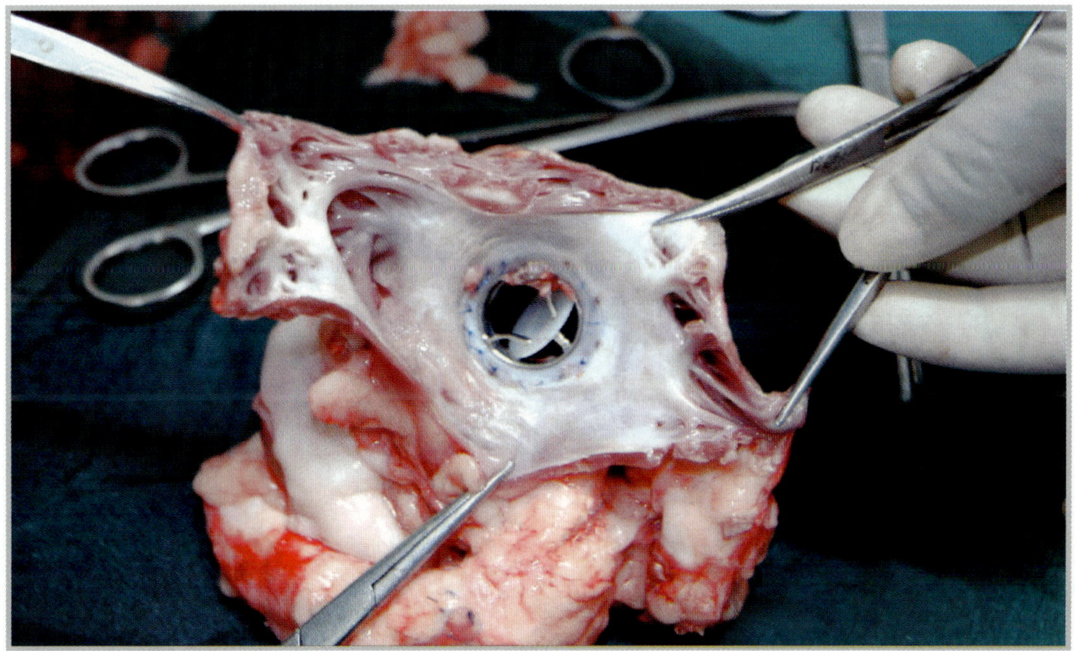

Figure 15B Mechanical heart valve. Gross image. Thrombus formation Thrombi adjacent to sewing ring

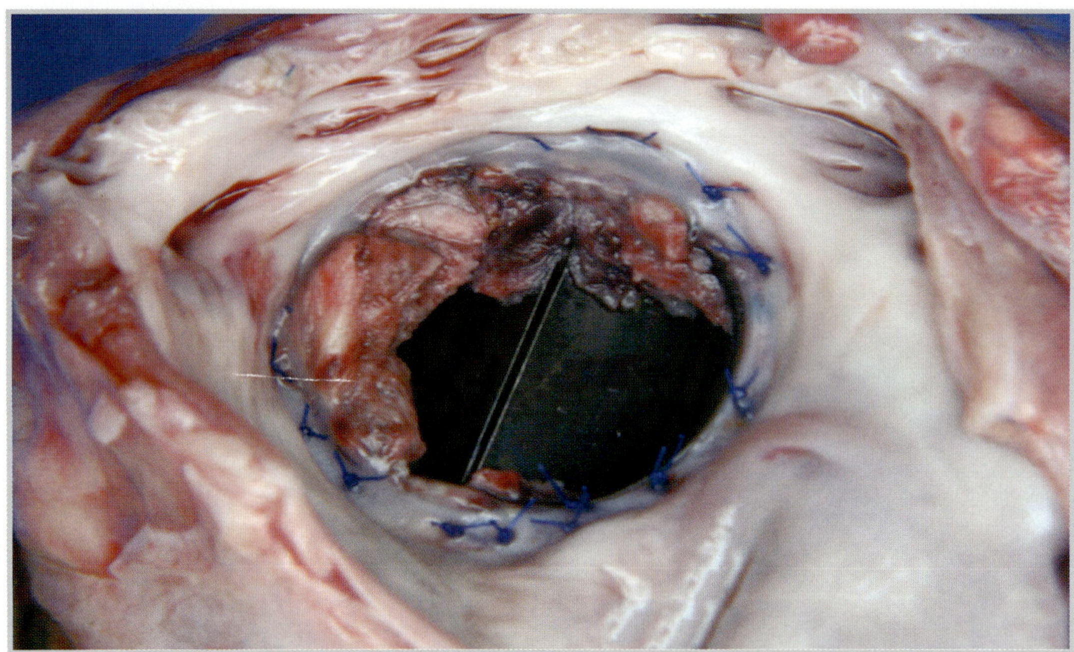

Figure 15C Mechanical heart valve. Gross image. Thrombus formation
Thrombi adjacent to sewing ring

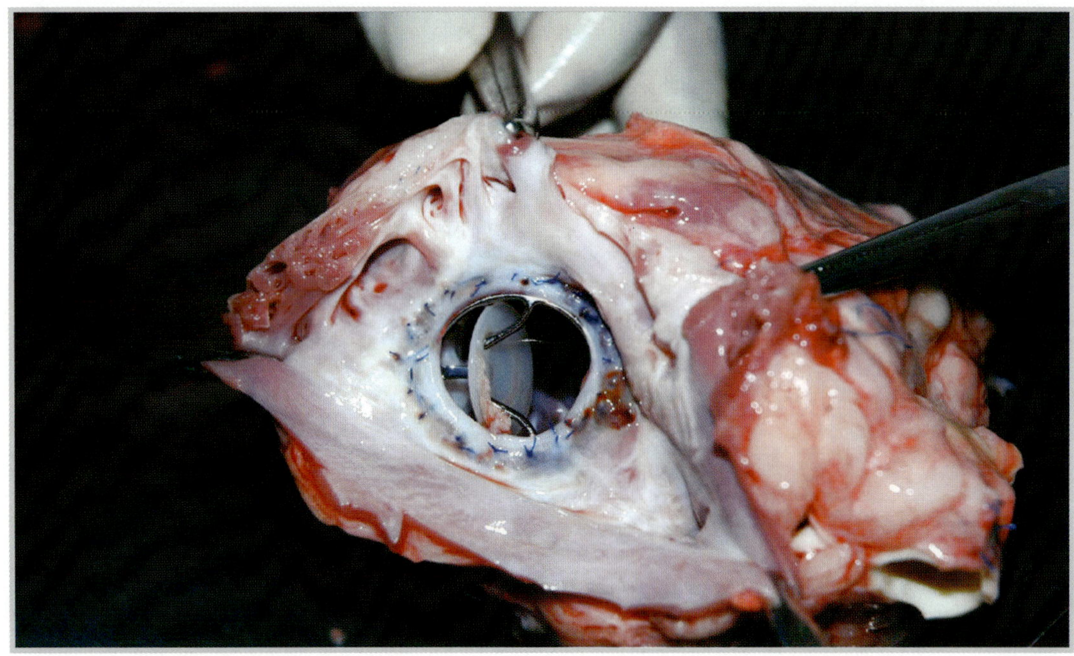

Figure 15D Mechanical heart valve. Gross image. Thrombus formation
Thrombi on valve disk. The thrombi are firm and pinkish white

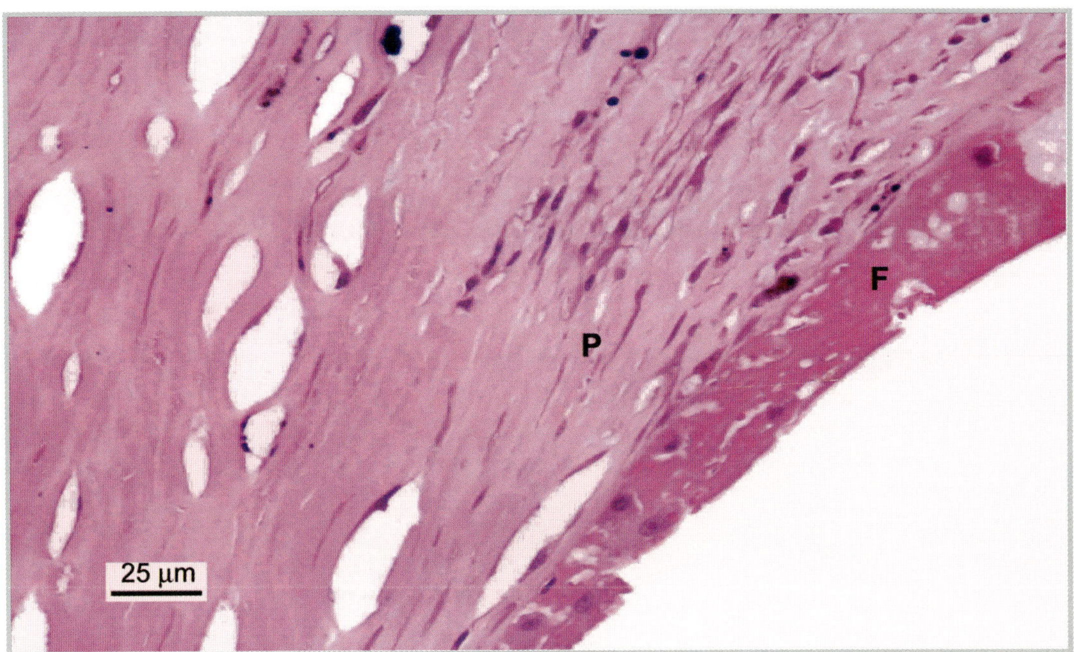

Figure 16 Mechanical heart valve. H & E x 40
Layer of fibrin (F) along edge of pannus (P)

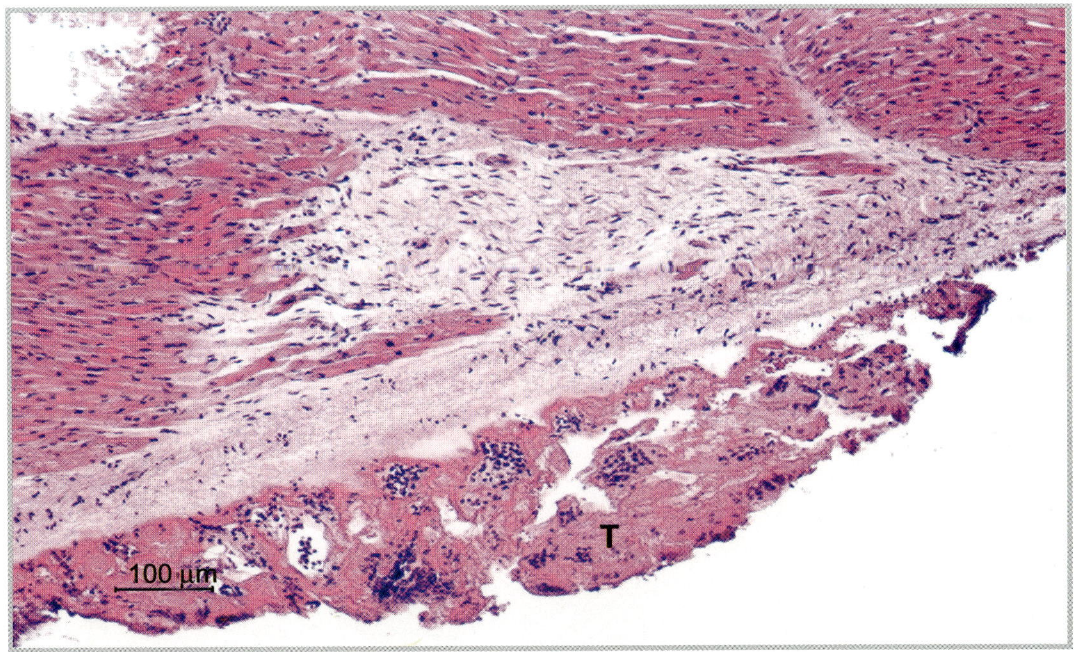

Figure 17A Mechanical heart valve. H & E x 10
Thrombus (T) on endocardium

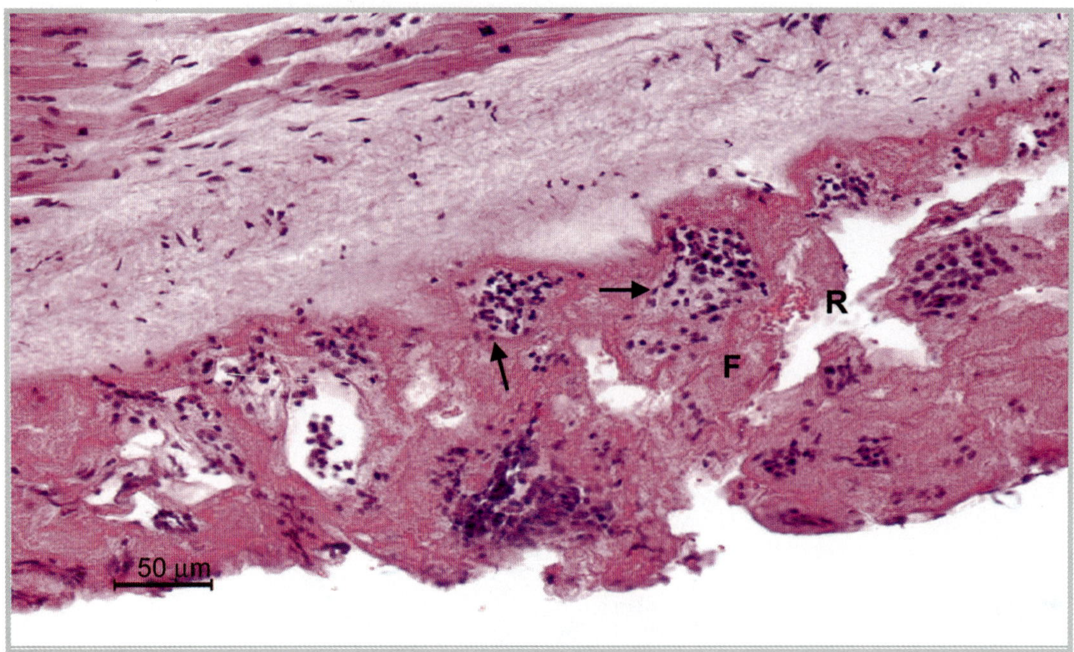

Figure 17B Mechanical heart valve. H & E x 20
Higher magnification of thrombus (T) on endocardium. Polymorphonuclear cells (↑) and red blood cells (R) enmeshed in fibrin (F)

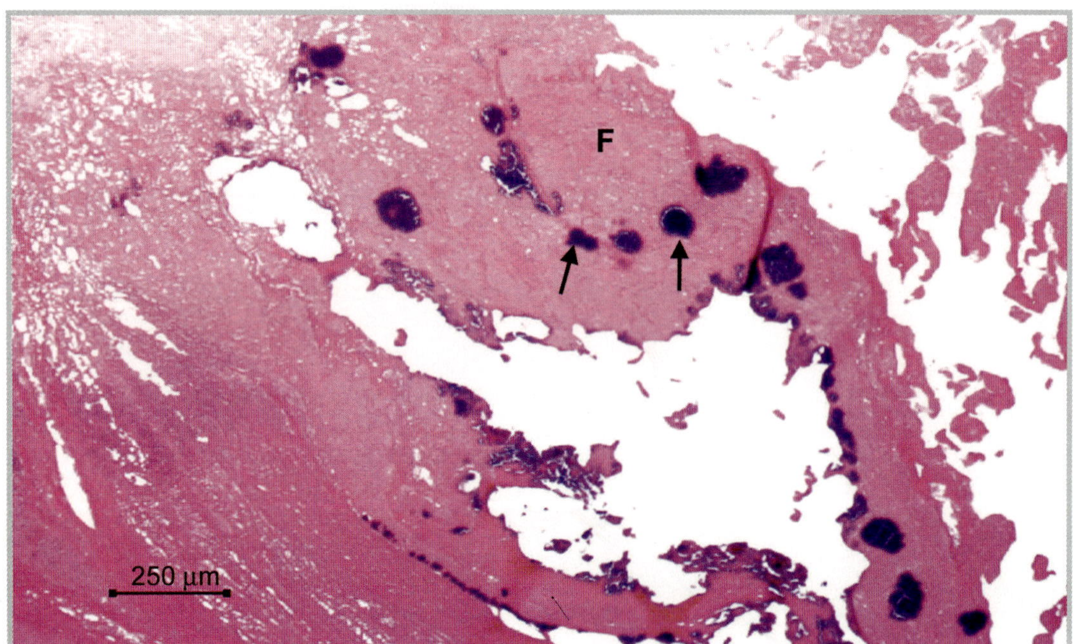

Figure 18 Mechanical heart valve. H & E x 4
Bacterial colonies (↑) in fibrin thrombus (F)

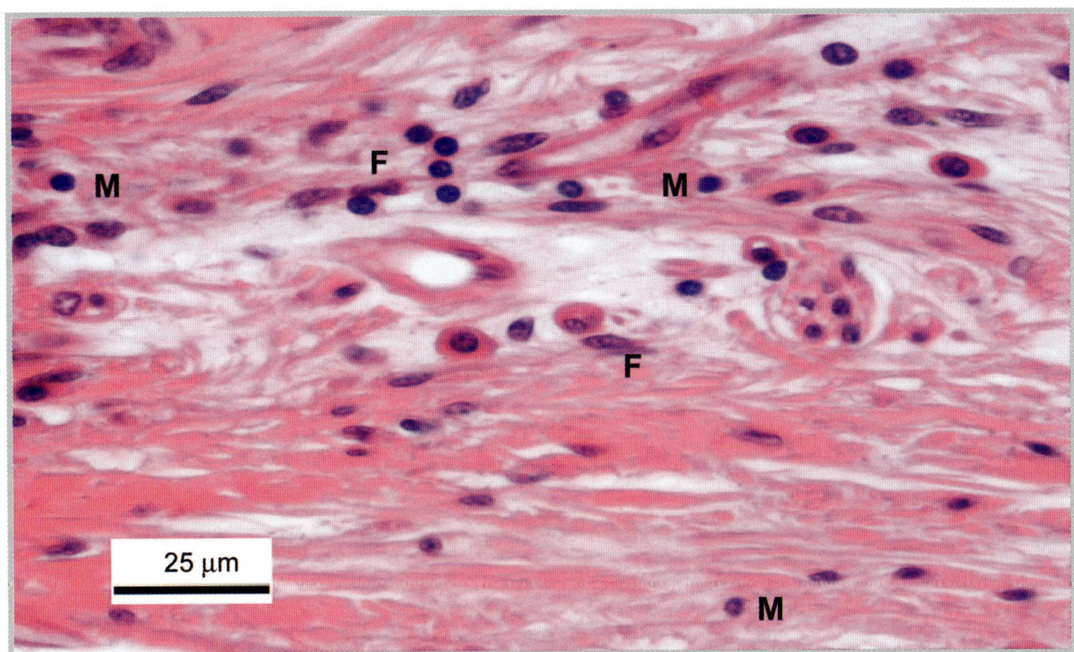

Figure 19 Mechanical heart valve. H & E x 40
Mononuclear cells (M) and fibroblasts (F) in tissue adjacent to sewing ring

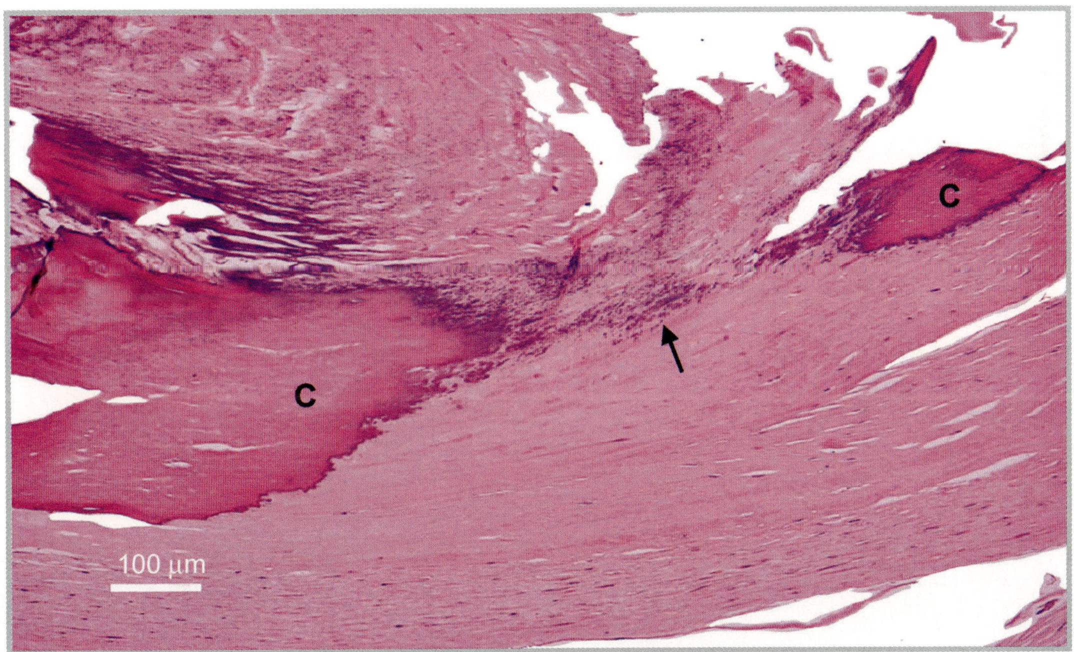

Figure 20A Mechanical heart valve. H & E x 10
Heavy (C) and spotty calcification (↑) adjacent to sewing ring

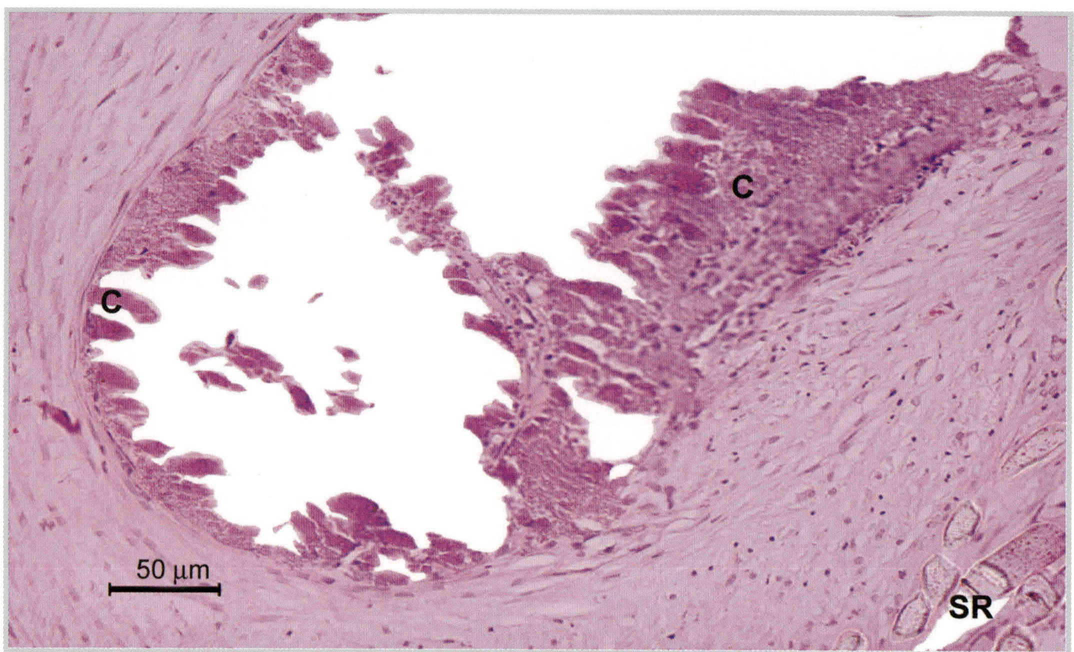

Figure 20B Mechanical heart valve. H & E x 20
Moderate calcification (C) in tissue adjacent to sewing ring (SR)

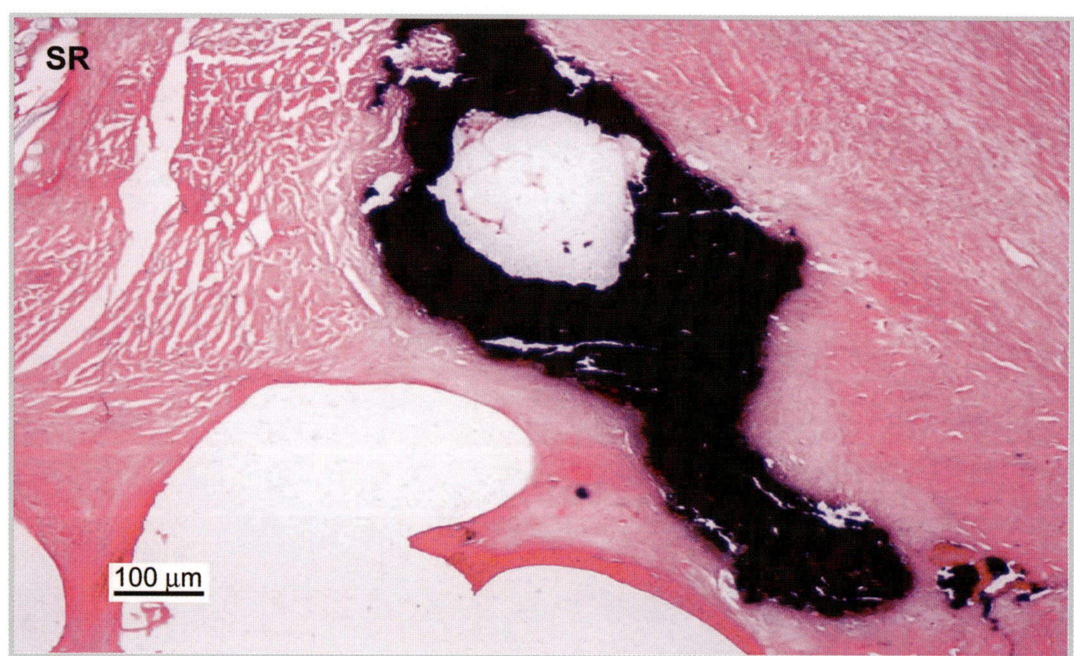

Figure 21 Mechanical heart valve. Von Kossa x 10
Calcific areas stained black adjacent to sewing ring (SR)

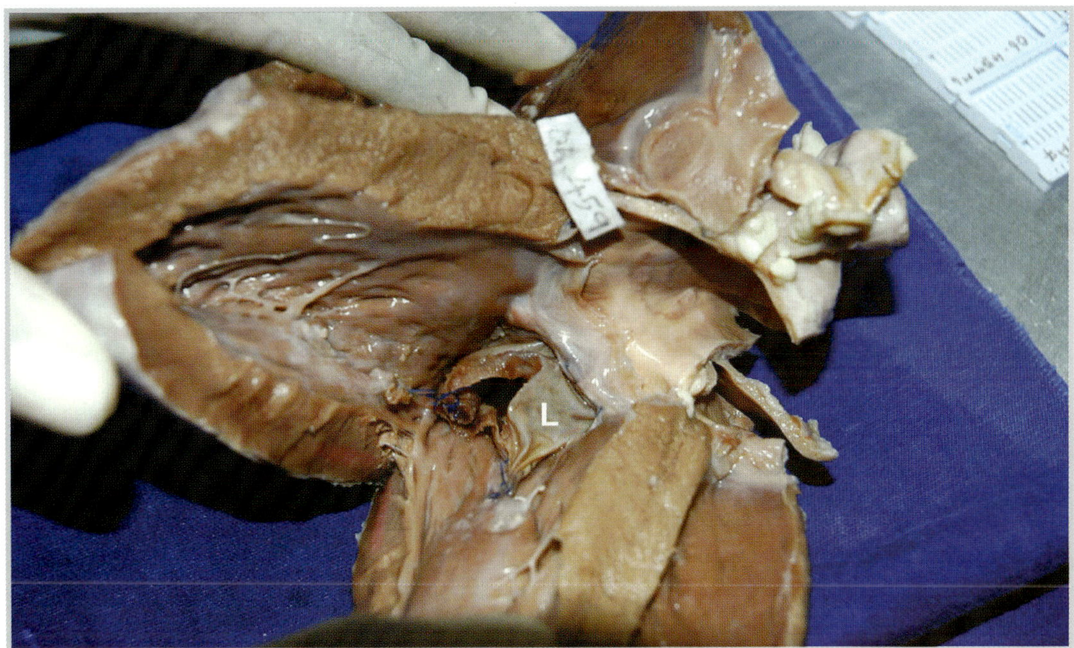

Figure 22 Bioprosthetic heart valve. Gross image
Bioprosthetic heart valve in situ in the heart. Leaflets (L) are soft and pliable

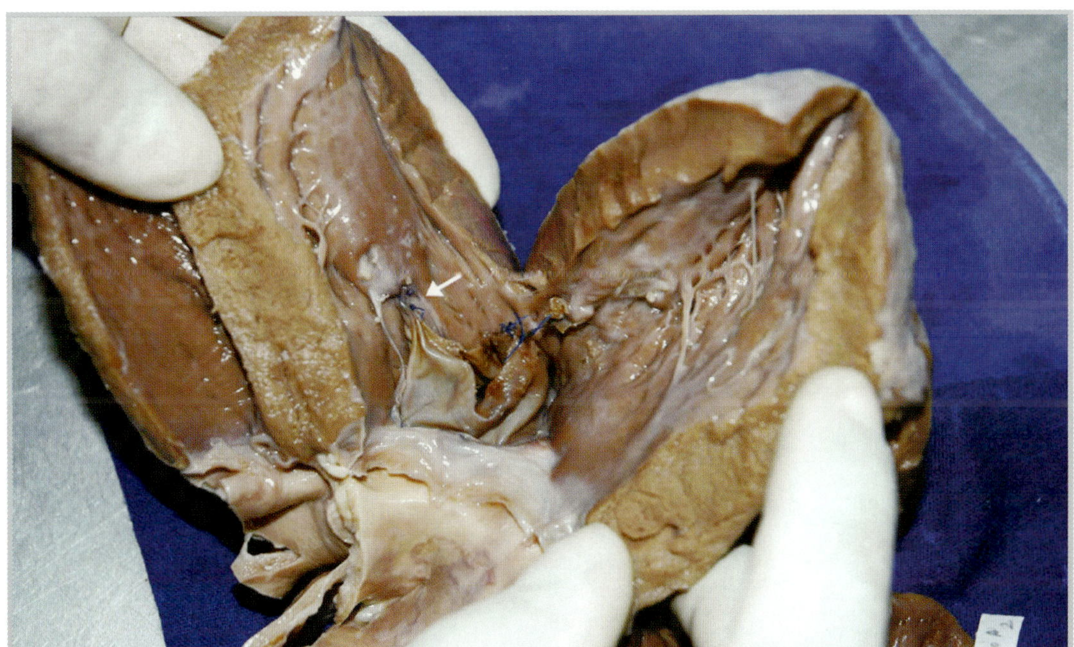

Figure 23 Bioprosthetic heart valve. Gross image
Bioprosthetic heart valve in situ in the heart. One of the leaflets end sutured to papillary muscle (↑) in left ventricle

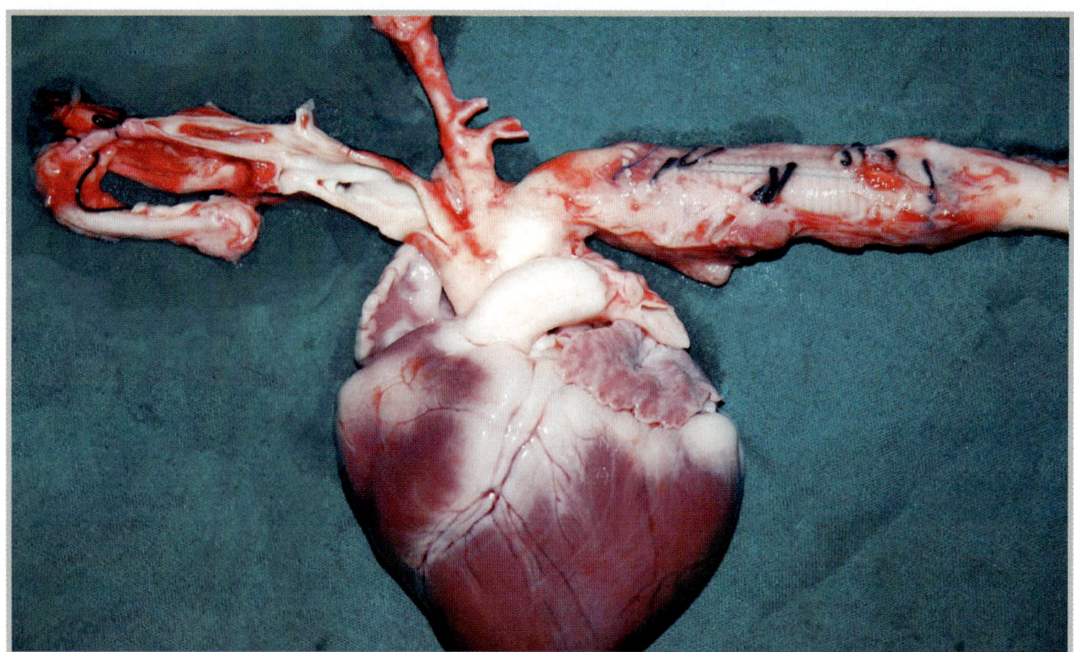

Figure 24A Large diameter prosthetic vascular graft in situ. Gross image
Heart with adjoining aorta with interposed graft

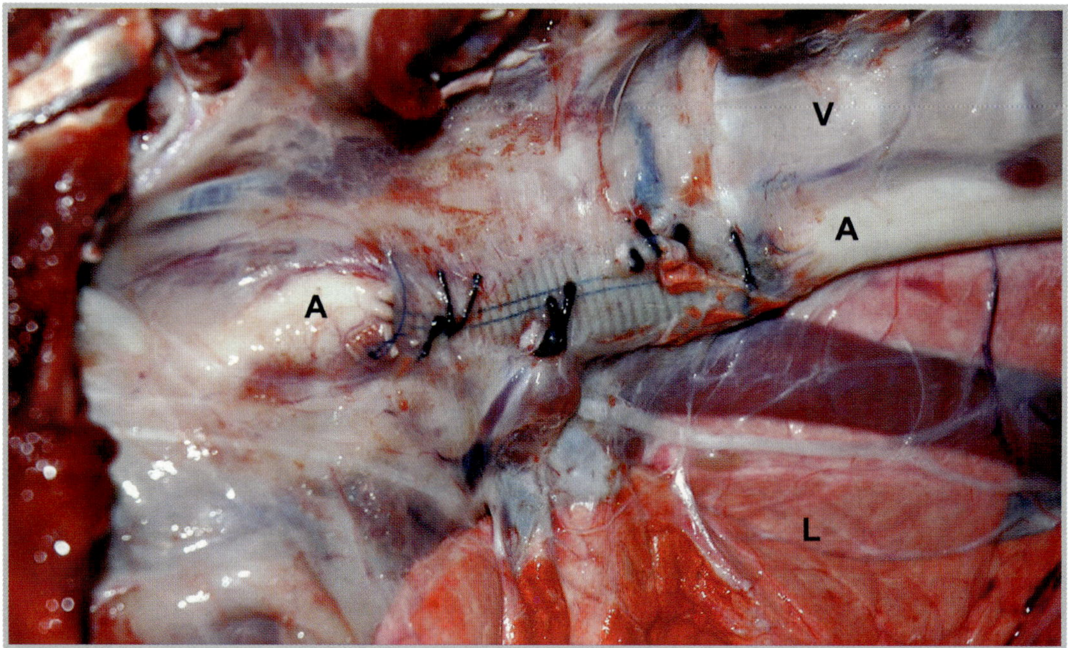

Figure 24B Large diameter prosthetic vascular graft in situ in thoracic cavity. Gross image
The aorta (A) has been cut and the graft interposed between the two cut ends. The cut ends are sutured at the anastomosis. Lung lobe (L), thoracic vertebra (V)

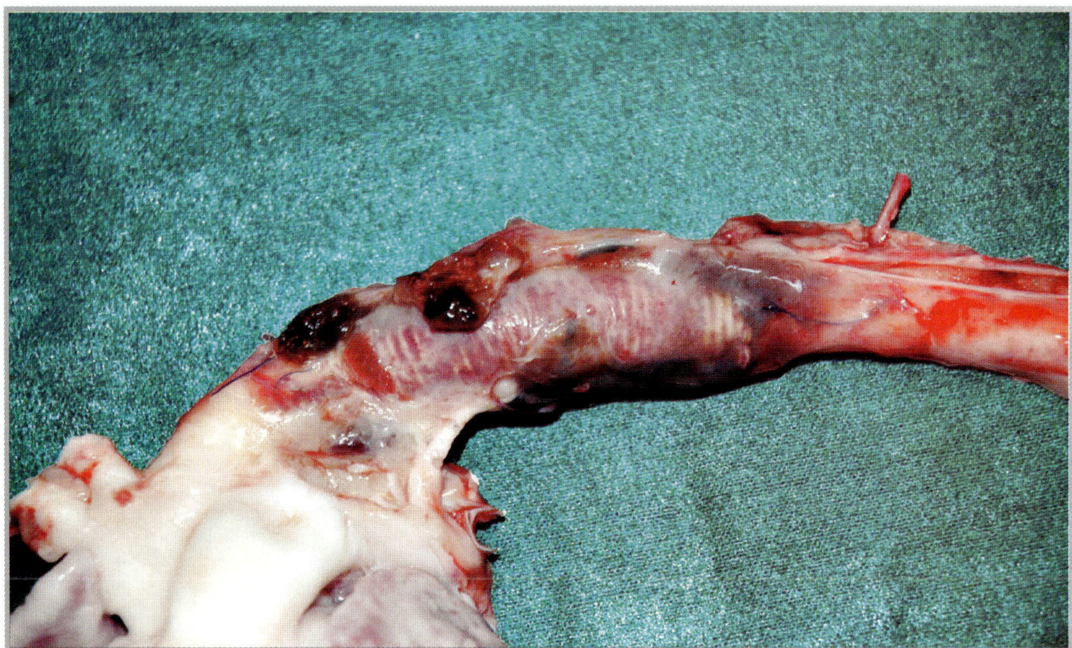

Figure 24C Large diameter prosthetic vascular graft in situ. Gross image

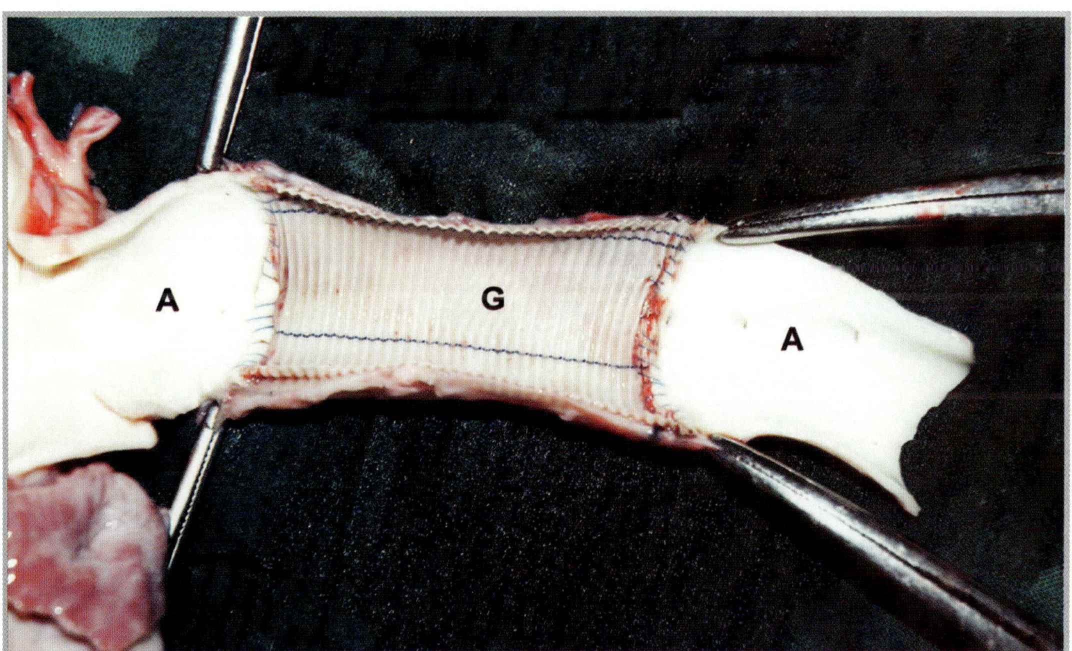

Figure 25 Large diameter prosthetic vascular graft in situ. Gross image.
The aorta (A) and graft (G) has been cut open longitudinally to expose the inner surface of the graft. The surgical technique of suturing at the anastomosis on either side is important as irregularity can cause eddies in flow resulting in thrombus formation

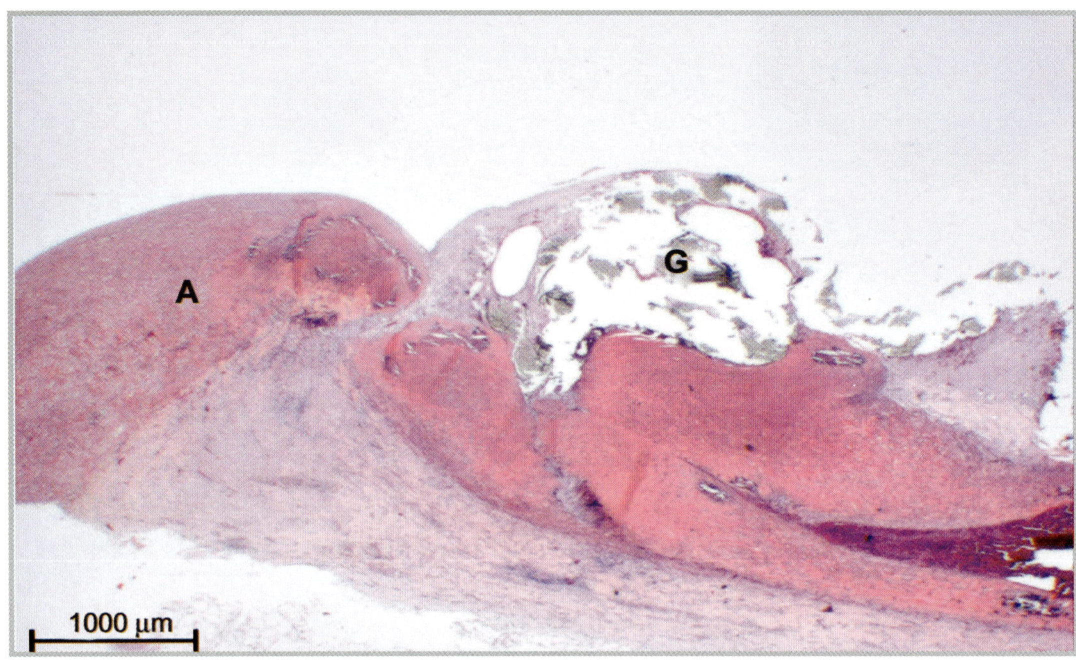

Figure 26A Large diameter prosthetic vascular graft. H & E x 1
Cross-sections through the graft (G) on the right and adjoining host aorta (A) on the left

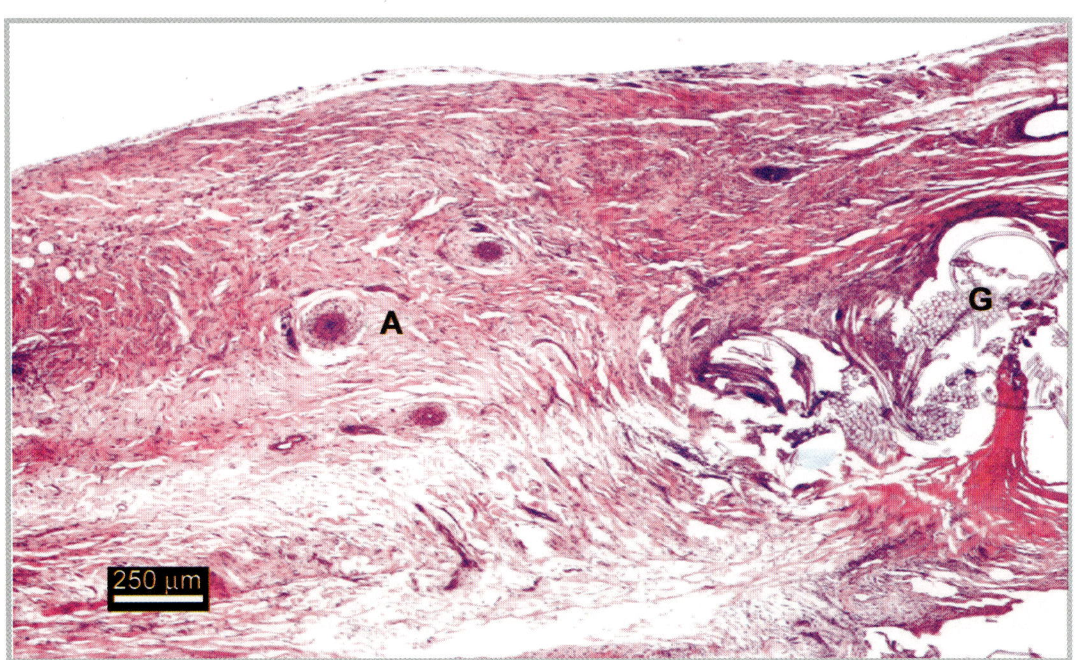

Figure 26B Large diameter prosthetic vascular graft. H & E x 4
Anastomosis of the graft (G) with adjoining aorta (A)

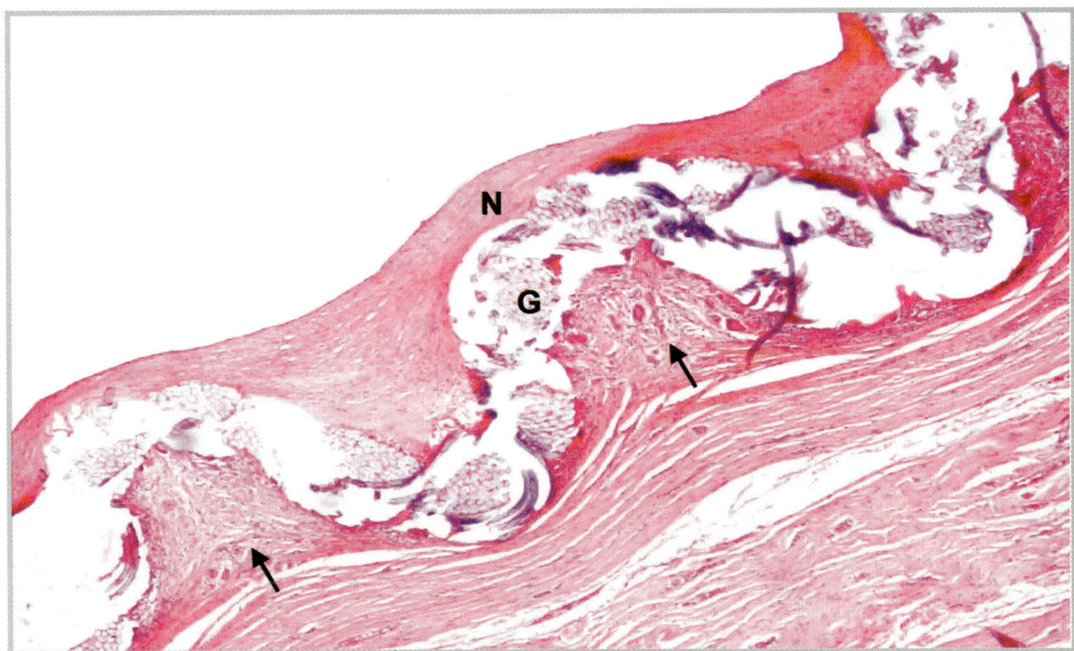

Figure 27 Large diameter prosthetic vascular graft. H & E x 4
Cross-sections through the graft (G). Tissue ingrowth (↑) from adventitia through pores of the graft is seen externally and neointima (N) is present along the inner surface

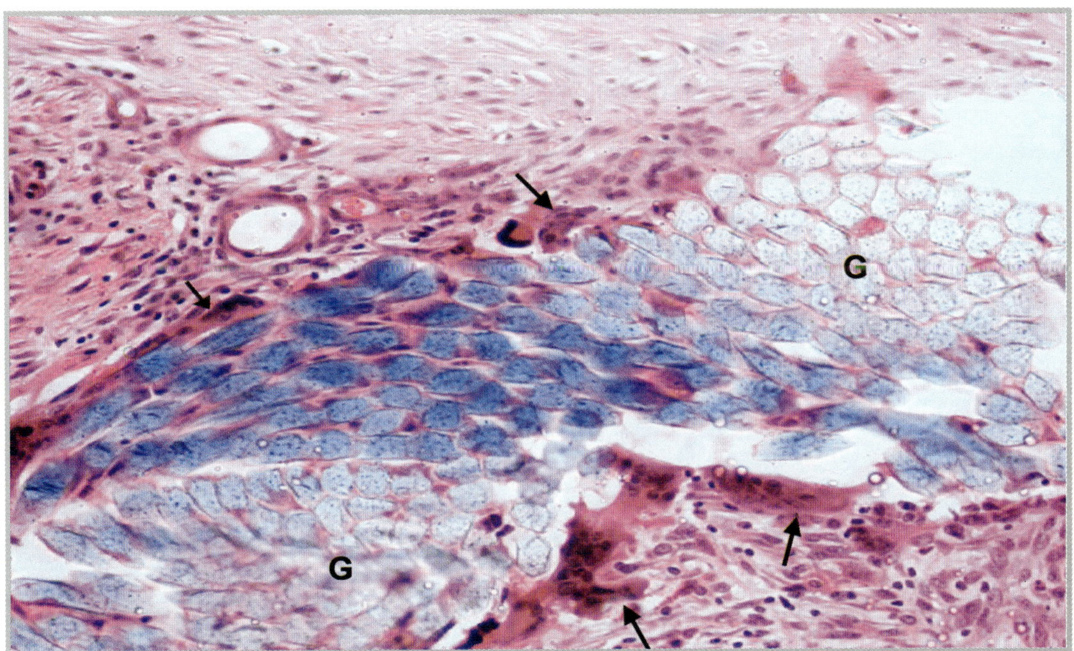

Figure 28 Large diameter prosthetic vascular graft. H & E x 40
Numerous foreign body type of giant cells (↑) and macrophages are seen in the interstices of the graft (G)

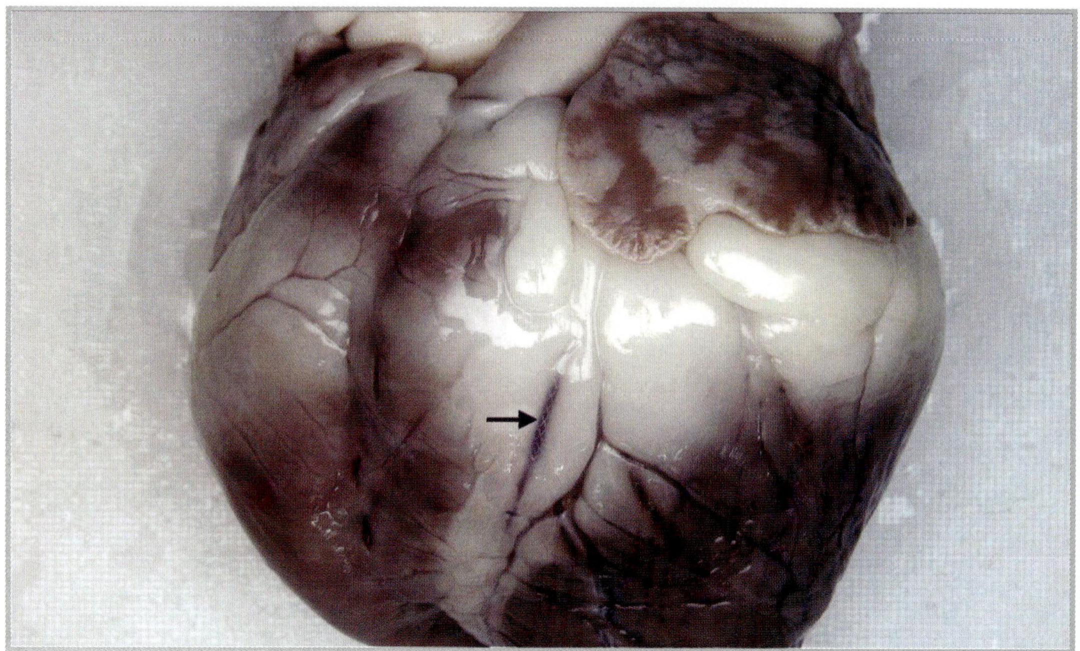

Figure 29A Vascular stent. Gross image
Metal stent (↑) in coronary blood vessel in heart

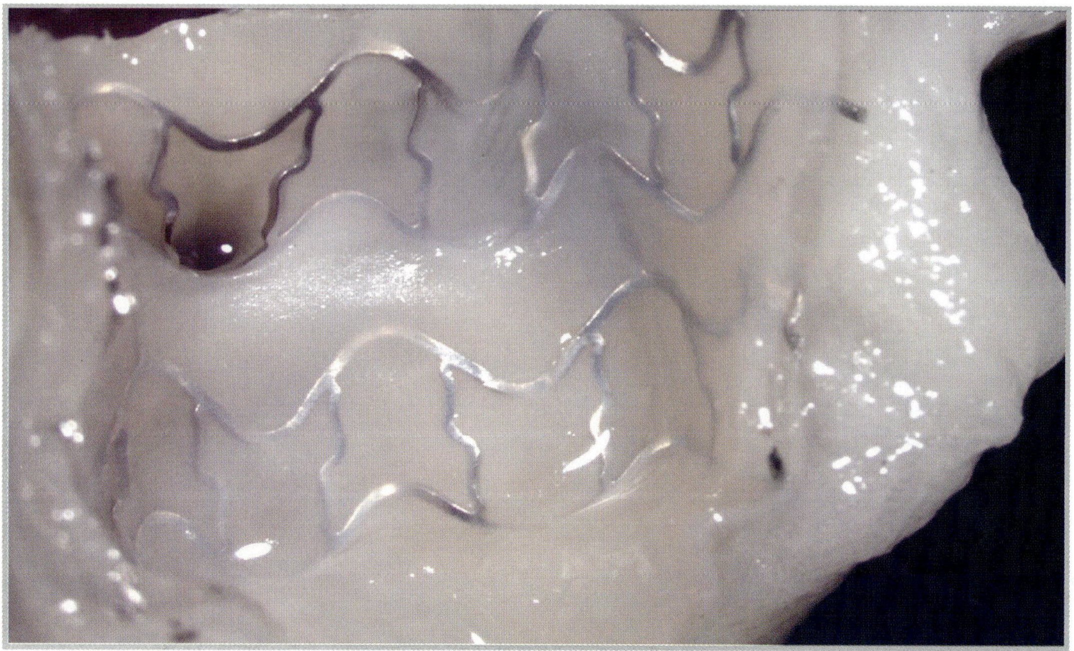

Figure 29B Vascular stent
Cut open coronary blood vessel with stent, examined under stereomicroscope neointima covering stent struts is seen

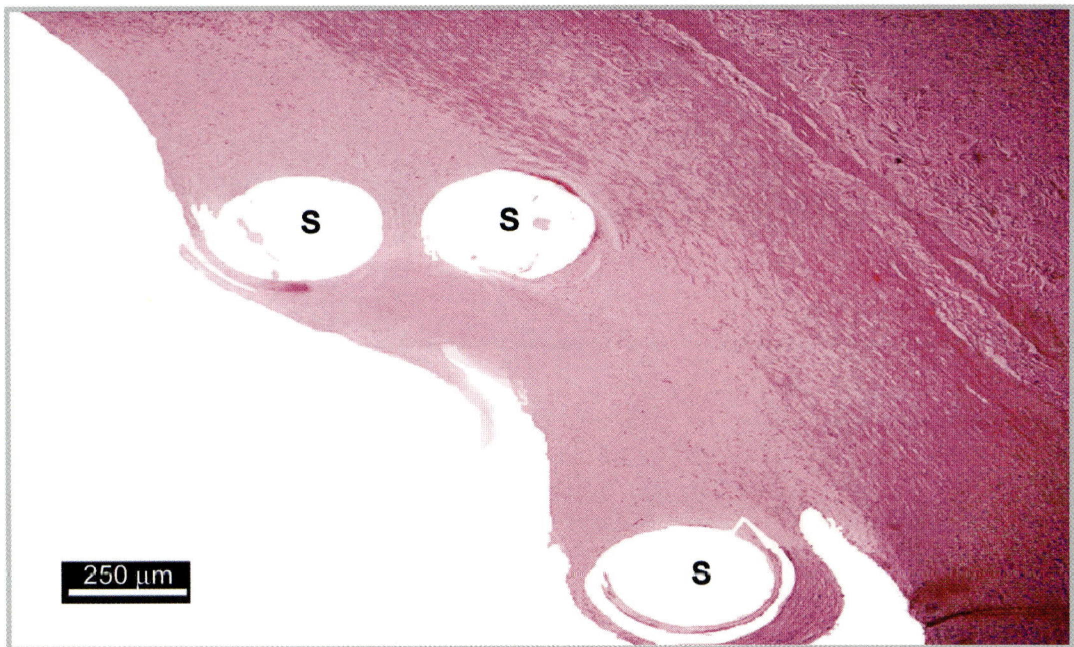

Figure 30A Vascular stent. H & E x 4
Overlapping stent strut sites (S) in cross-section of coronary artery. Blood vessel cut open longitudinally, stent carefully removed from the vessel wall and cross-sections of the blood vessel processed

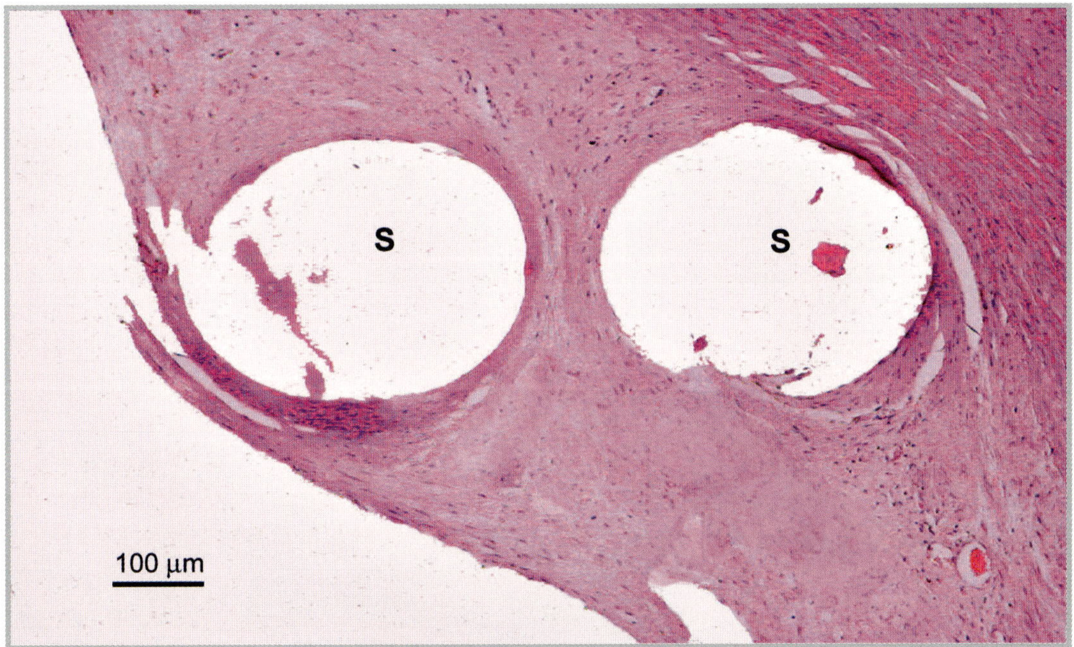

Figure 30B Vascular stent. H & E x 10
Higher magnification of overlapping stent strut sites (S) in cross-section of coronary artery

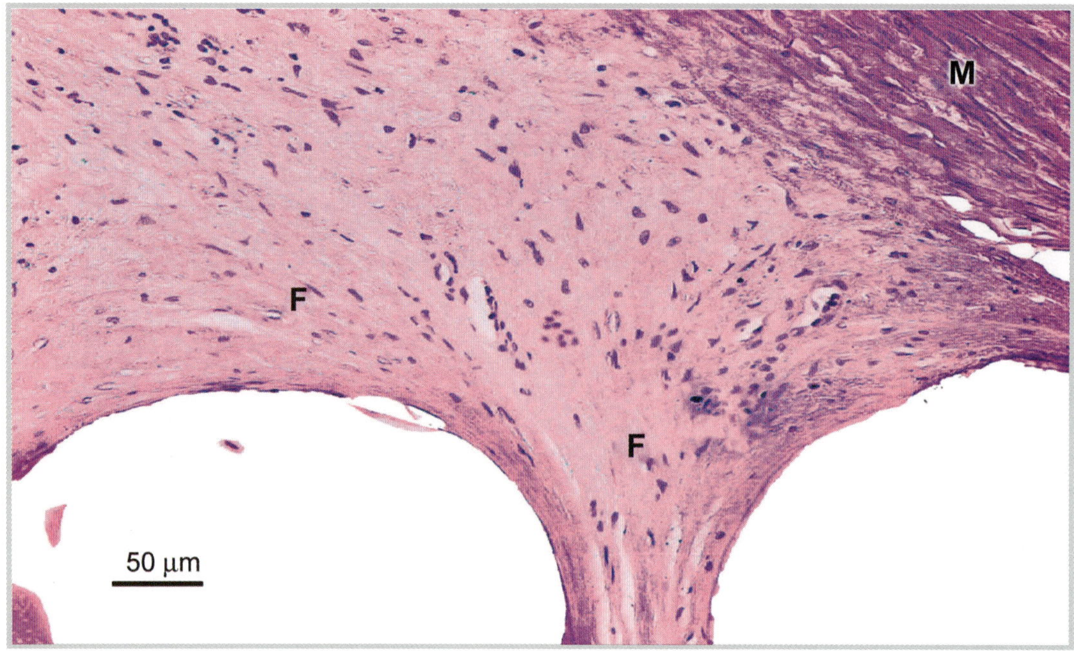

Figure 31 Vascular stent. H & E x 20
Fibrocytes (F) at stent site-tissue interface. (M) Denotes smooth muscle cells in medial layer of vessel wall

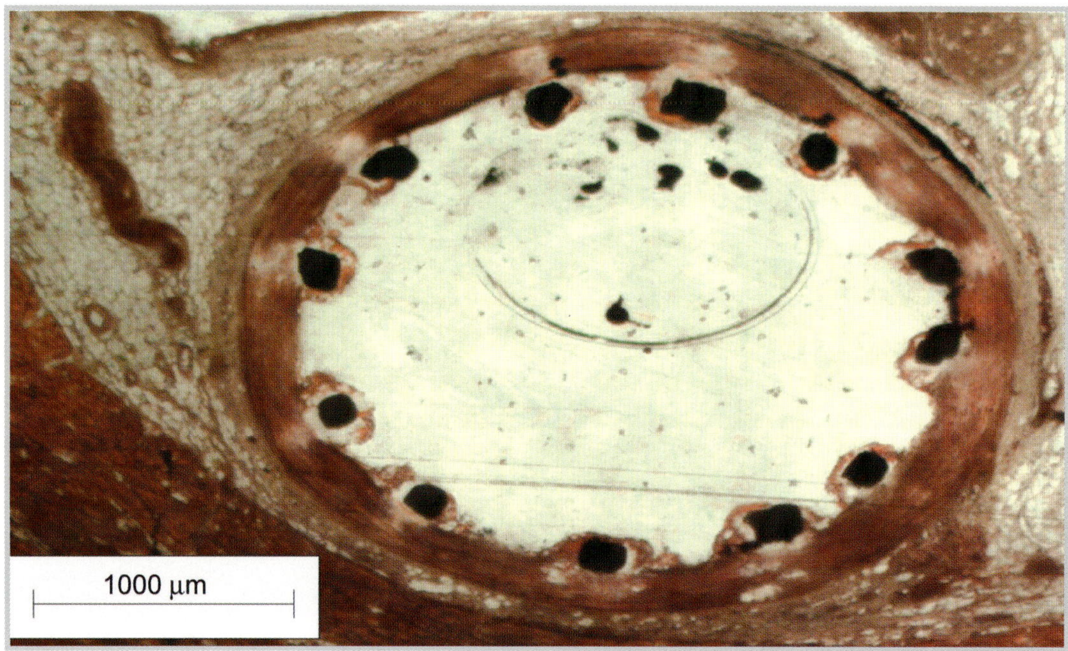

Figure 32A Vascular stent at 7 days. Resin H & E x 1
Cross-section of coronary artery with expanded stent at 7 days post-deployment
Stent struts seen as black areas embedded in the wall. Scant tissue is seen at the strut interface

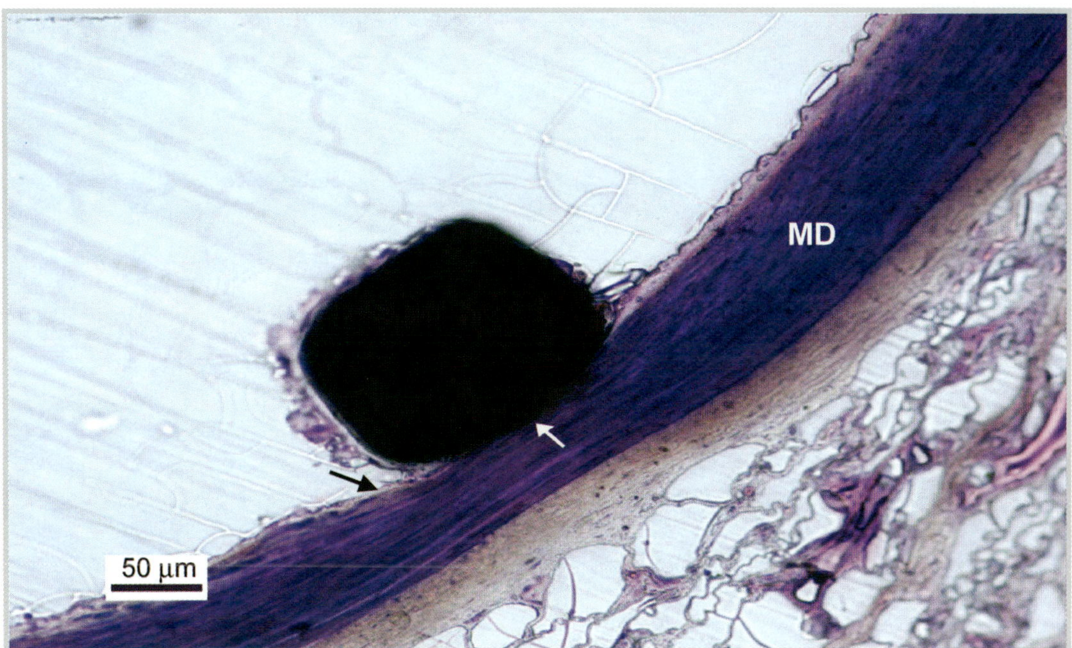

Figure 32B Vascular stent at 7 days. Resin H & E x 20
Higher magnification showing intact intimal layer of vessel wall (↑) in the interstrut space which is injured at strut. The medial layer (MD) is compressed

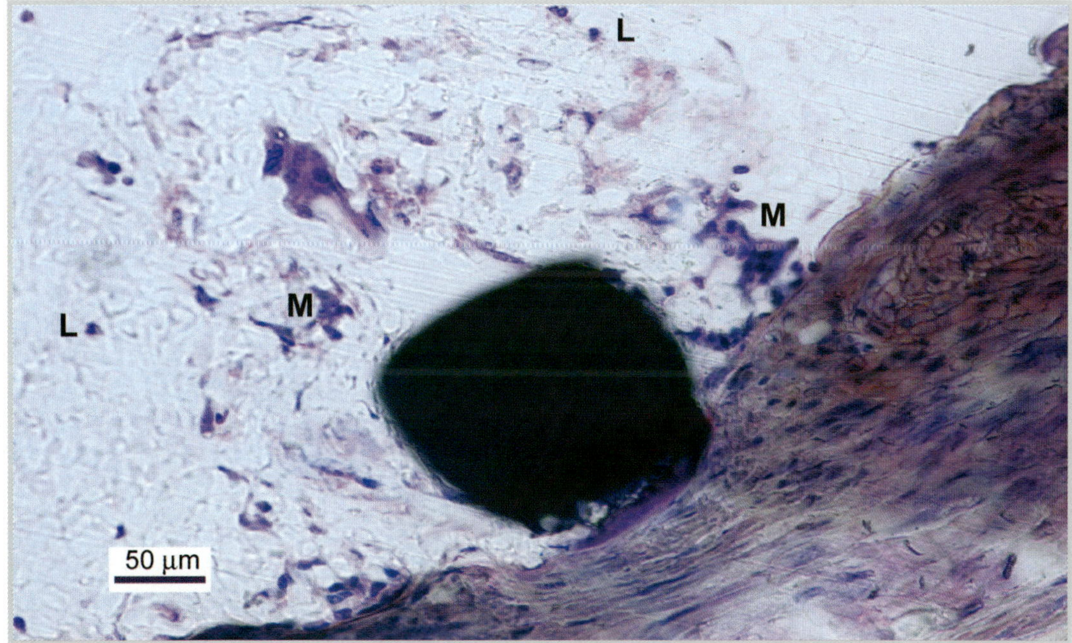

Figure 32C Vascular stent at 7 days. Resin H & E x 20
Cross-section of coronary artery with expanded stent at 7 days post-deployment
Macrophages (M) and occasional lymphocytes (L) are present

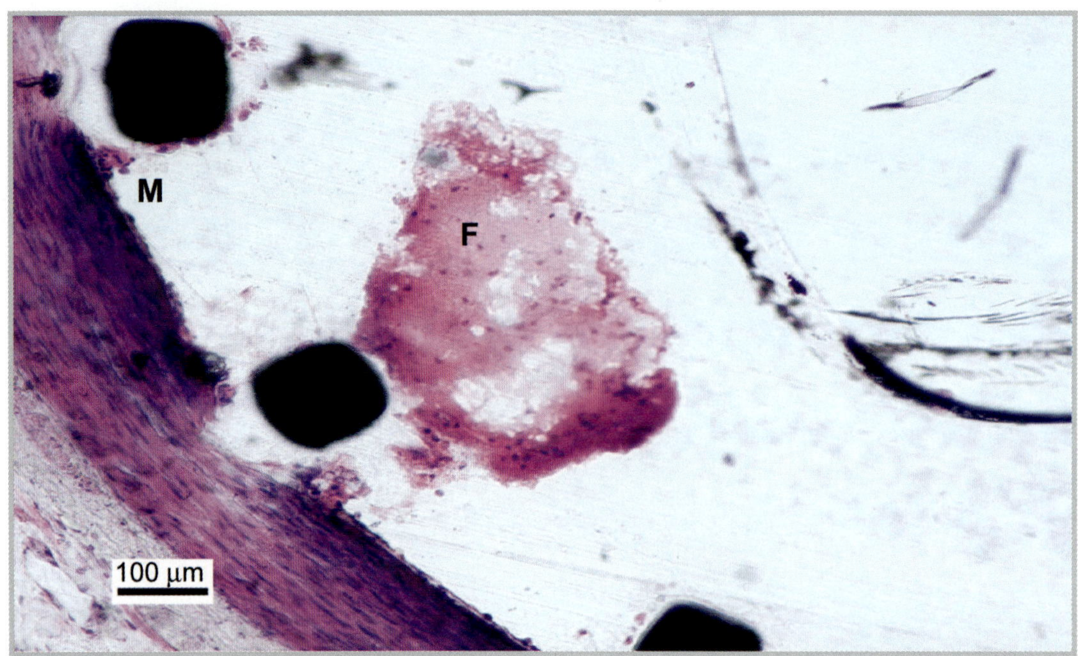

Figure 32D Vascular stent at 7 days. Resin H & E x 10
Fibrin (F), macrophages (M) and occasional lymphocytes are present

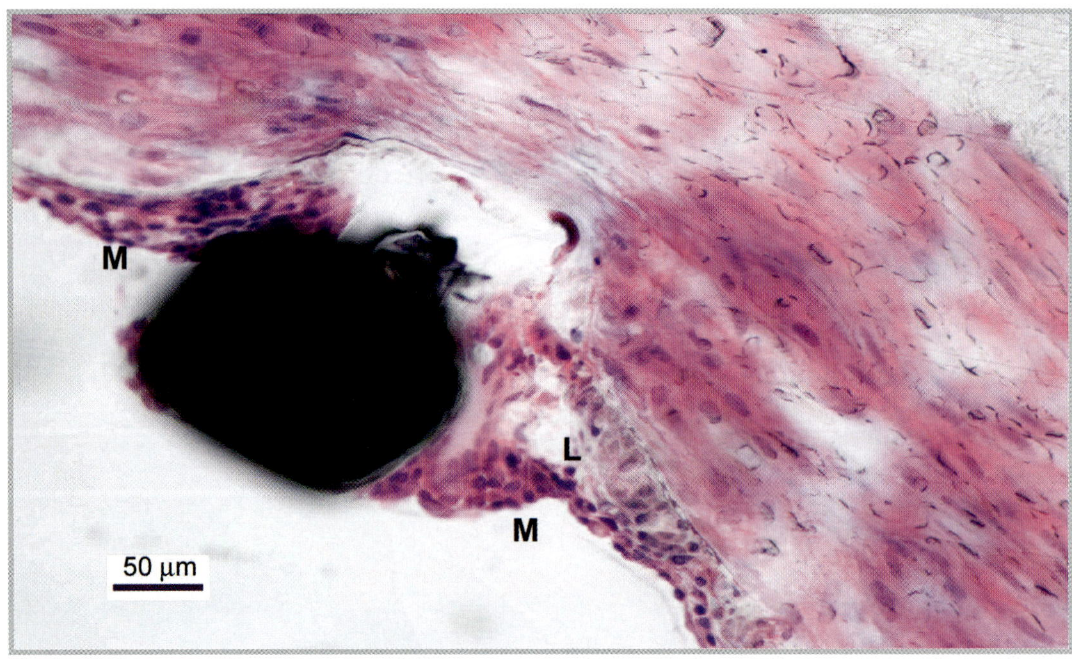

Figure 32E Vascular stent at 7 days. Resin H & E x 20
Fibrin (F), macrophages (M) and occasional lymphocytes (L) are present

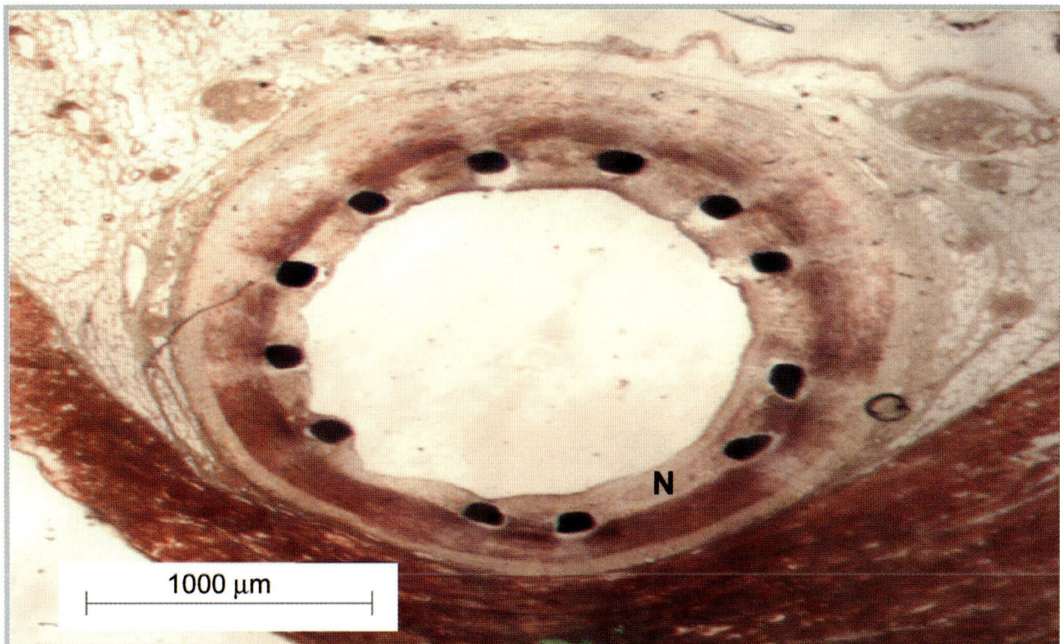

Figure 33A Vascular stent at 4 weeks. Resin H & E x 1
At this magnification the expansion of the stent can be assessed with respect to wall damage due to over expansion. A layer of neointima (N) is present

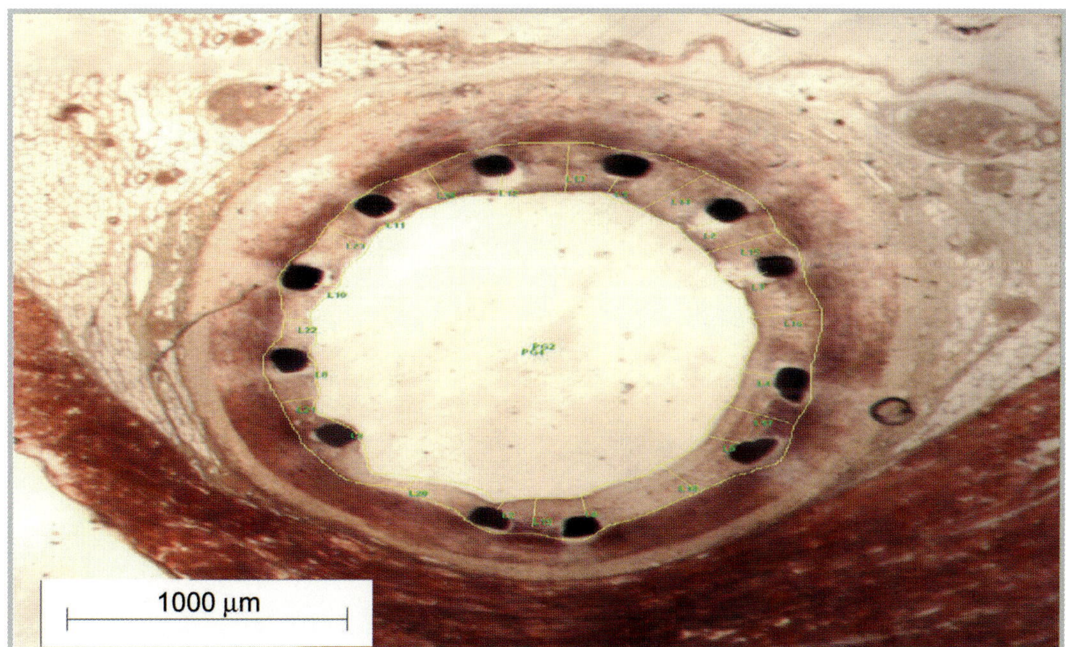

Figure 33B Vascular stent at 4 weeks. Resin H & E x 1
Cross-section of coronary artery with expanded stent 4 weeks post-deployment. Measurements of the thickness of the neointimal layer at strut and interstrut points, original area within the medial wall and present luminal area within the neointima are made

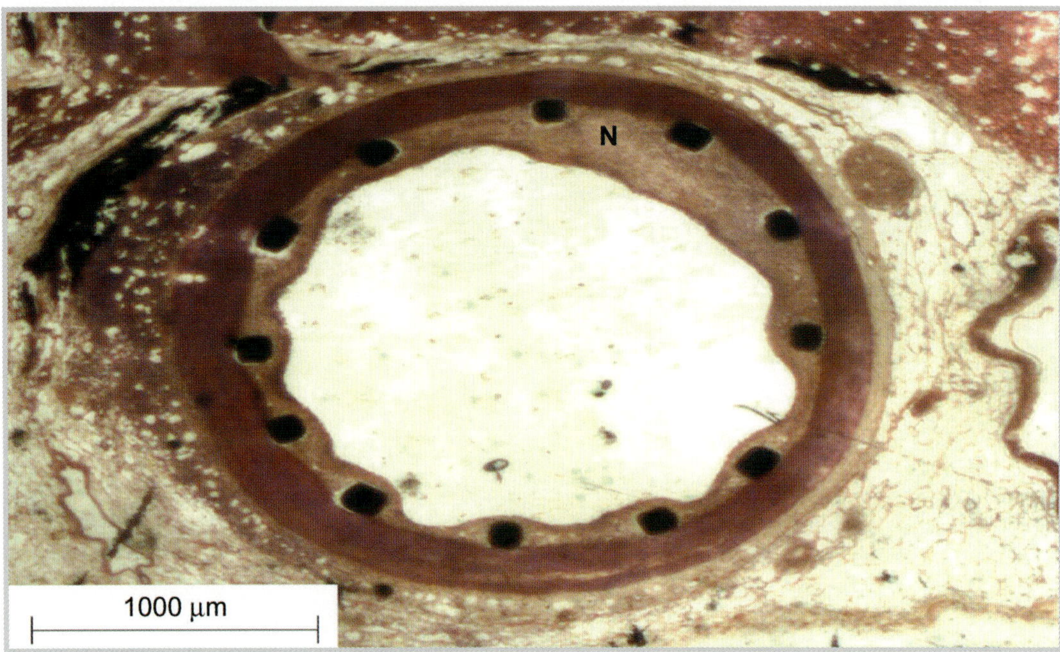

Figure 33C Vascular stent at 4 weeks. Resin H & E x 1
Cross-section of coronary artery with expanded stent 4 weeks post-deployment
Focal thicker neointima (N) is seen

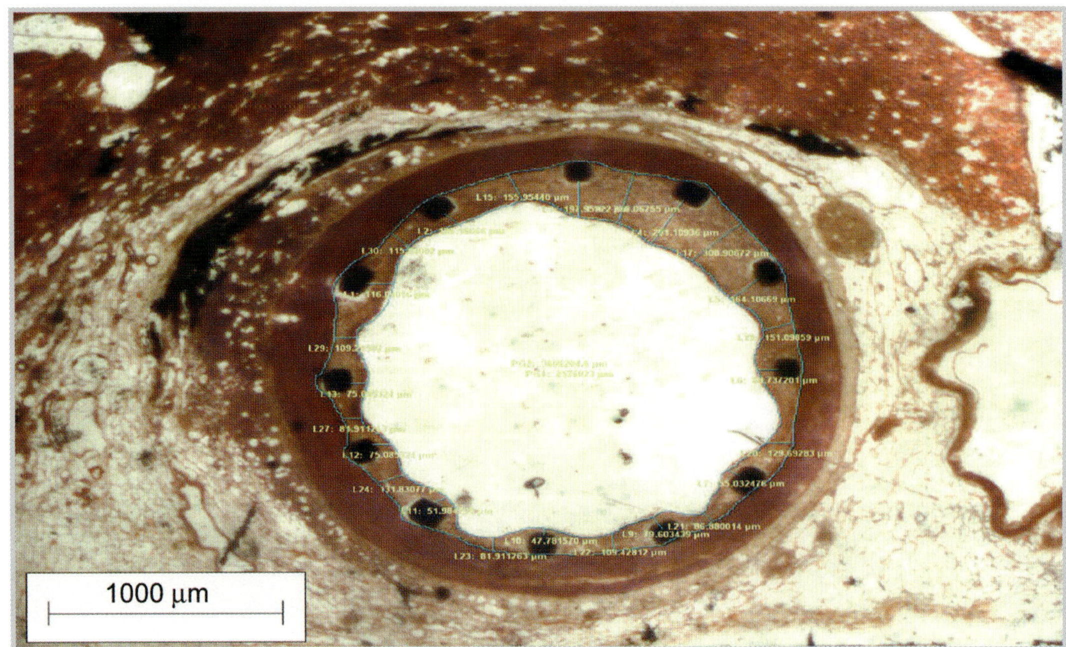

Figure 33D Vascular stent at 4 weeks. Resin H & E x 1
Cross-section of coronary artery with expanded stent 4 weeks post-deployment.
Focal thicker neointima with measurements

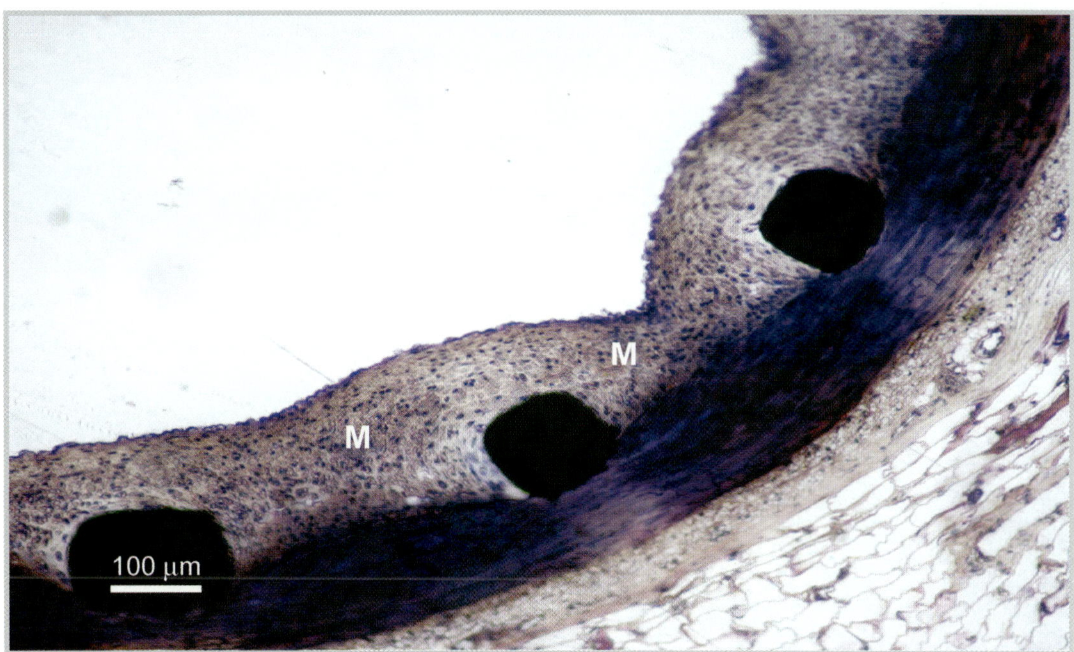

Figure 33E Vascular stent at 4 weeks. Resin H & E x 10
Cross-section of coronary artery with expanded stent 4 weeks post-deployment
Macrophages (M) are present in the neointima

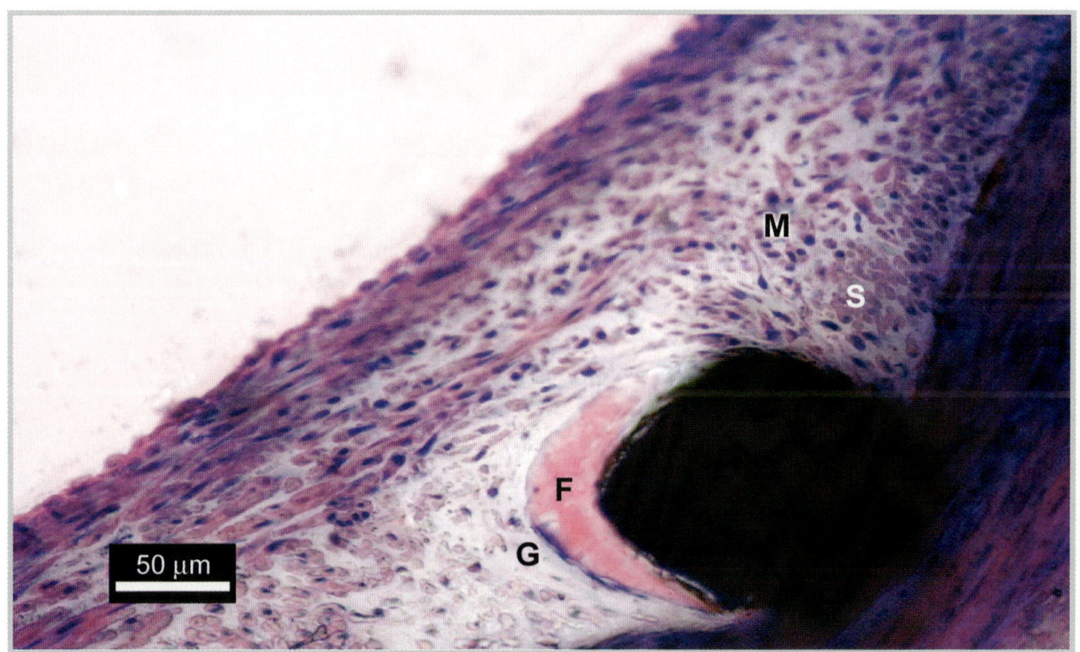

Figure 33F Vascular stent at 4 weeks. Resin H & E x 20
Cross-section of coronary artery with expanded stent 4 weeks post-deployment
Occasional giant cells (G), macrophages (M), smooth muscle cells (S) and fibrin (F) at the strut interface

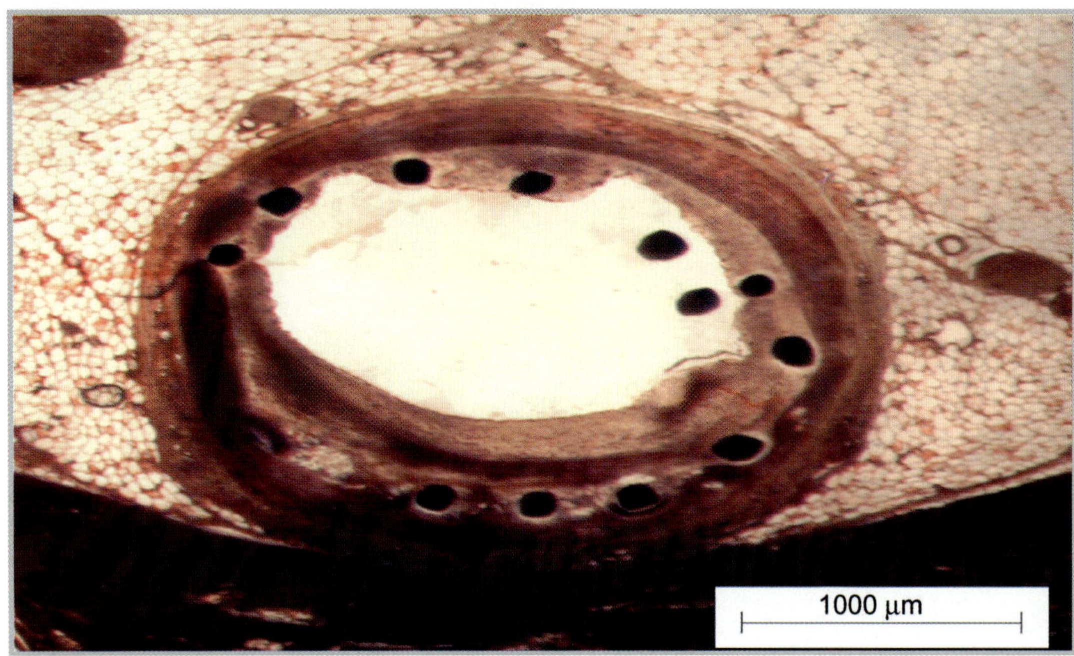

Figure 34A Vascular stent at 26 weeks. Resin H & E x 1
Cross-section of coronary artery with expanded stent.
The neointima increases in thickness with time and decreases due to tissue remodeling. Loose struts in lumen due to failure in stent expansion

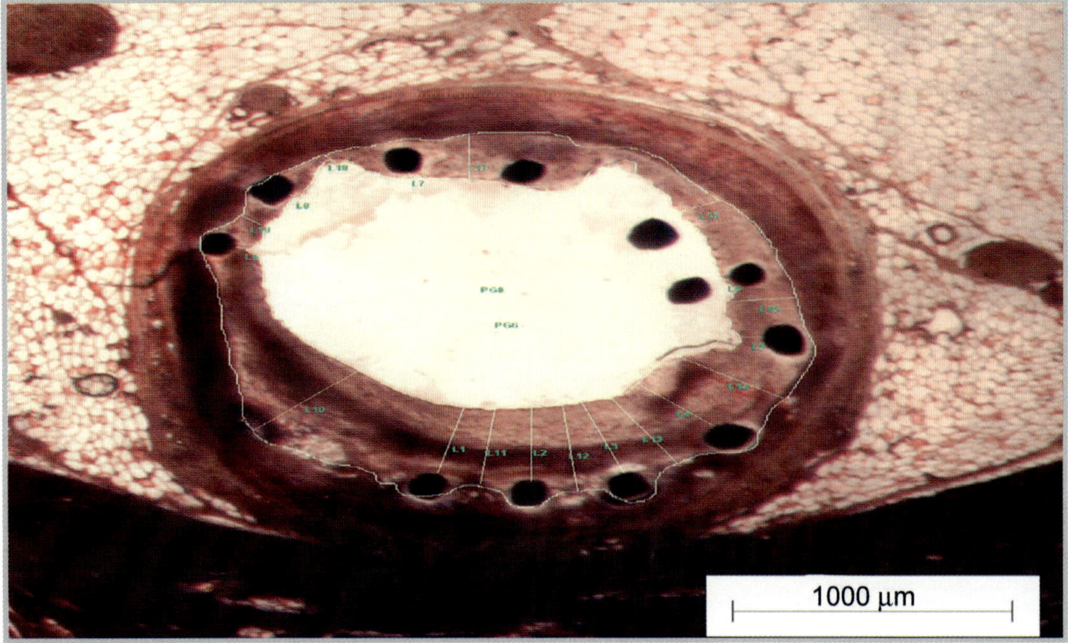

Figure 34B Vascular stent at 26 weeks. Resin H & E x 1
Cross-section of coronary artery with expanded stent 26 weeks post-deployment
Measurements in proximal segment

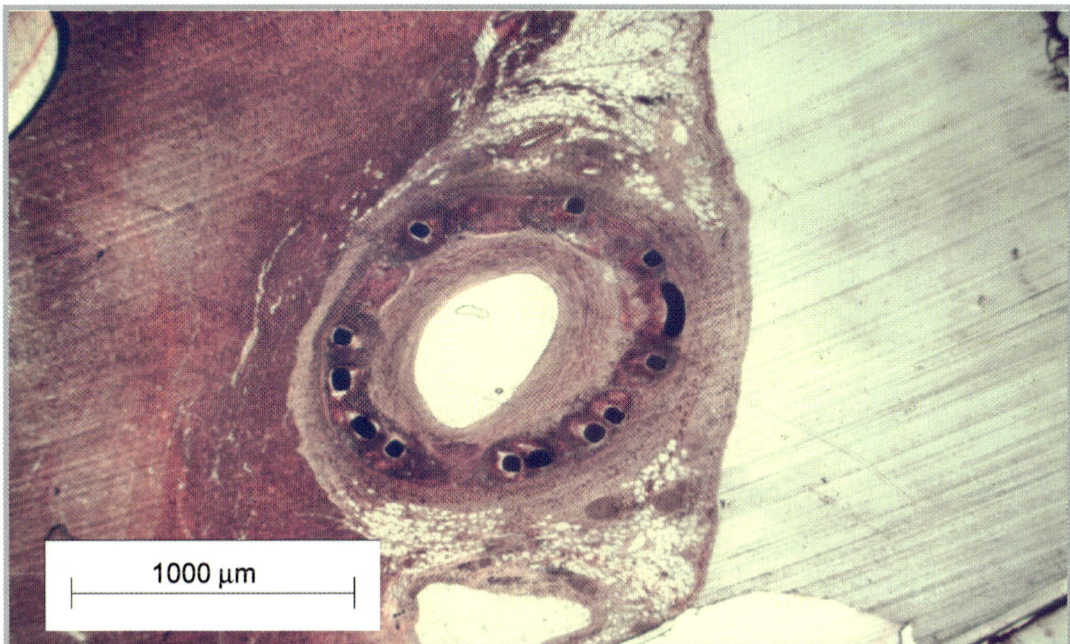

Figure 34C Vascular stent at 26 weeks. Resin H & E x 1
Cross-section of coronary artery with expanded stent 26 weeks post-deployment
Thick neointima in proximal segment

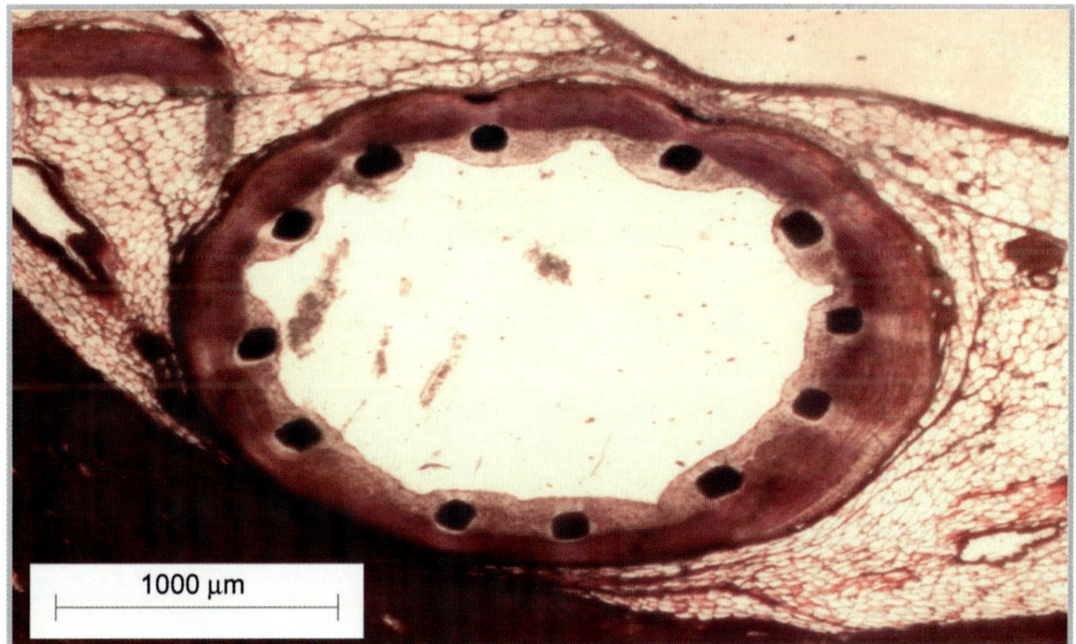

Figure 34D Vascular stent at 26 weeks. Resin H & E x 1
Cross-section of coronary artery with expanded stent 26 weeks post-deployment
Middle segment

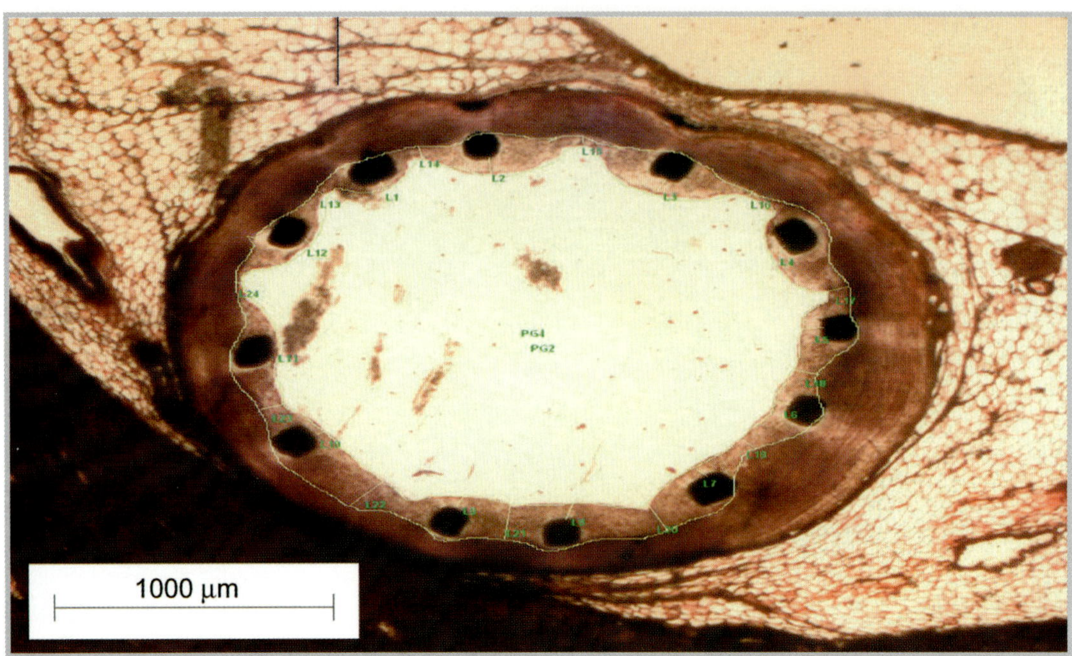

Figure 34E Vascular stent at 26 weeks. Resin H & E x 1
Cross-section of coronary artery with expanded stent 26 weeks post-deployment
Measurements in middle segment

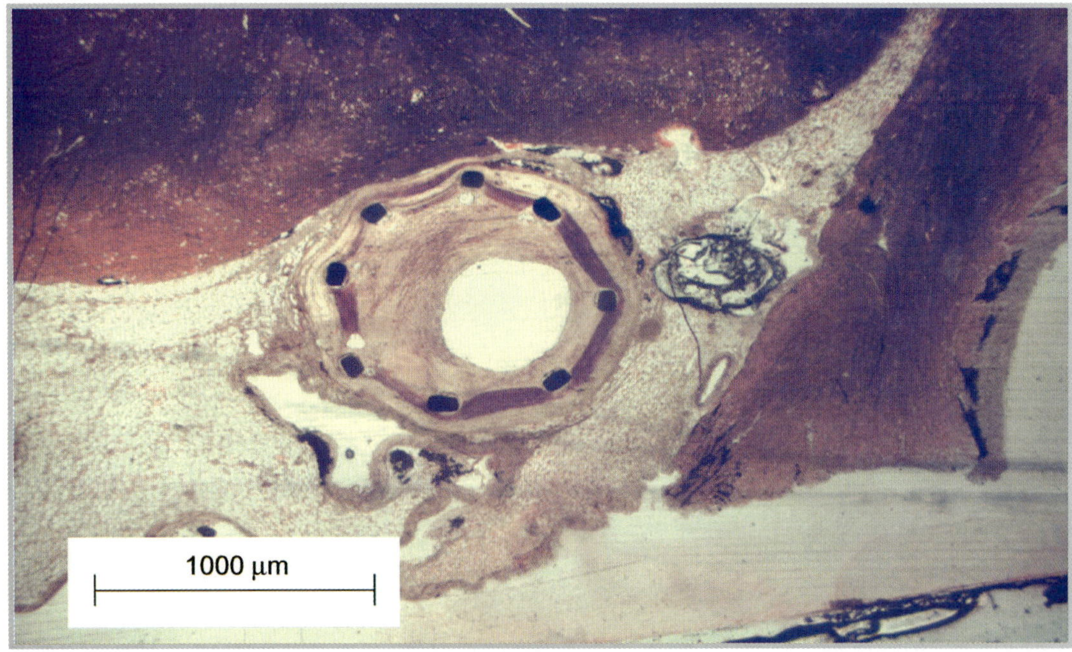

Figure 34F Vascular stent at 26 weeks. Resin H & E x 1
Cross-section of coronary artery with expanded stent 26 weeks post-deployment
Thick neointima along one wall of stent in comparison to the neointima on the opposite wall

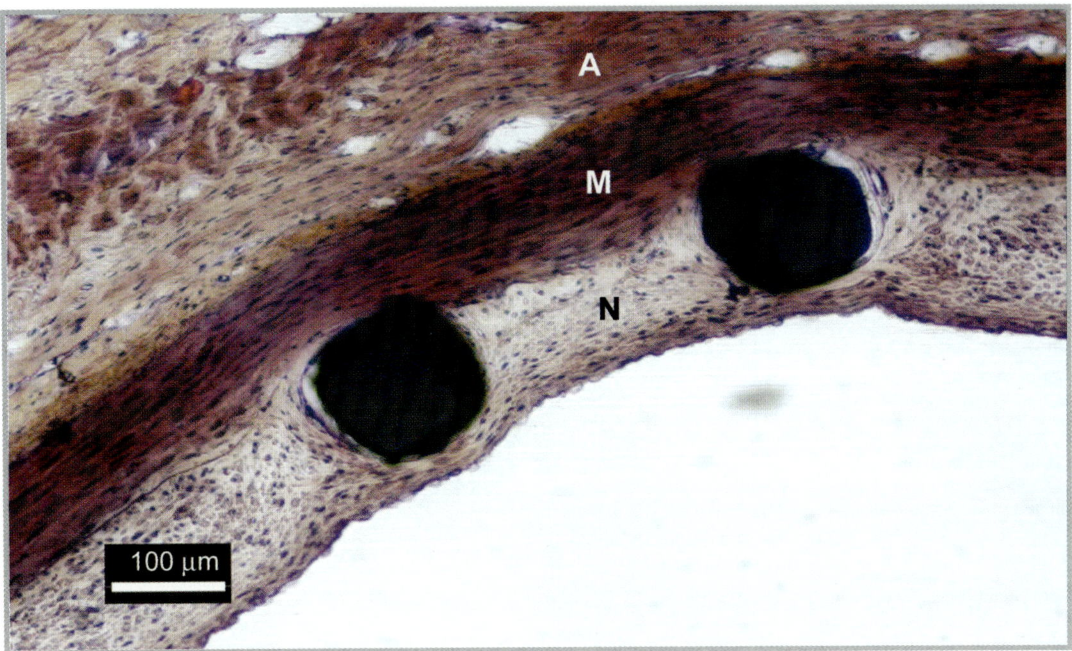

Figure 35A Vascular stent at 26 weeks. Resin H & E x 10
Cross-section of coronary artery with expanded stent 26 weeks post-deployment
Well-defined neointima (N), media (M) and adventitia (A)

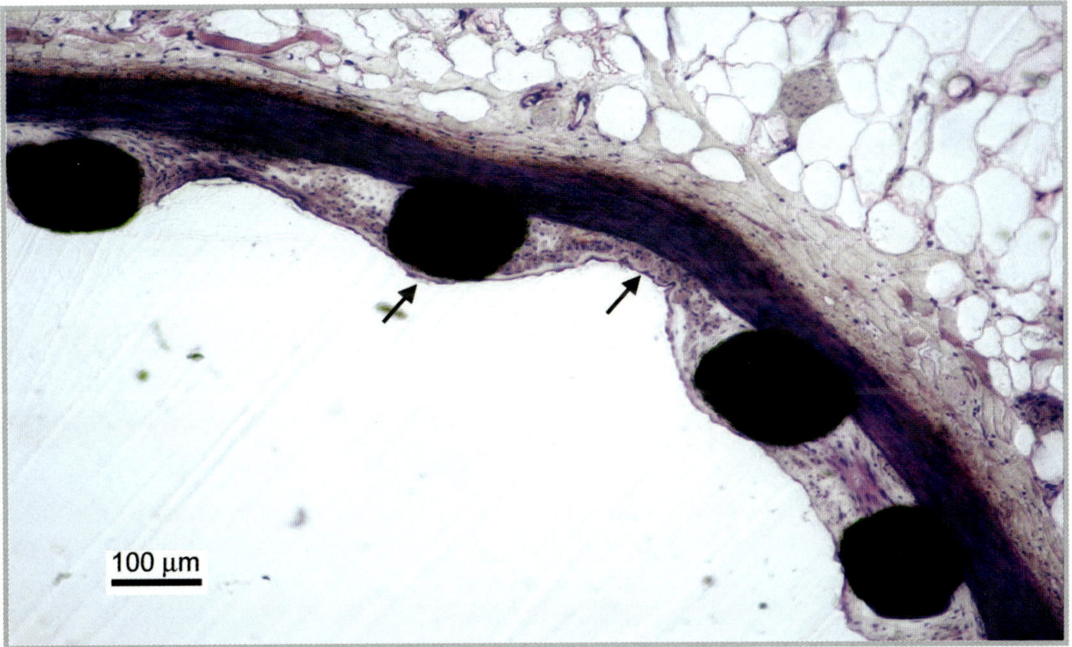

Figure 35B Vascular stent at 26 weeks. Resin H & E x 10
Cross-section of coronary artery with expanded stent 26 weeks post-deployment
Neointima is very thin over struts and interstrut areas

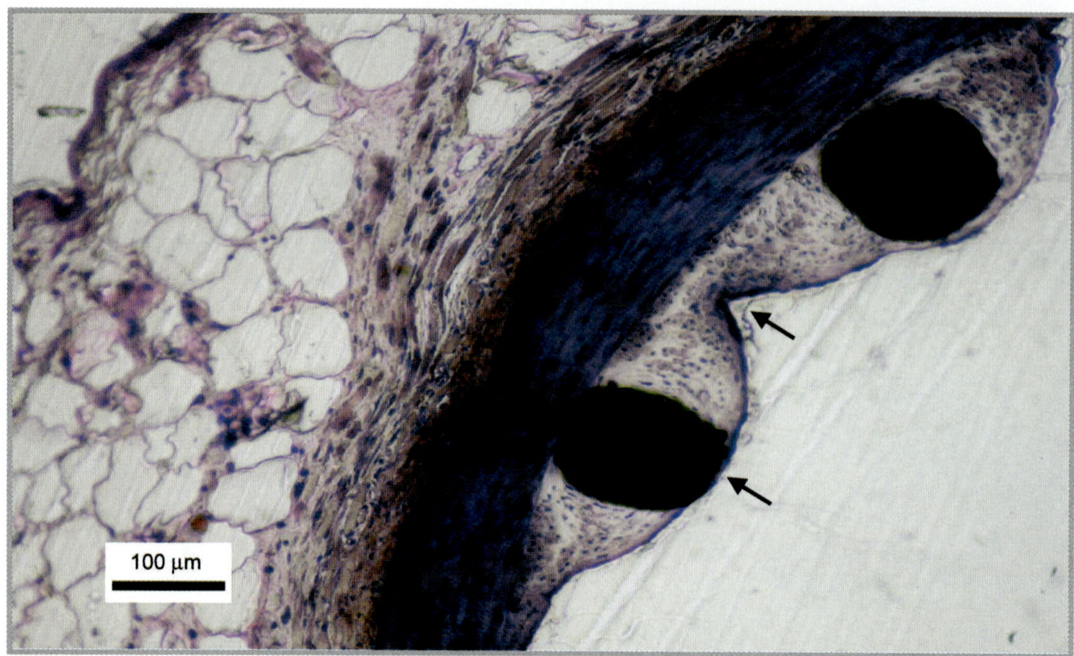

Figure 35C Vascular stent at 26 weeks. Resin H & E x 10
Cross-section of coronary artery with expanded stent 26 weeks post-deployment
Neointima (↑) is very thin over struts and interstrut areas

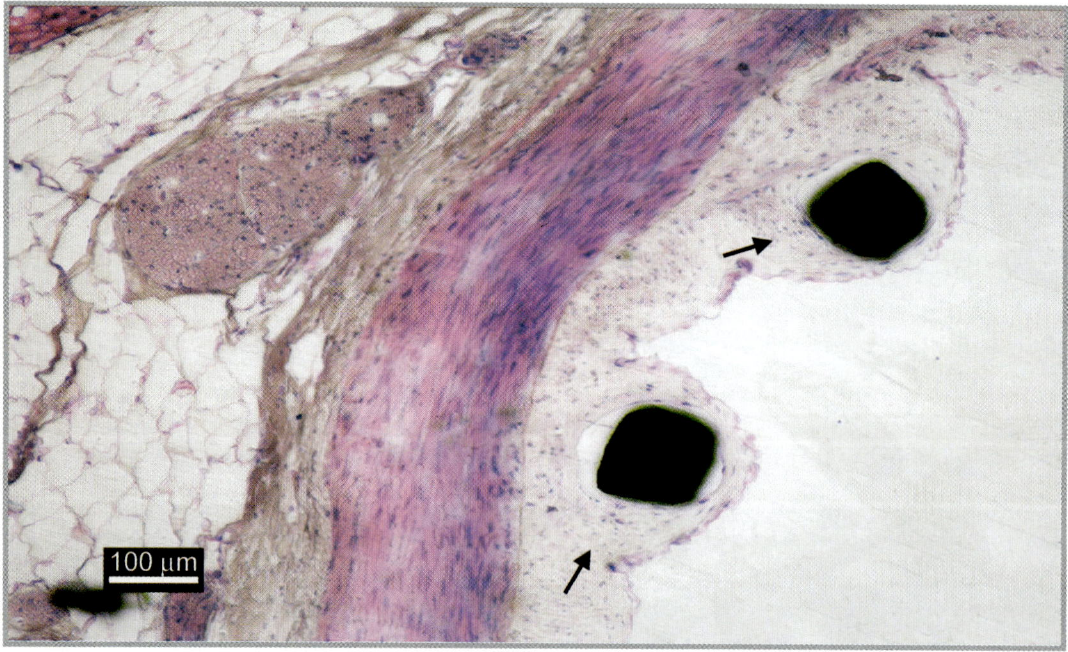

Figure 36A Vascular stent at 26 weeks. Resin H & E x 10
The morphological characteristics of the neointima (↑) depends upon the surface characteristics of the stent material, whether it is bare metal or coated with a degradable polymer impregnated with a drug

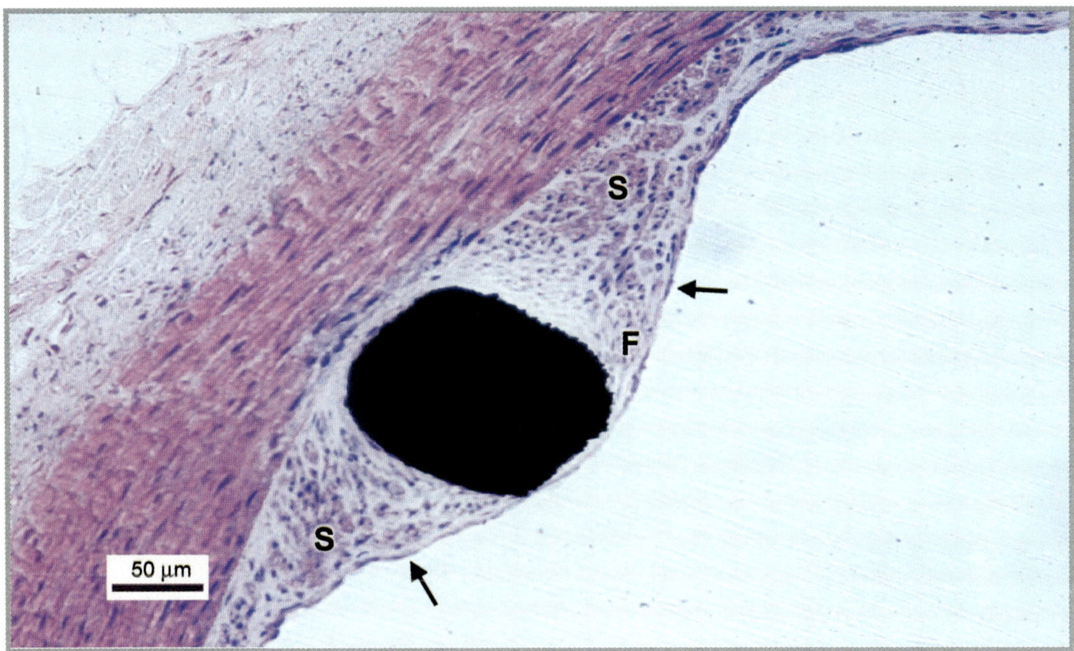

Figure 36B Vascular stent at 26 weeks. Resin H & E x 20
Cross-section of coronary artery with expanded stent 26 weeks post-deployment
Moderate smooth muscle cells (S) and fibrocytes (F) in the neointima with endothelial like cells (↑) at the luminal surface

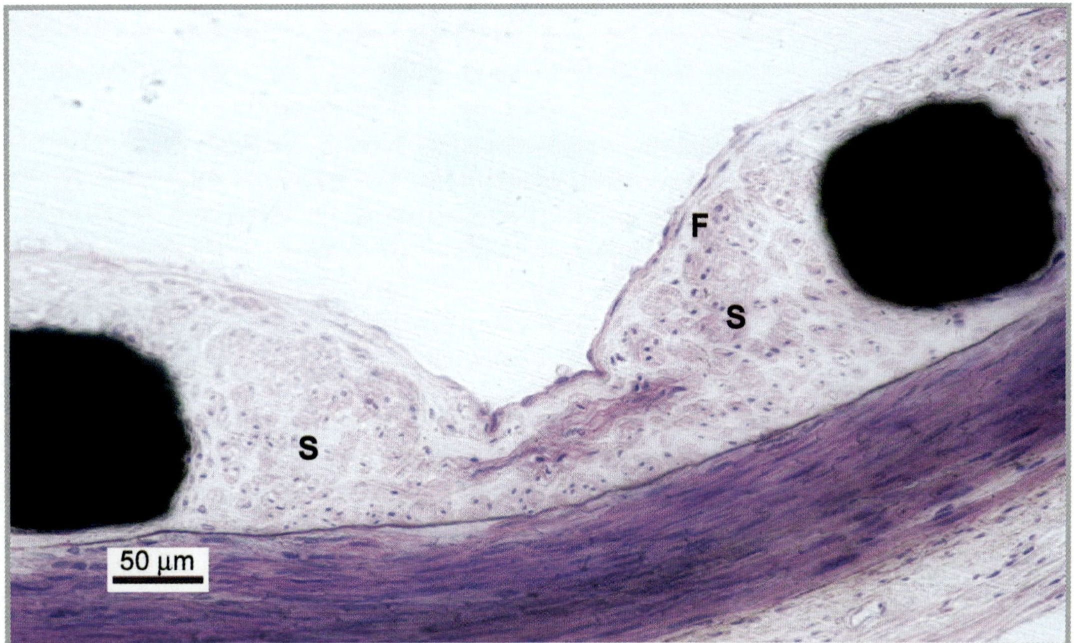

Figure 36C Vascular stent at 26 weeks. Resin H & E x 20
Cross-section of coronary artery with expanded stent 26 weeks post-deployment
Moderate smooth muscle cells (S) and fibrocytes (F) in the neointima

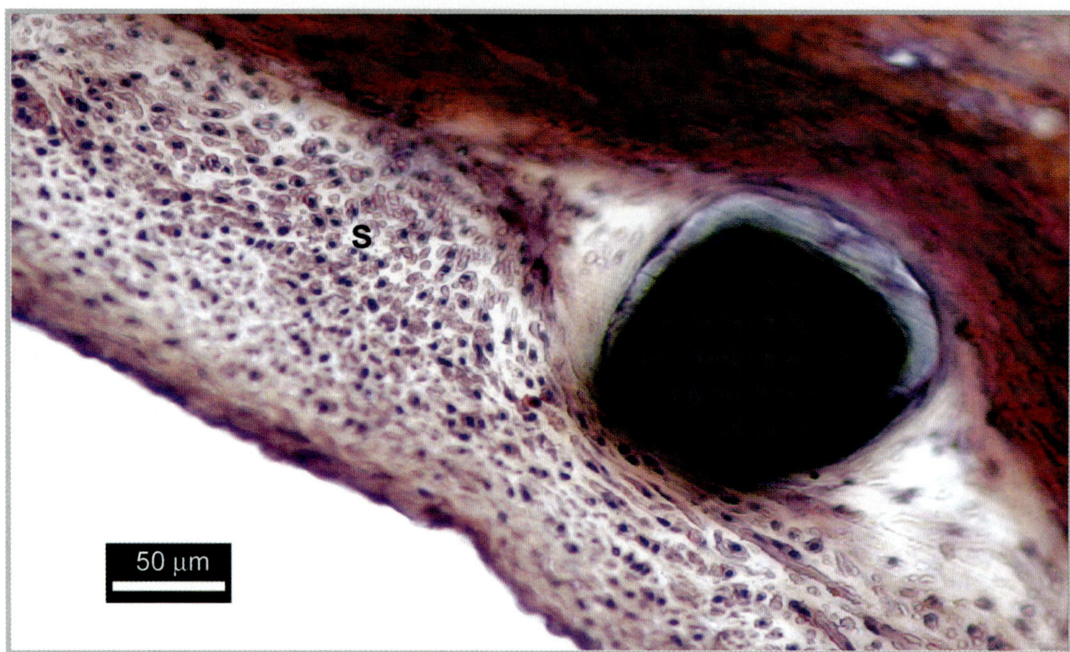

Figure 36D Vascular stent at 26 weeks. Resin H & E x 20
Cross-section of coronary artery with expanded stent 26 weeks postdeployment
Compact neointima with predominant smooth muscle cells (S)

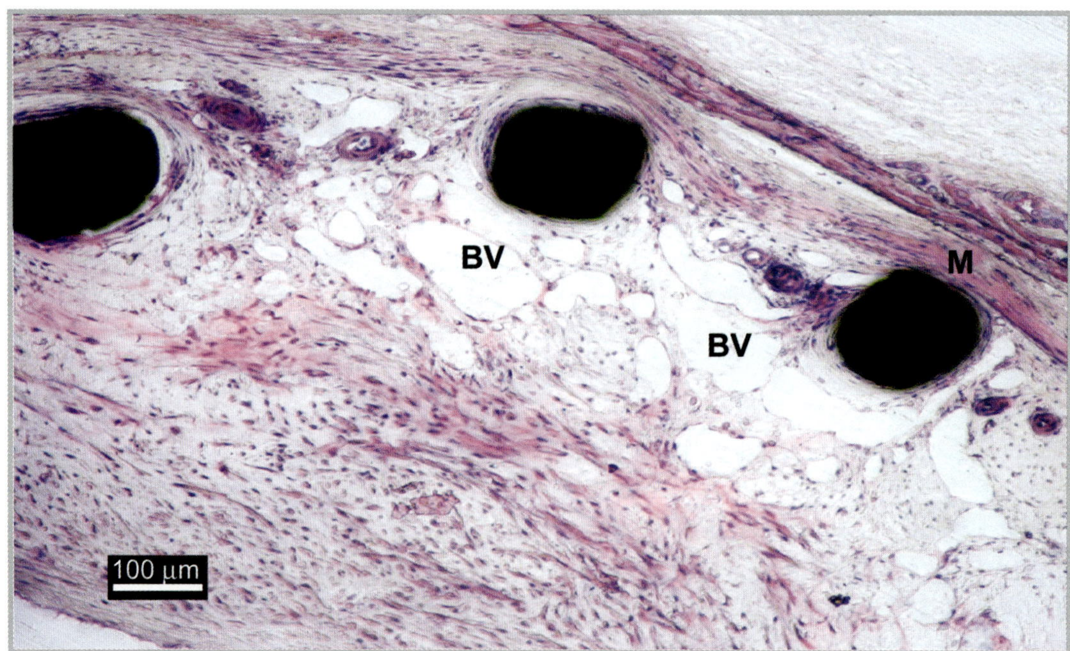

Figure 37A Vascular stent at 26 weeks. Resin H & E x 10
Cross-section of coronary artery with expanded stent 26 weeks post-deployment
Numerous thin walled blood vessels (BV) in the neointima

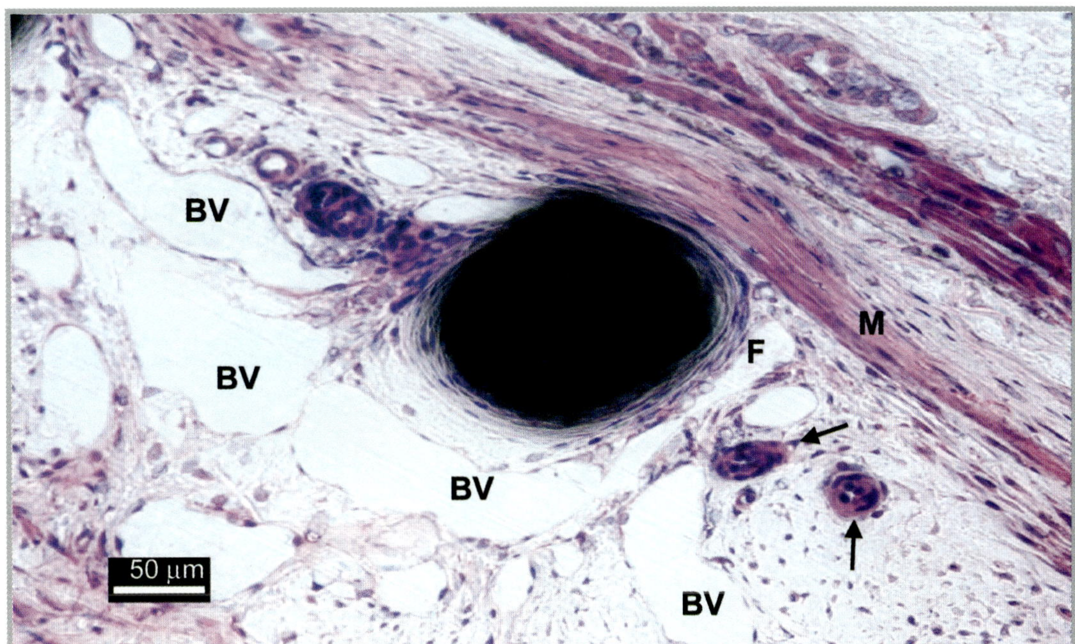

Figure 37B Vascular stent at 26 weeks. Resin H & E x 20
Higher magnification of blood vessels (BV) and arteriales (↑). Fibrocytes (F) and medial layer (M) are also seen

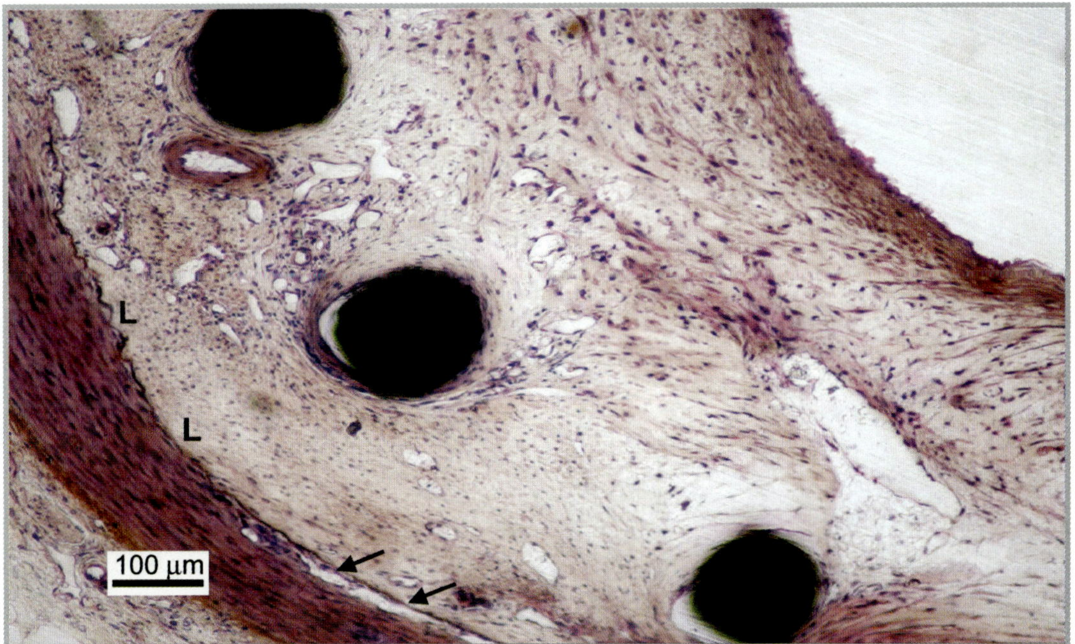

Figure 37C Vascular stent at 26 weeks. Resin H & E x 10
Cross-section of coronary artery with expanded stent 26 weeks post-deployment
Internal elastic lamina (L) stretched (↑) intermittently

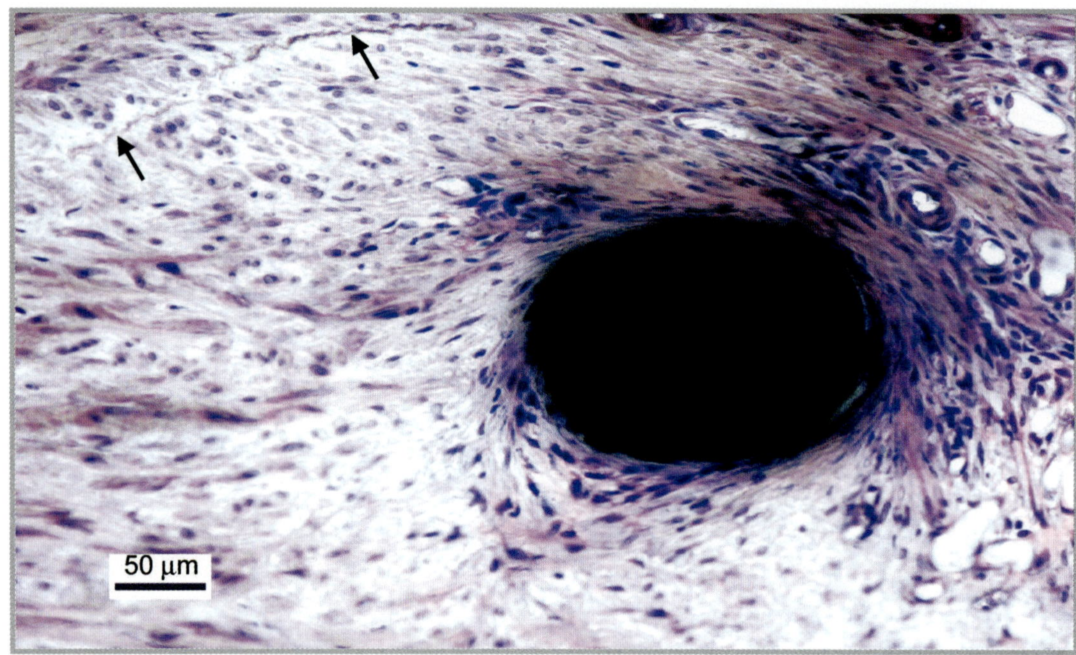

Figure 37D Vascular stent at 26 weeks. Resin H & E x 20
Cross-section of coronary artery with expanded stent 26 weeks post-deployment
Fragments of damaged elastic lamina (↑)

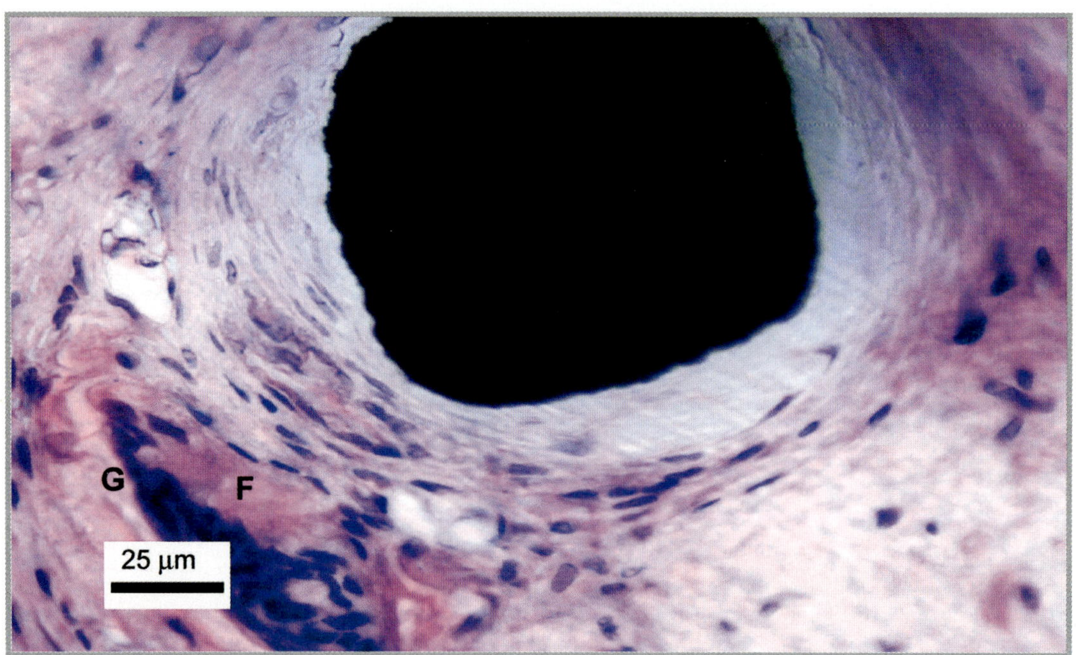

Figure 38 Vascular stent at 26 weeks. Resin H & E x 40
Fibrin (F) and foreign body giant cell (G) below stent strut

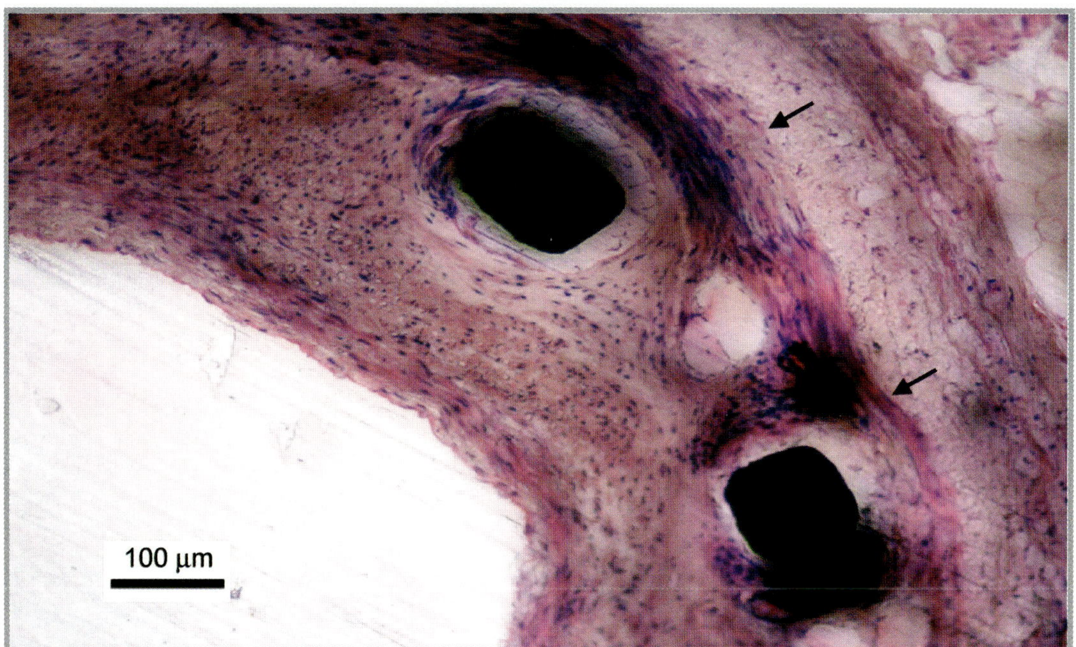

Figure 39A Vascular stent at 26 weeks. Resin H & E x 10
Severe compression of the media (↑) is seen

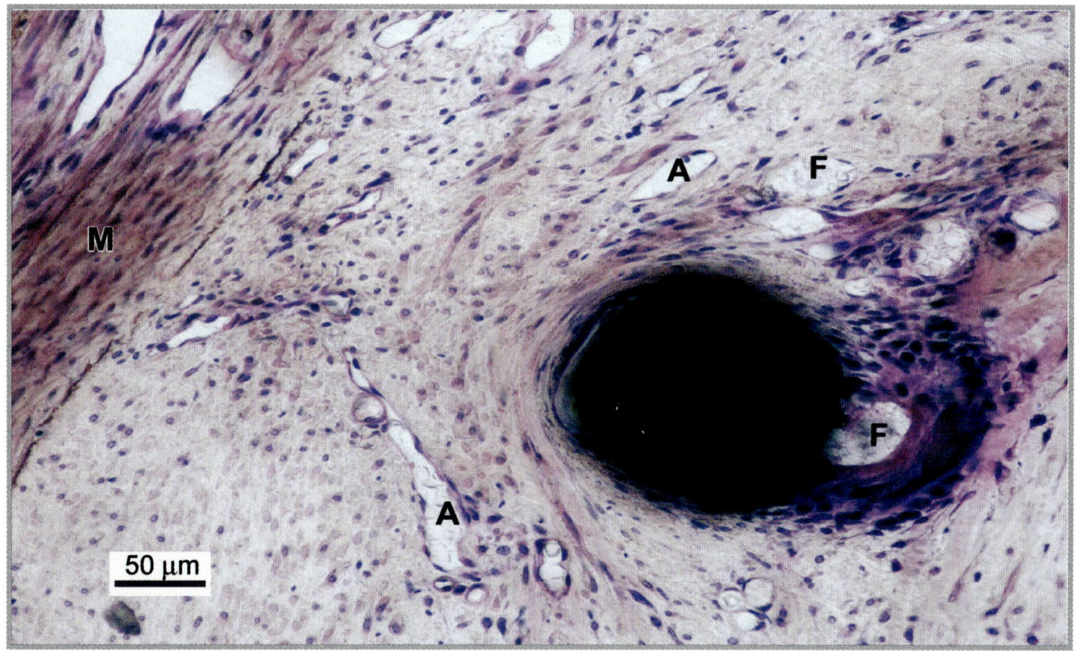

Figure 39B Vascular stent at 26 weeks. Resin H & E x 20
Intact media. Foamy areas (F), smooth muscle cells and fibrocytes are present
Angiogenesis (A) is also seen

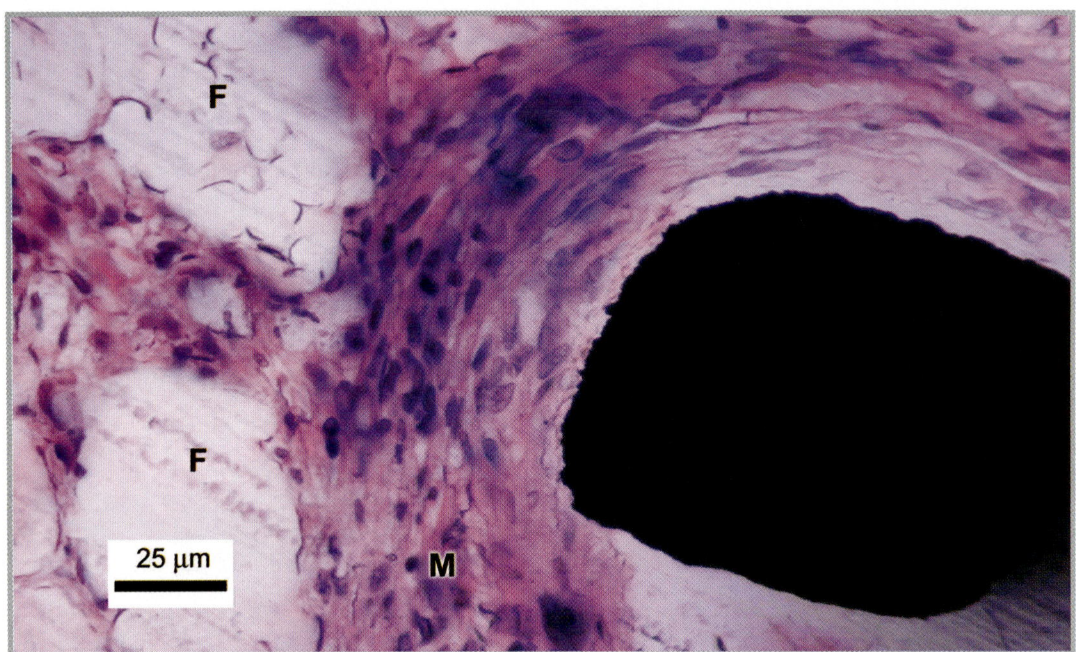

Figure 39C Vascular stent at 26 weeks. Resin H & E x 40
Foamy areas (F) are seen occasionally at the strut interface

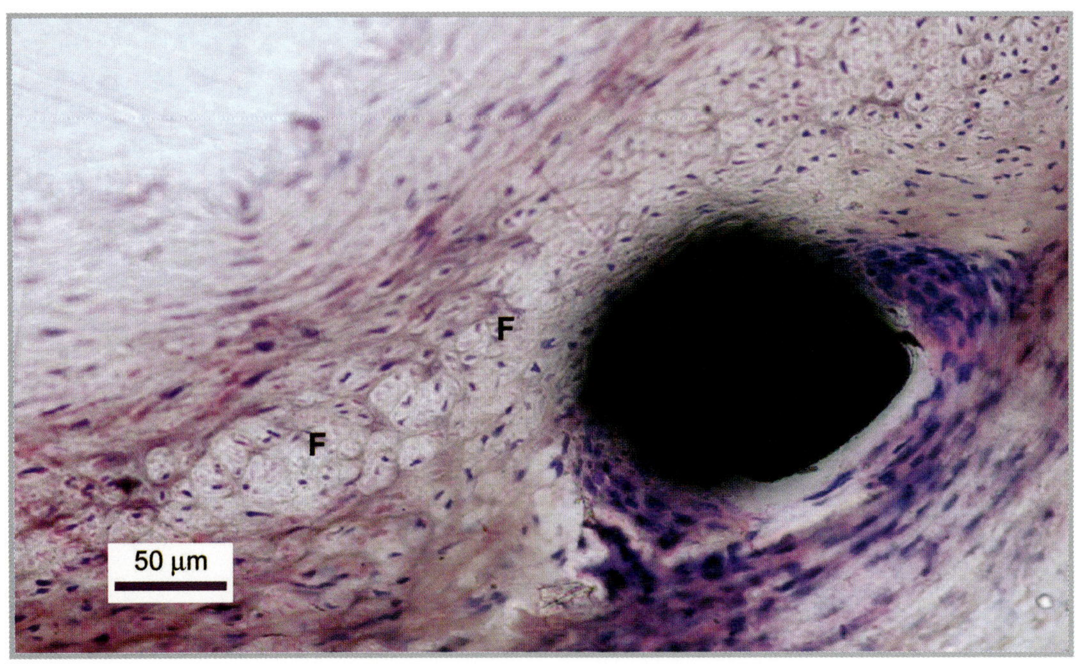

Figure 39D Vascular stent at 26 weeks. Resin H & E x 20
Foamy area (F)

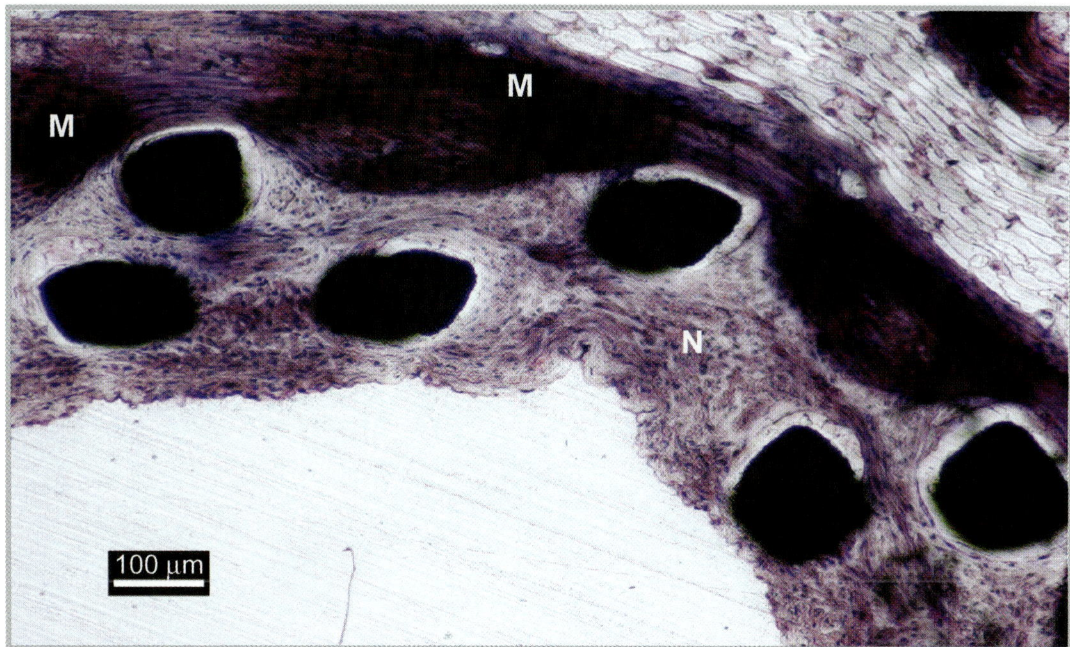

Figure 40A Vascular stent at 26 weeks. Resin H & E x 10
Cross-section of coronary artery with expanded overlapping stents
Media (M) is intact and compressed. Neointima (N) seen

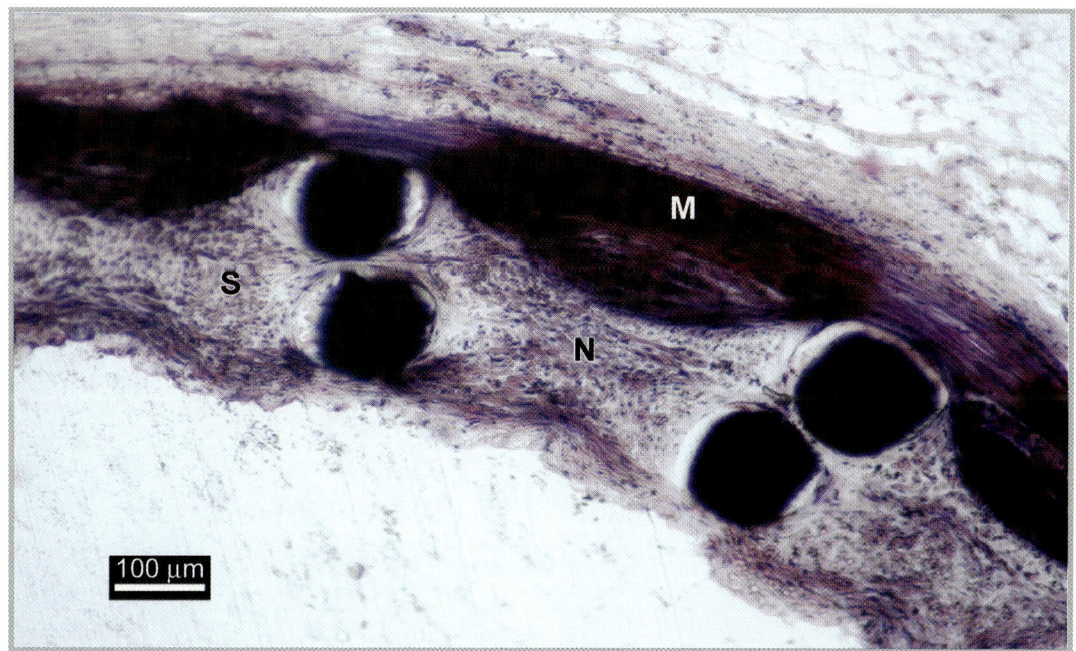

Figure 40B Vascular stent at 26 weeks. Resin H & E x 10
Cross-section of coronary artery with expanded overlapping stents
Moderately thick neointima (N) with smooth muscle cell (S) proliferation and compressed media (M) is present

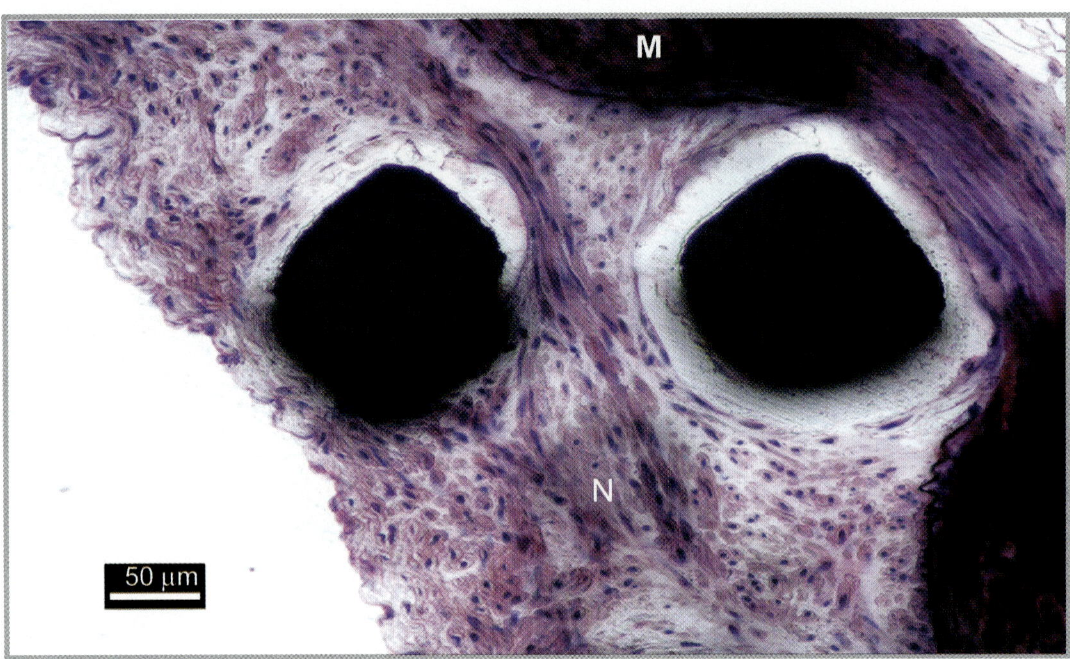

Figure 40C Vascular stent at 26 weeks. Resin H & E x 20
Higher magnification of neointima (N) and media (M)

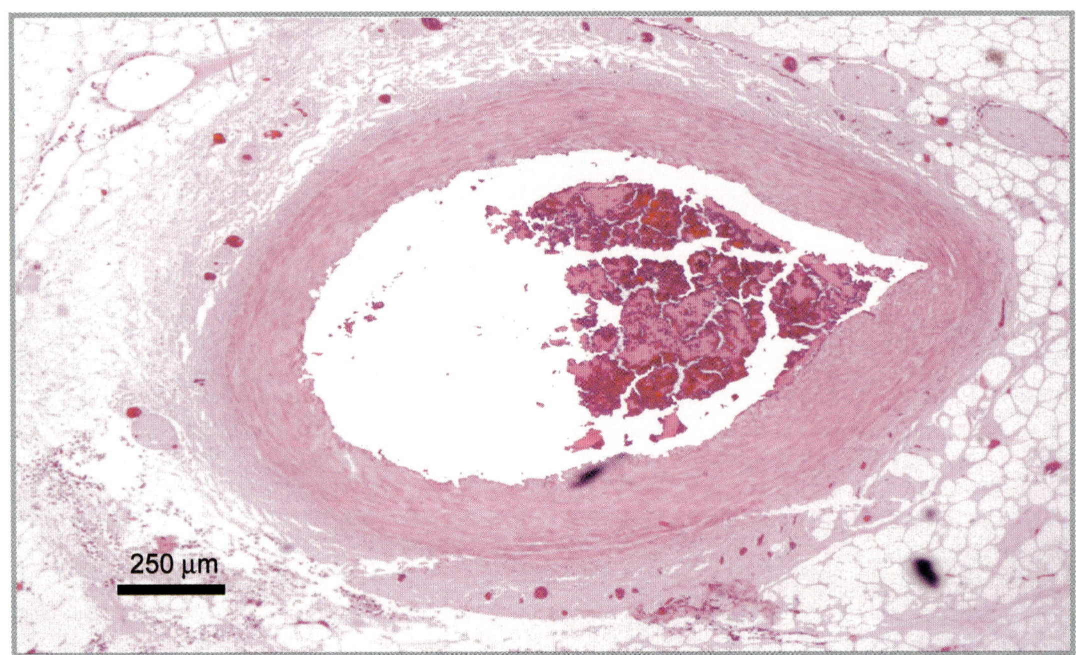

Figure 41A Vascular stent. Paraffin H & E x 4
Fresh thrombus in lumen of non-stented segment of blood vessel

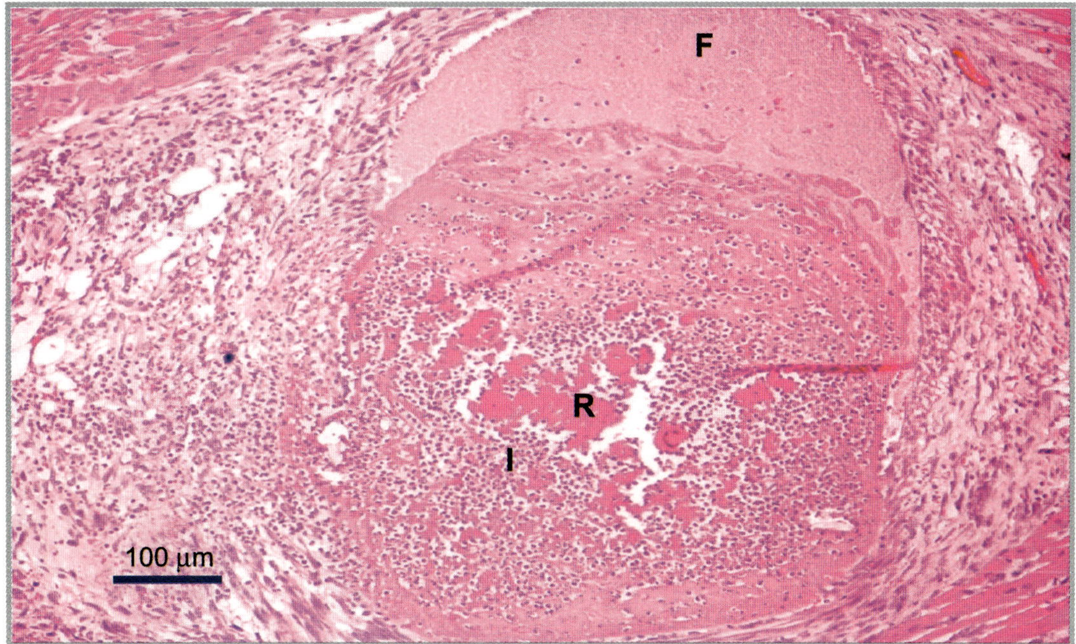

Figure 41B Vascular stent. Paraffin H & E x 10
Thrombus composed of fibrin (F) identified as homogenous pink material, red cells (R) and inflammatory cells (I) in non-stented segment of blood vessel

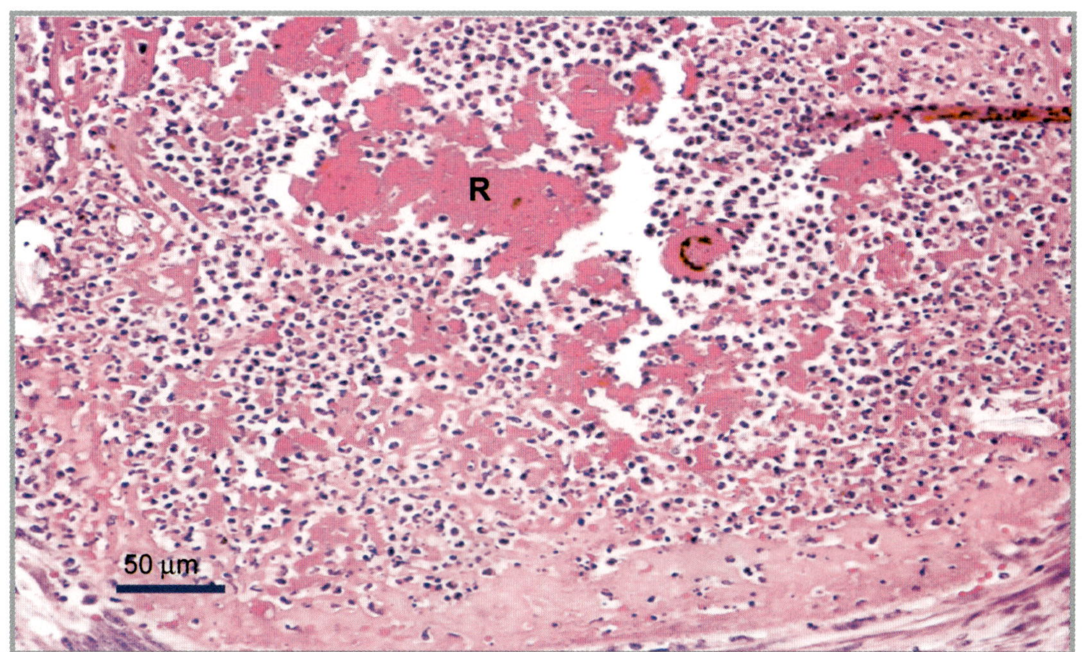

Figure 41C Vascular stent. Paraffin H & E x 20
Higher magnification of thrombus with red cells (R) and inflammatory cells

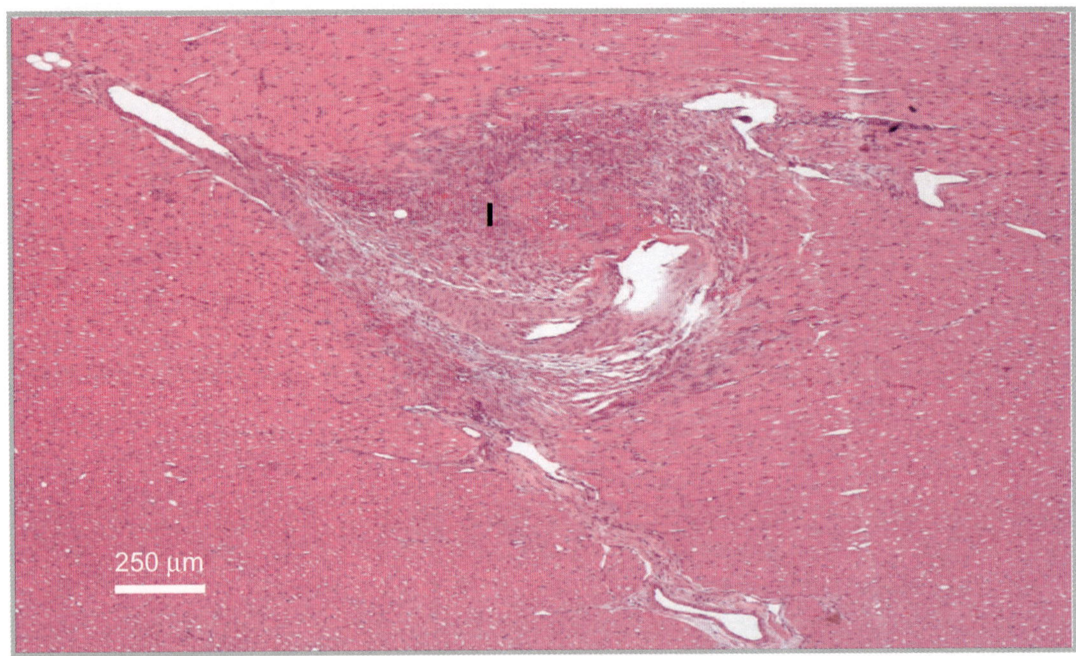

Figure 42 Vascular stent. Paraffin H & E x 4
Supply area of myocardium. Infarct (I) due to thrombus in the stented vessel

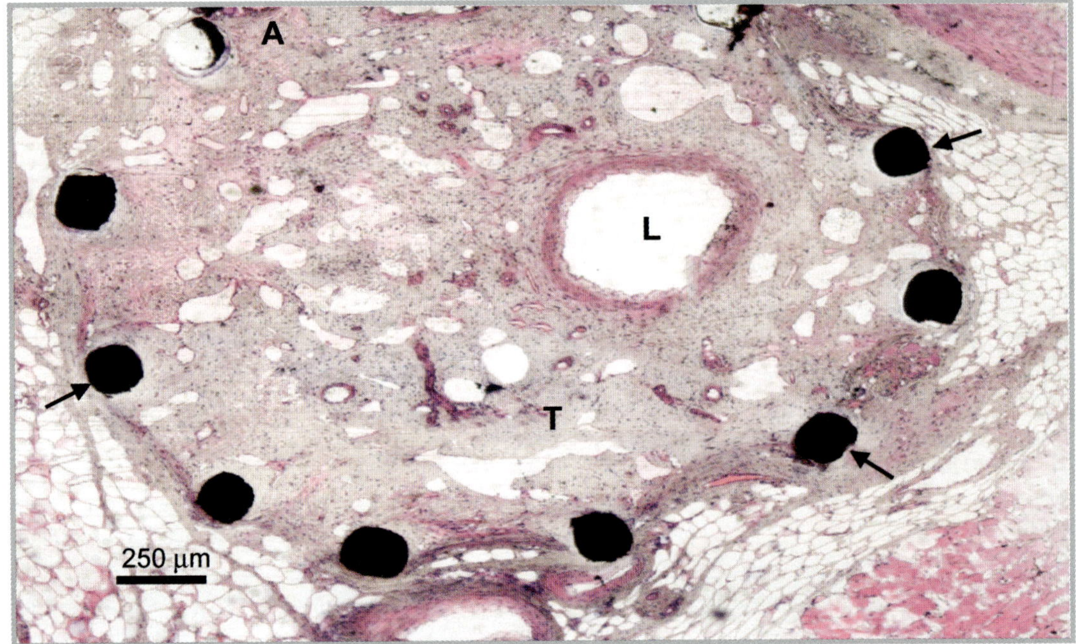

Figure 43A Vascular stent. Resin H & E x 4
Cross-section of coronary artery with over expanded stent
The stent has expanded into adventitia (A) with complete injury (↑) to the media. Organized thrombus (T) with small lumen (L) is seen

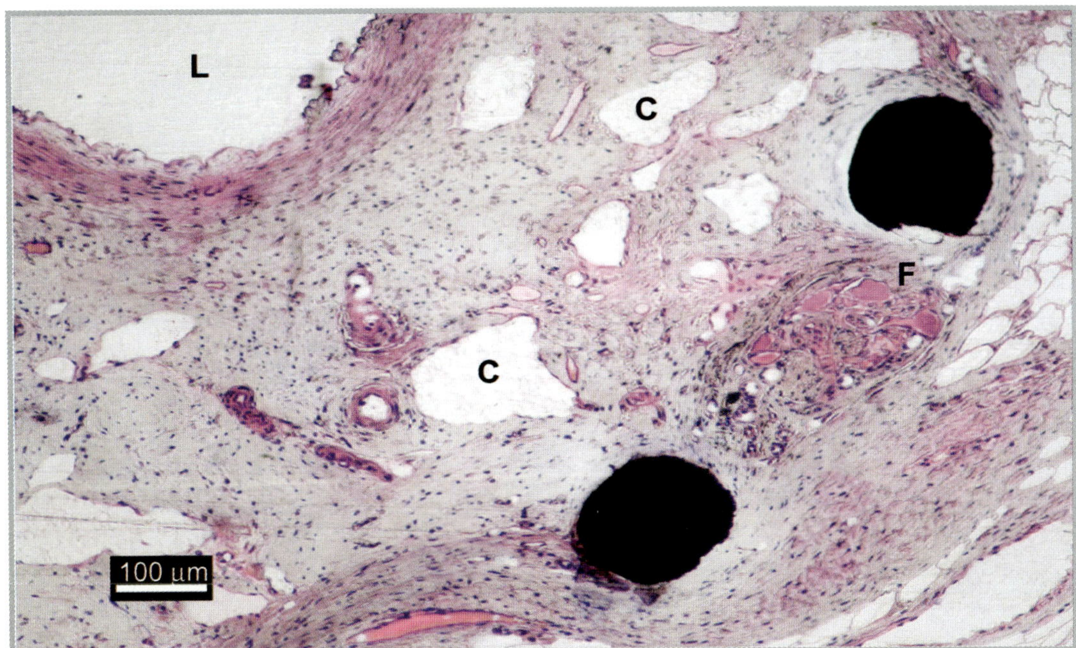

Figure 43B Vascular stent. Resin H & E x 10
Cross-section of coronary artery with over expanded stent.
The thrombus is organized with granulation tissue and collagen deposition. Newly formed blood vessels (C), fibroblasts and fibrocytes and fibrin (F) are present

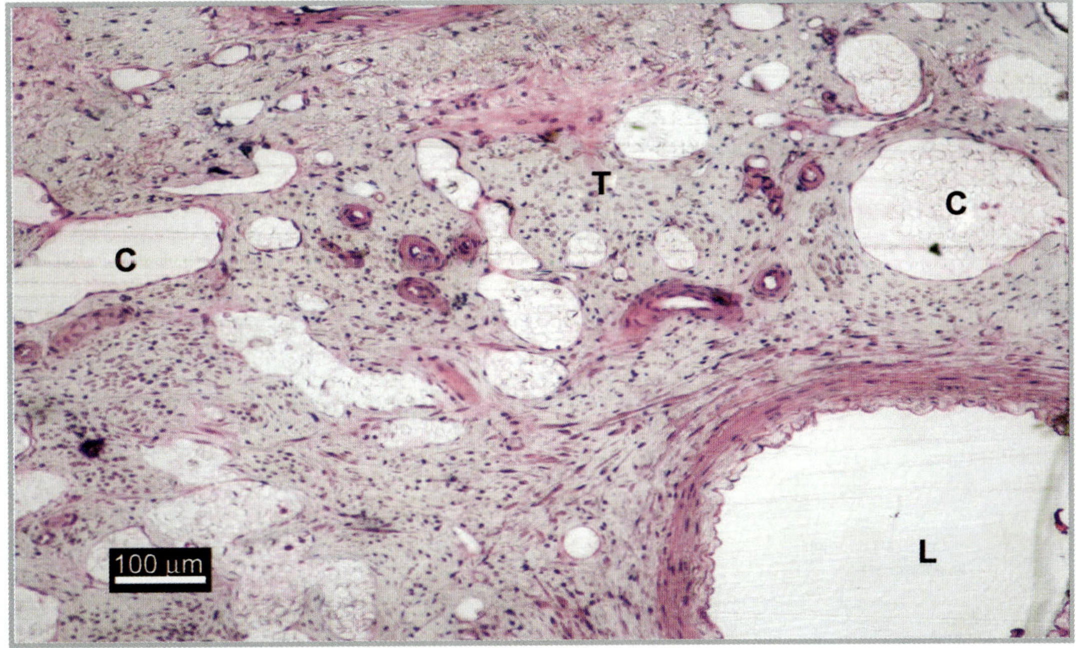

Figure 43C Vascular stent. Resin H & E x 10
Cross-section of coronary artery with over expanded stent
The thrombus (T) is recanalized with a lumen (L) and newly formed blood vessels (C)

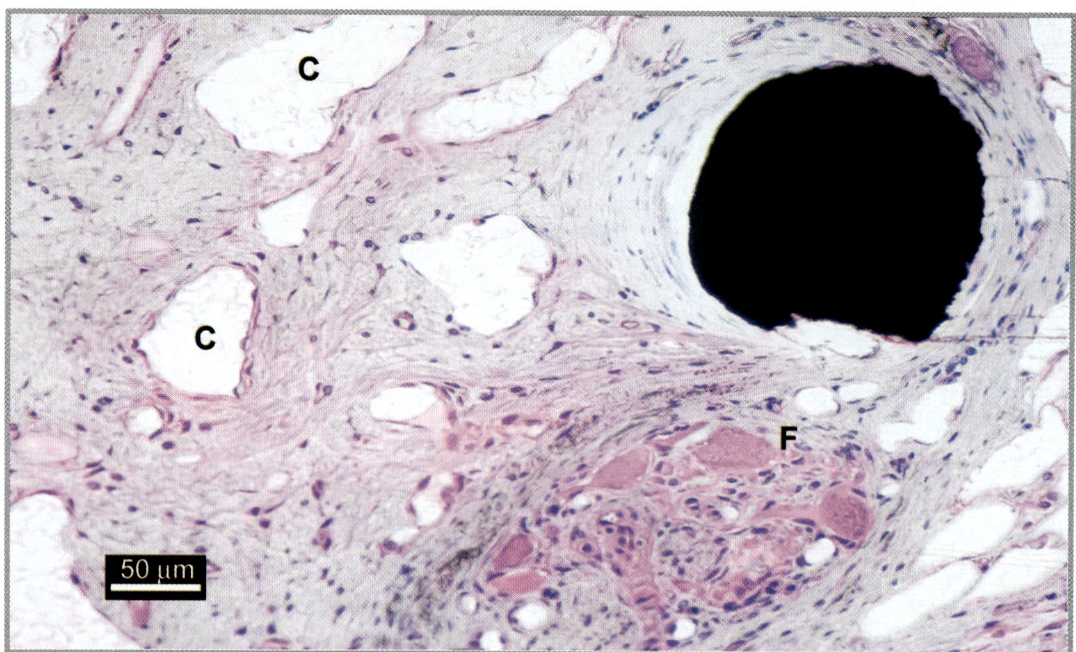

Figure 43D Vascular stent. Resin H & E x 20
Cross-section of coronary artery with over expanded stent and thrombus
Fibrin (F) deposits persist. Newly formed blood vessels (C) seen

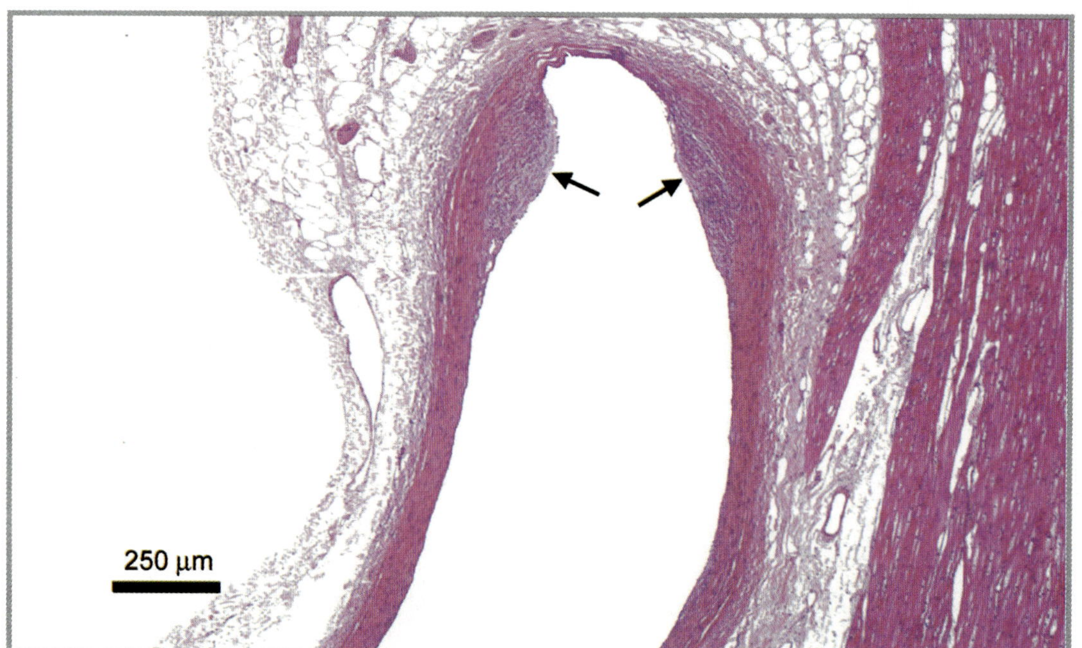

Figure 44 Vascular stent. Paraffin H & E x 4
Focal proliferation of cells (↑) in the intimal layer of vessel distal to stent in coronary artery

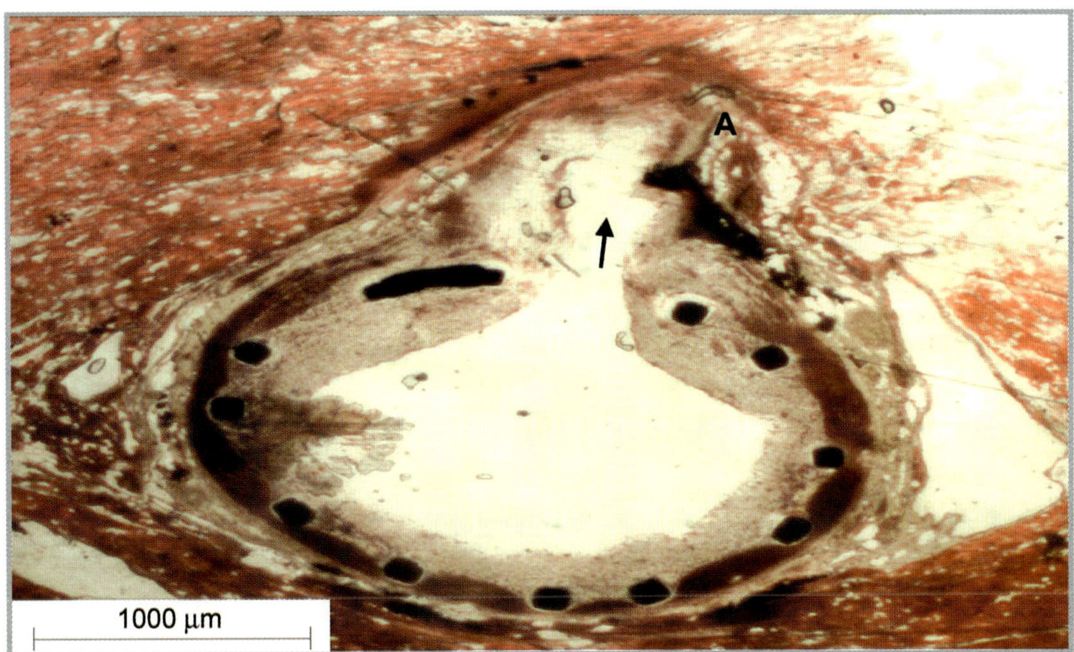

Figure 45 Vascular stent. Resin H & E x 1
Cross-section through stented vessel at lateral branch point (↑). Adventitia (A) is seen

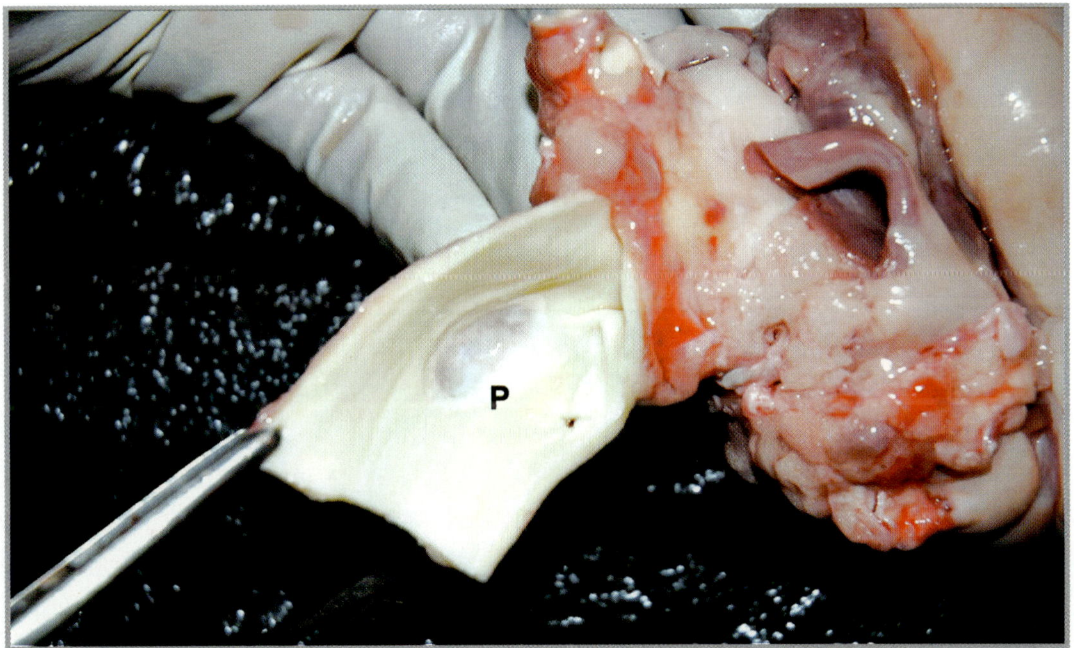

Figure 46A Biological prosthesis. Gross image
Decellularized pericardial tissue implanted as a circular patch (P) in defect created in wall of large blood vessel, the aorta

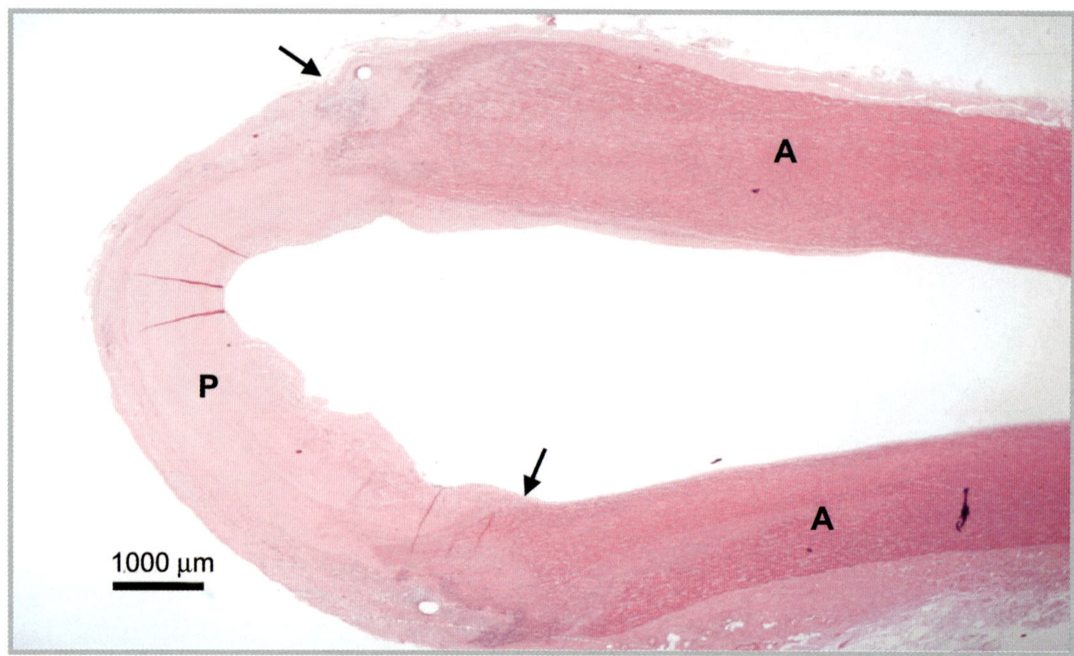

Figure 46B Biological prosthesis. H & E x 1
Cross-section of the vessel wall with the patch (P) sutured (↑) in between host aortic wall tissue (A) on both sides

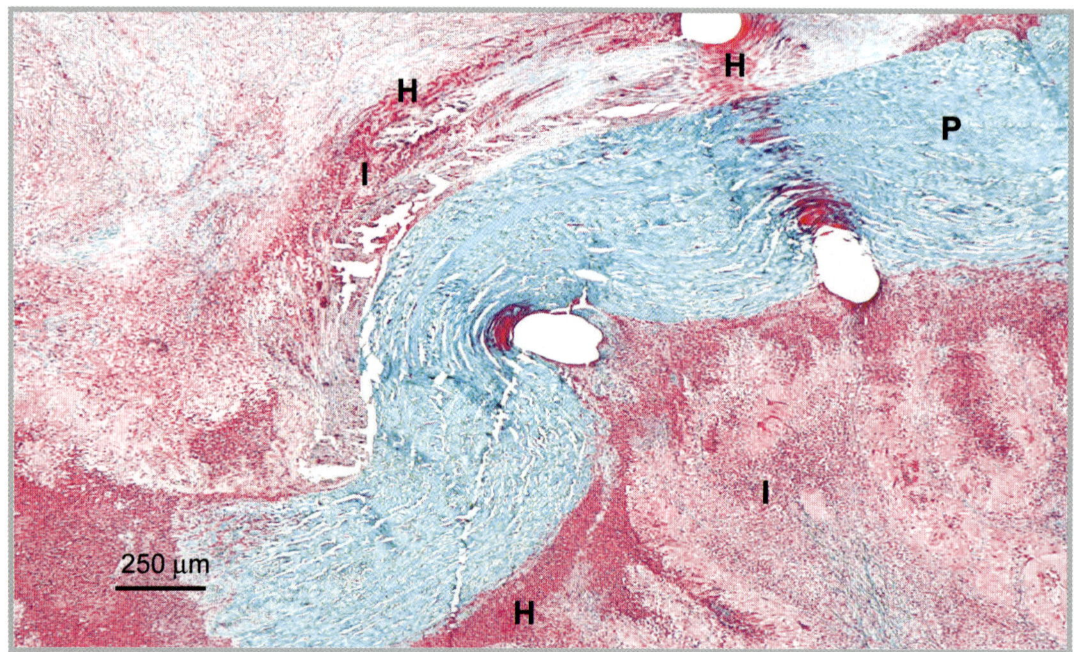

Figure 46C Biological prosthesis. Masson's trichrome x 4
Cross-section of the vessel wall with the patch (P). Suture spaces with adjacent inflammation (I) and hemorrhage (H) at the interface

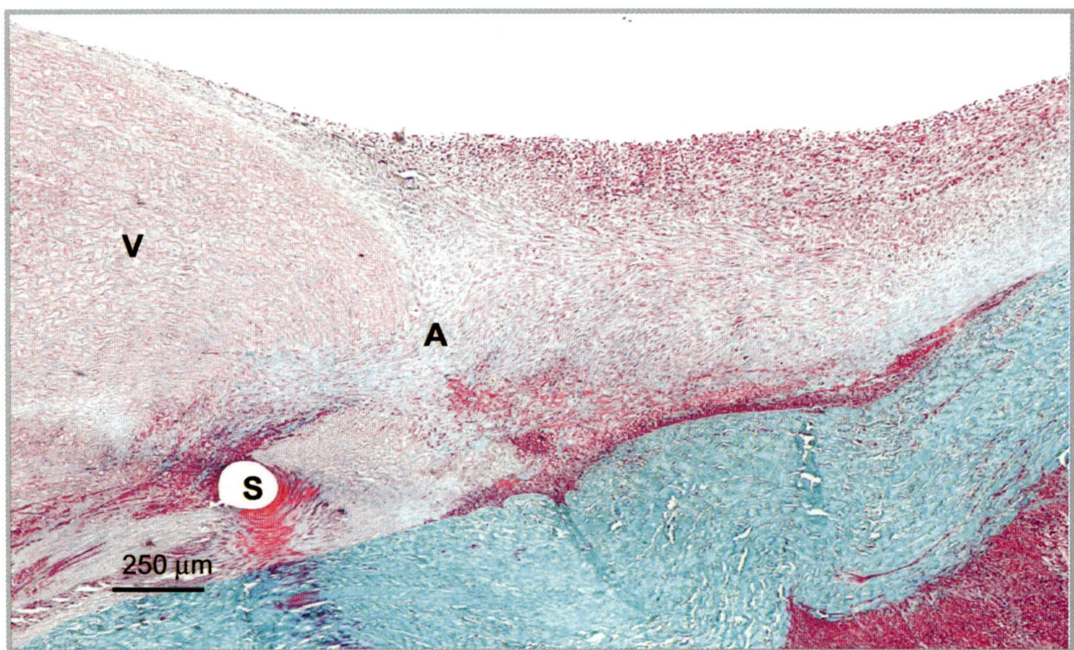

Figure 47 Biological prosthesis. Masson's trichrome x 4
Decellularized pericardial tissue implanted as a circular patch in defect created in wall of large blood vessel, the aorta. Cross-section of the site of anastomosis (A) to vessel wall (V) with suture sites (S)

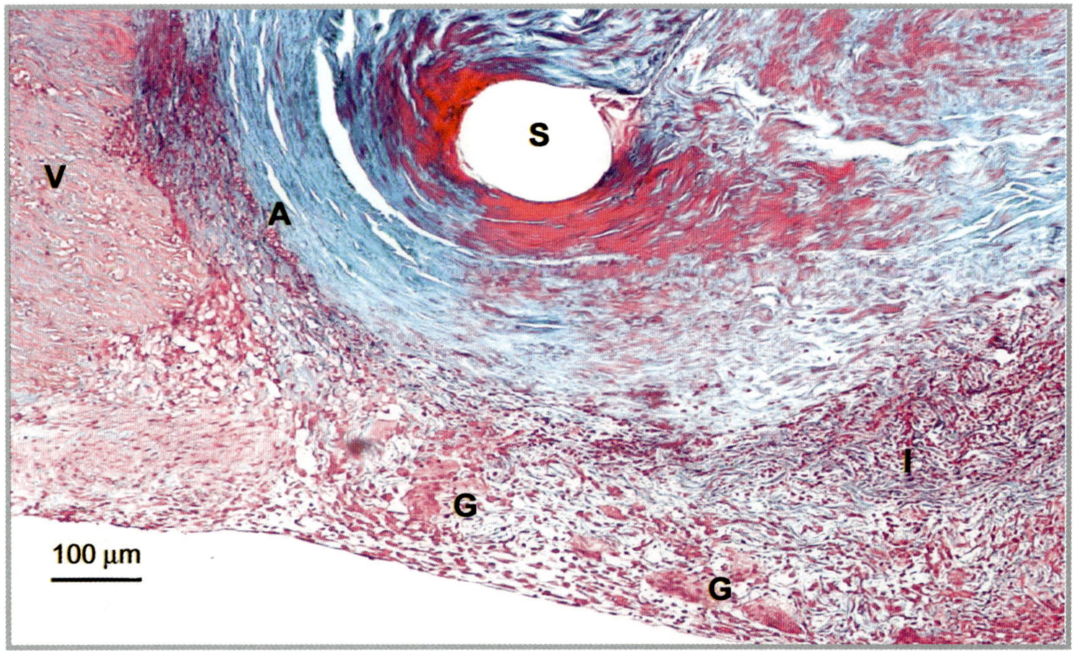

Figure 48 Biological prosthesis. Masson's trichrome x 10
Decellularized pericardial tissue implanted as a circular patch in defect created in wall of large blood vessel, the aorta. Early inflammation (I) with numerous foreign body type of giant cells (G) at the anastomosis (A)

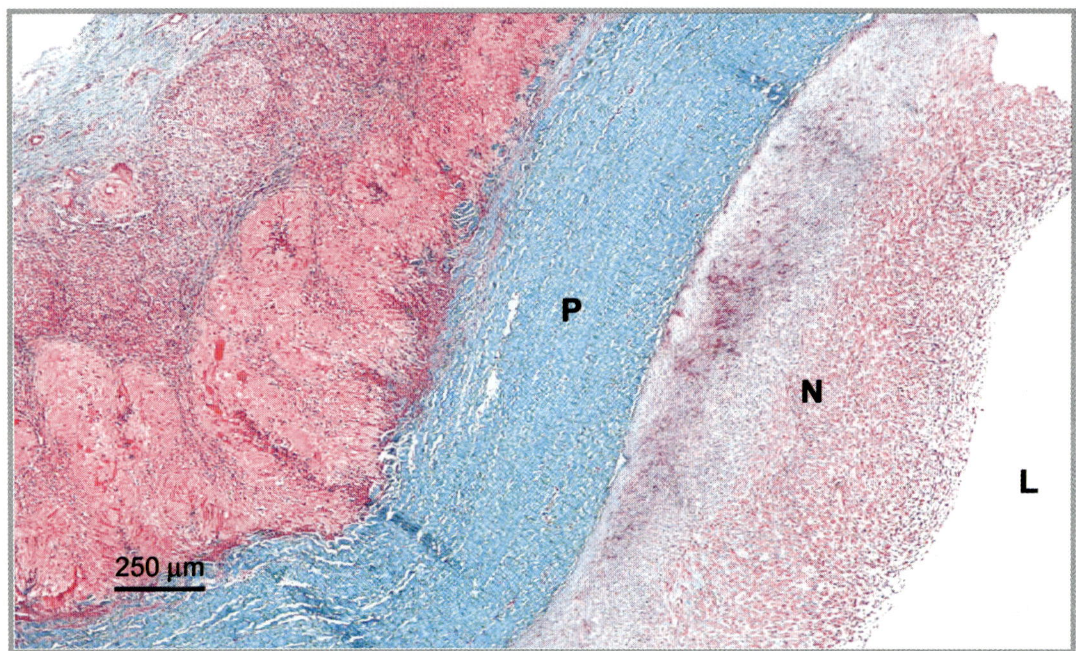

Figure 49A Biological prosthesis. Masson's trichrome x 4
Decellularized pericardial tissue implanted as a circular patch in defect created in wall of large blood vessel, the aorta
Neointima (N) formation on the luminal (inner) surface (L) of the patch (P)

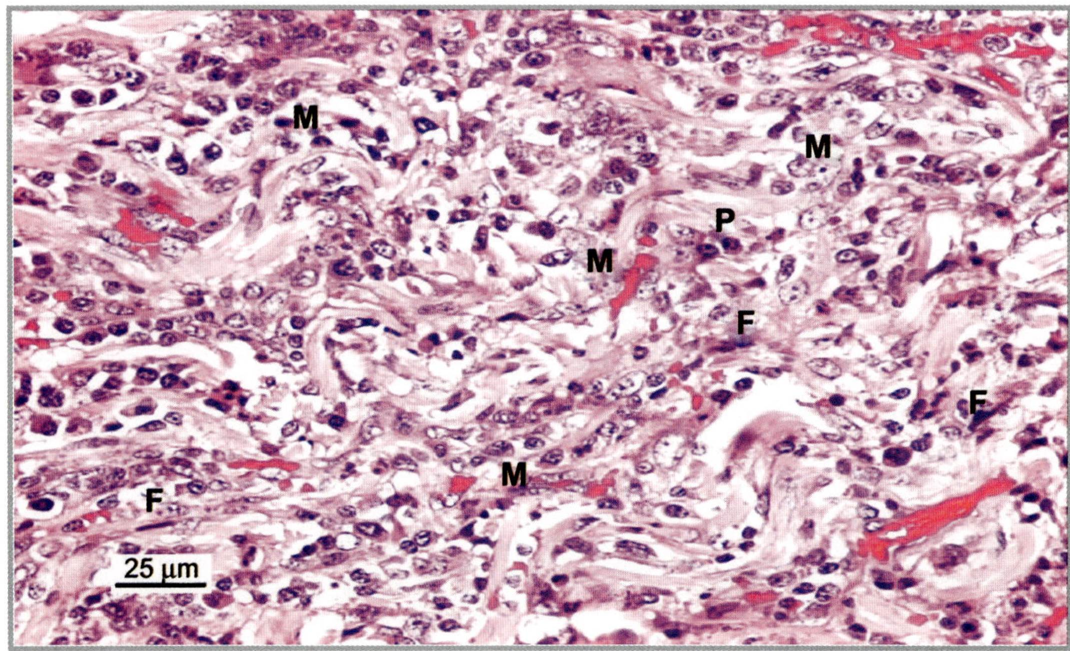

Figure 49B Biological prosthesis. H & E x 40
Early inflammation with macrophages (M), few plasma cells (P) and fibrocytes (F) in the neointima

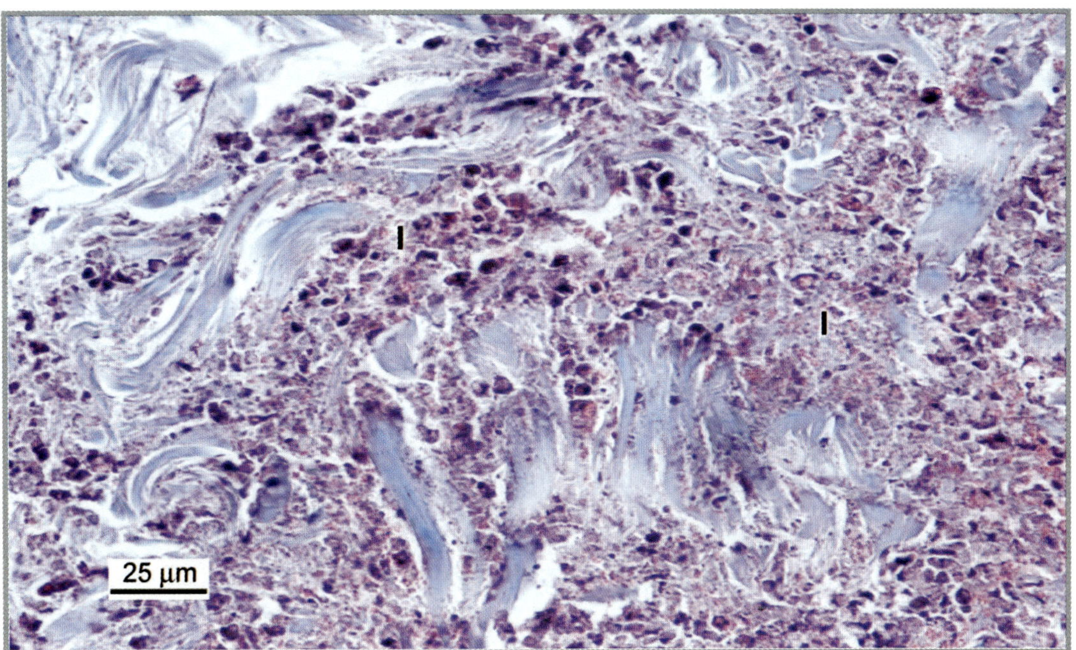

Figure 50 Biological prosthesis. Masson's trichrome x 40
Severe inflammation (I) seen in between the decellularized tissue fibers which stain blue

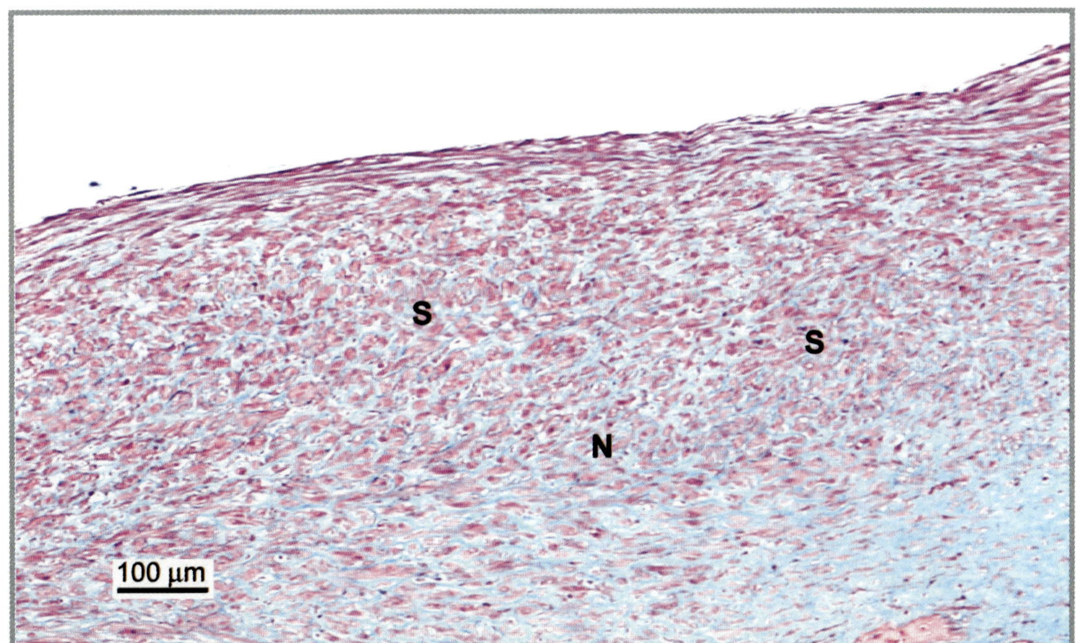

Figure 51 Biological prosthesis. Masson's trichrome x 10
Decellularized pericardial tissue implanted as a circular patch in defect created in wall of large blood vessel, the aorta. Healing with smooth muscle cell (S) proliferation in neointima (N)

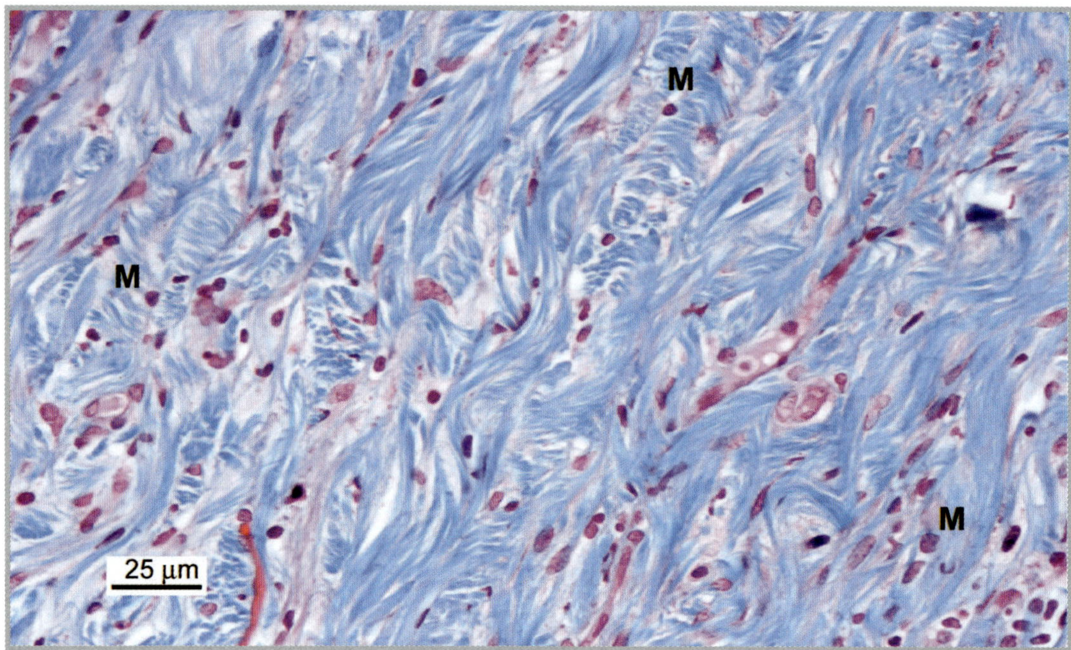

Figure 52 Biological prosthesis. Masson's trichrome x 40
Decellularized pericardial tissue implanted as a circular patch in defect created in wall of large blood vessel, the aorta. Reduction of macrophage (M) infiltration with healing

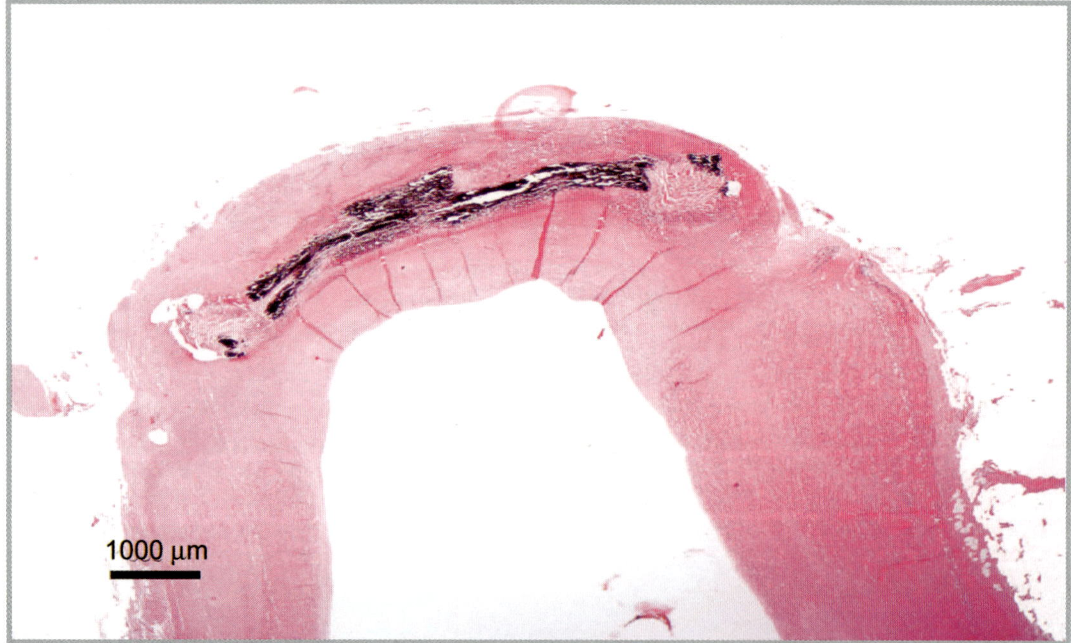

Figure 53A Biological prosthesis. Von Kossa x 1
Areas of late calcification (stained black) in the midgraft of implanted decellularized pericardial tissue

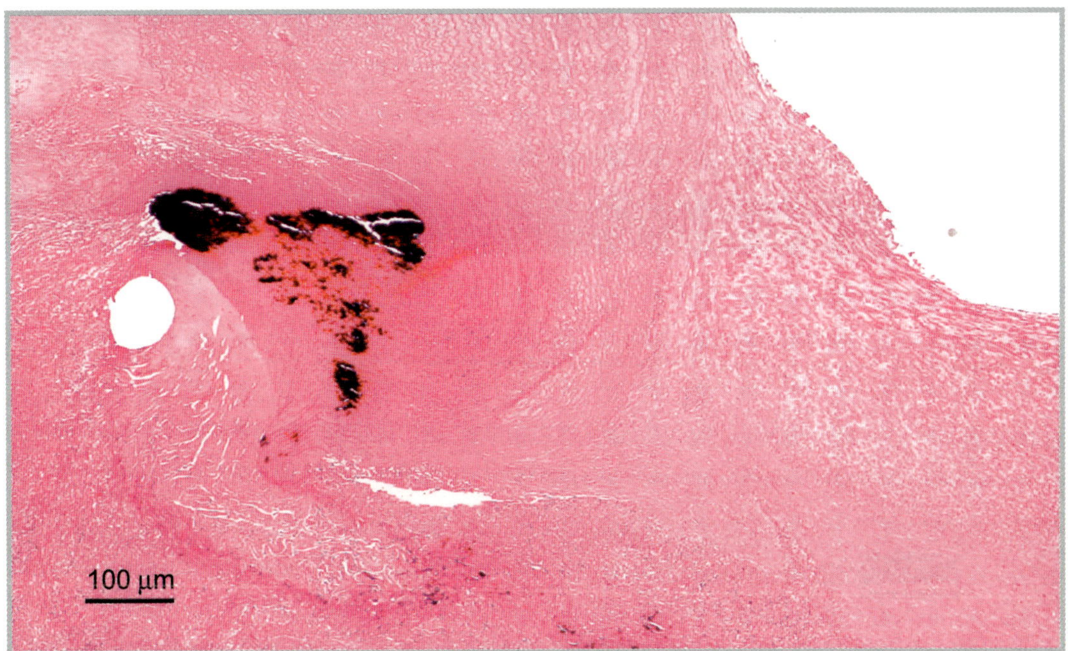

Figure 53B Biological prosthesis. Von Kossa x 10
Areas of late calcification (stained black) at the anastomosis site of the implanted decellularized pericardial tissue

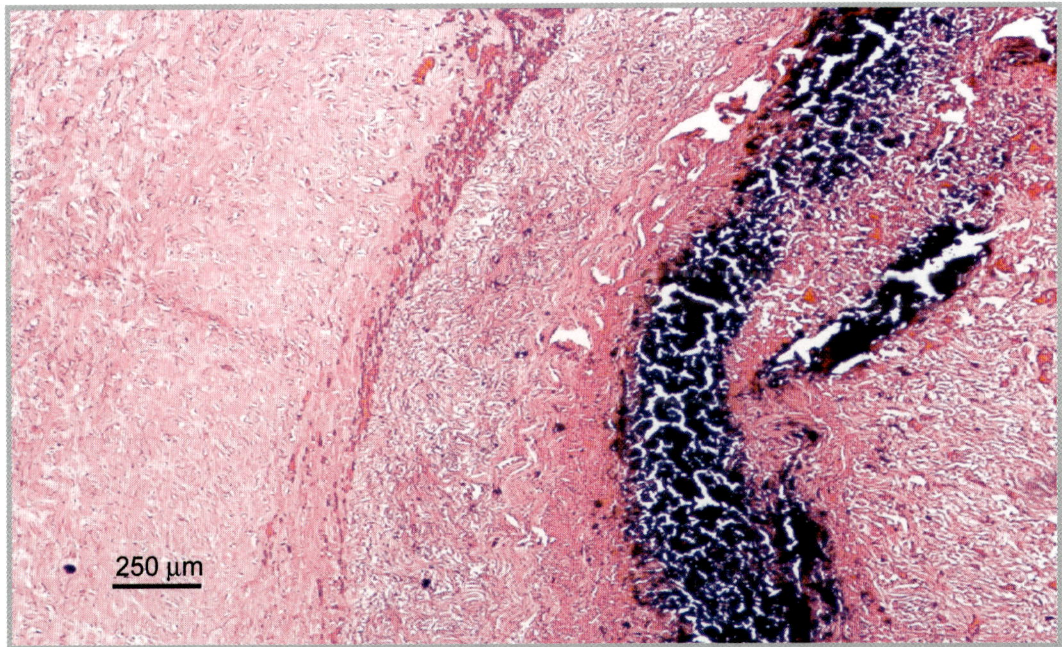

Figure 53C Biological prosthesis. Von Kossa x 4
Heavy late calcification (stained black) in the implanted decellularized pericardial tissue

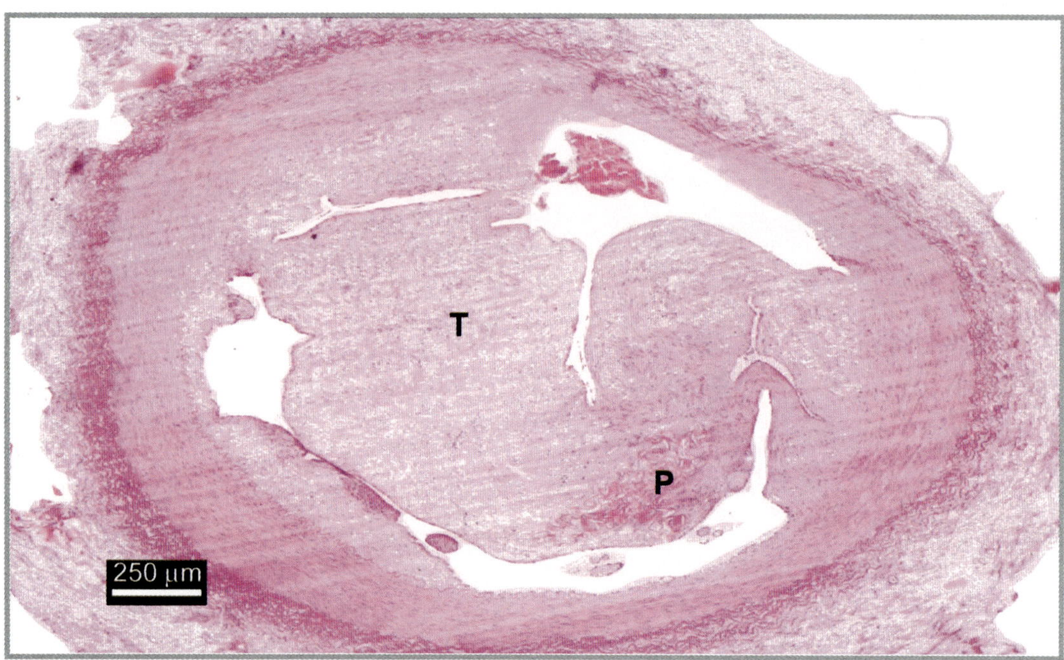

Figure 54A Endovascular embolization technique for aneurysms. H & E x 4
Organization of dense collagenous tissue (T) around an embolus of degrading polymer (P) lodged in the lumen of a blood vessel

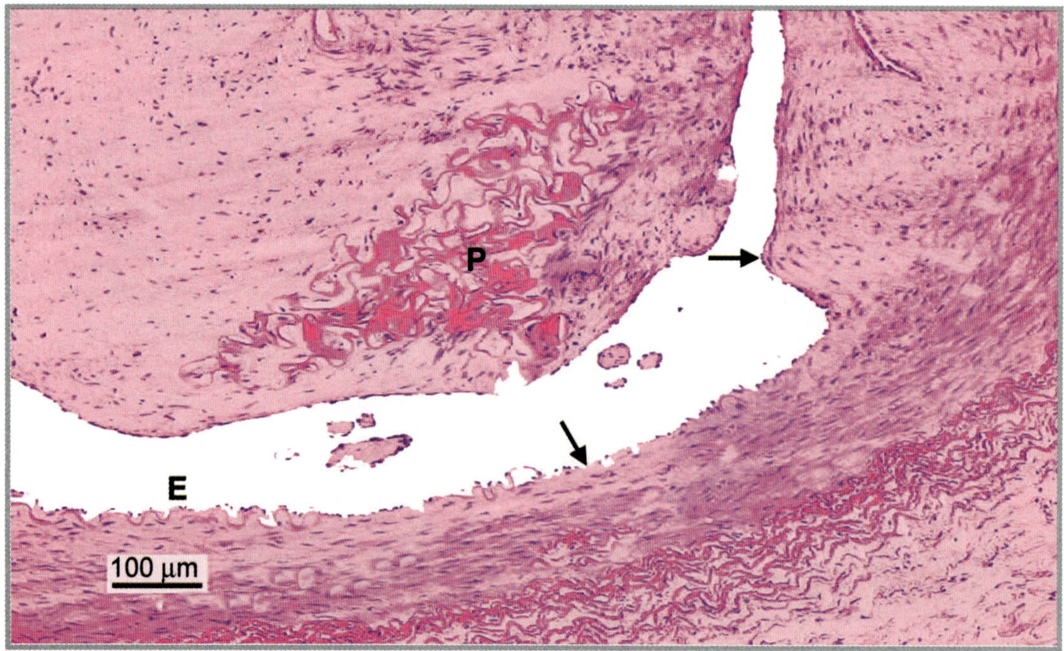

Figure 54B Endovascular embolization technique for aneurysms. H & E x 10
The tissue is gradually expected to fill the whole lumen and block blood supply to the aneurysm. Injury of endothelial layer (↑) of vessel wall during impaction of polymer (P) embolus. Wavy translucent internal elastic lamina (E) of the vessel wall is seen

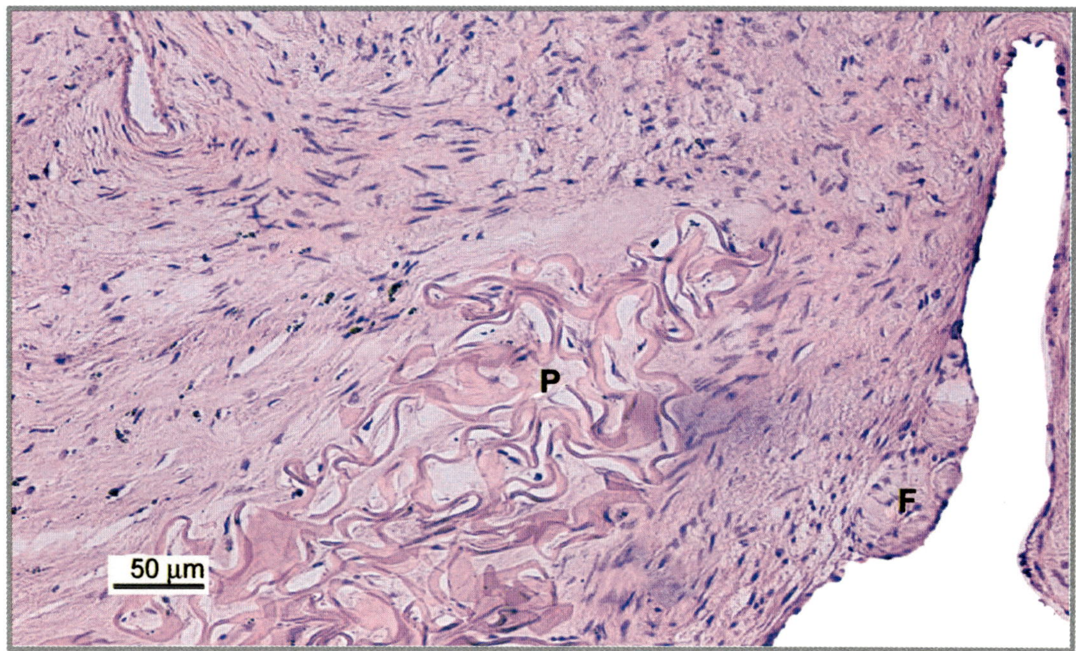

Figure 54C Endovascular embolization technique for aneurysms. H & E x 20
Inflammation is absent. This is desirable and indicates biocompatibility of the material (P) as it degrades. Fibrin thrombus (F) is seen

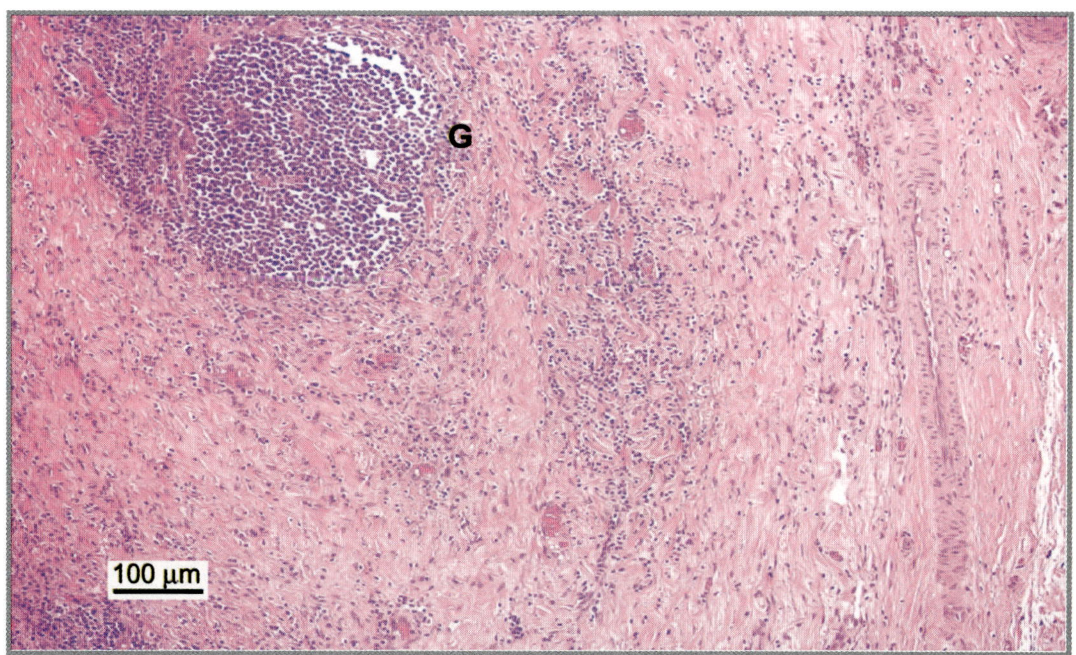

Figure 55 Myocardium. H & E x 10
Granuloma (G) in myocardium with collection of mononuclear cells

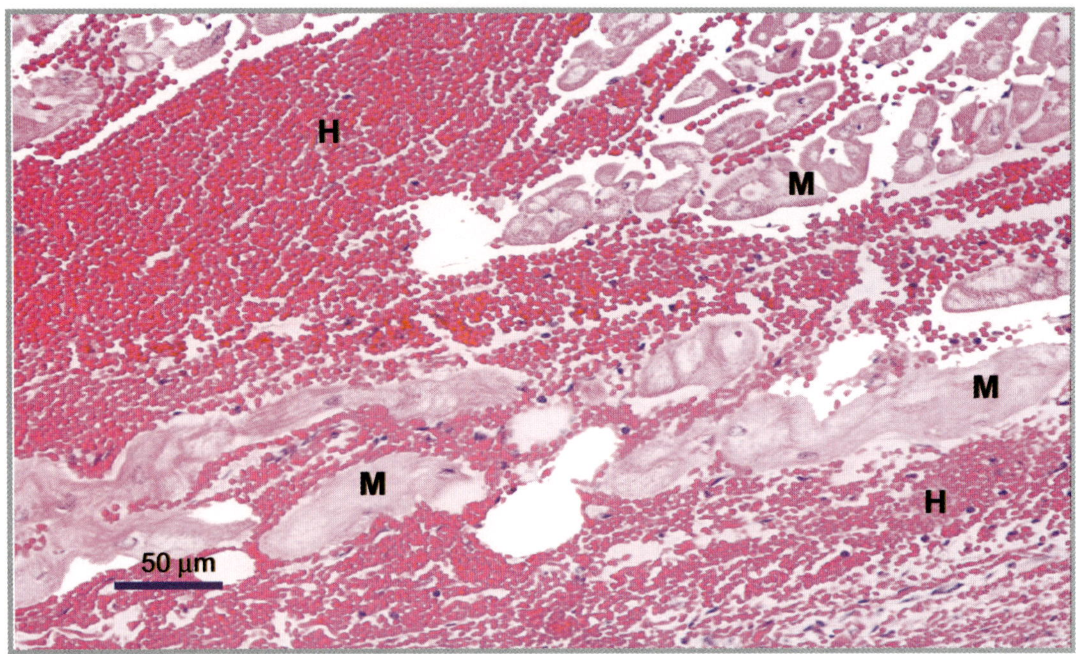

Figure 56 Myocardium. H & E x 20
Severe hemorrhage (H) in myocardium with myolysis (M) of muscle fibers

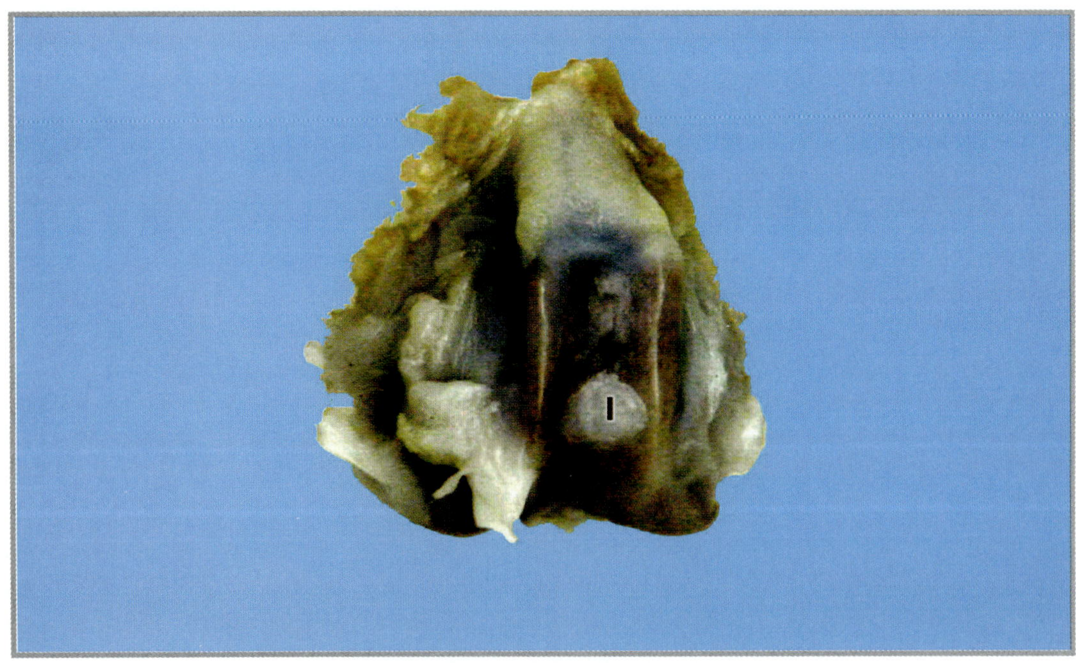

Figure 57A Knee joint cartilage implant. Gross image
Implant (I) in condylar region

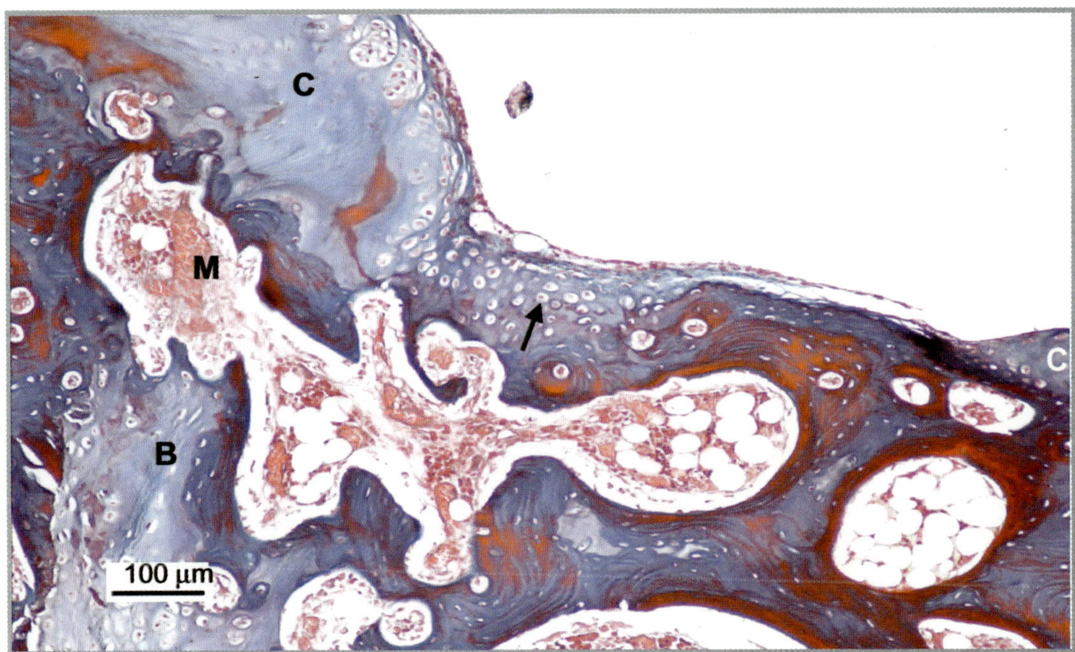

Figure 57B Knee joint cartilage implant. Masson's trichrome x 10
Newly formed chondrocytes (↑) in articular surface defect with host cartilage (C) on either side and bone (B) with marrow (M) below

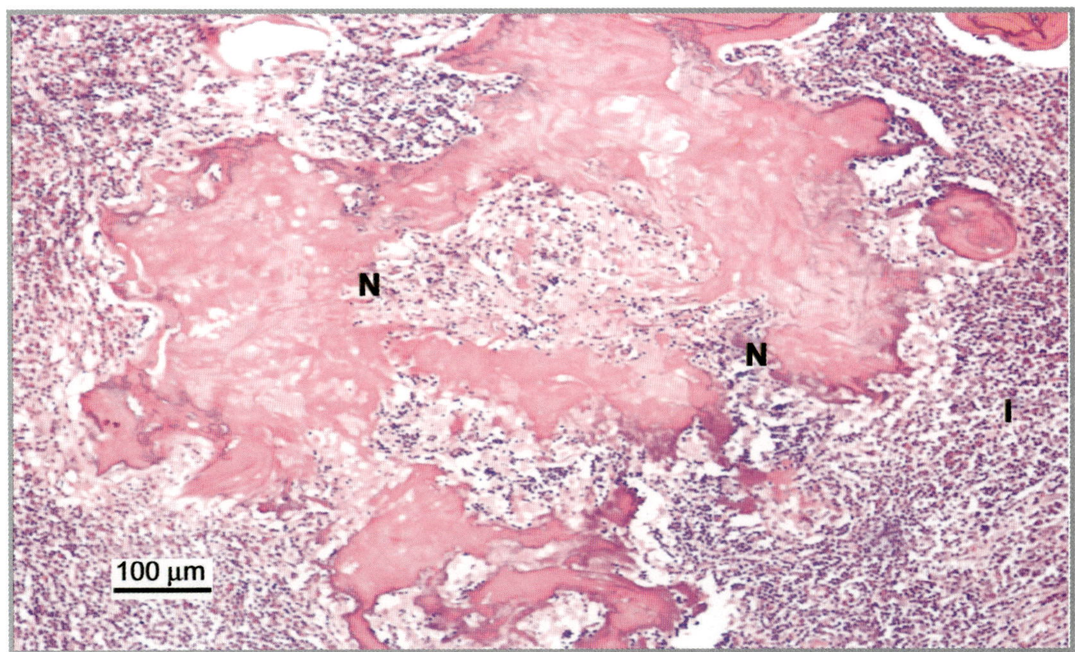

Figure 58A Knee joint cartilage implant. H & E x 10
Necrosis (N) of underlying bone and inflammation (I)

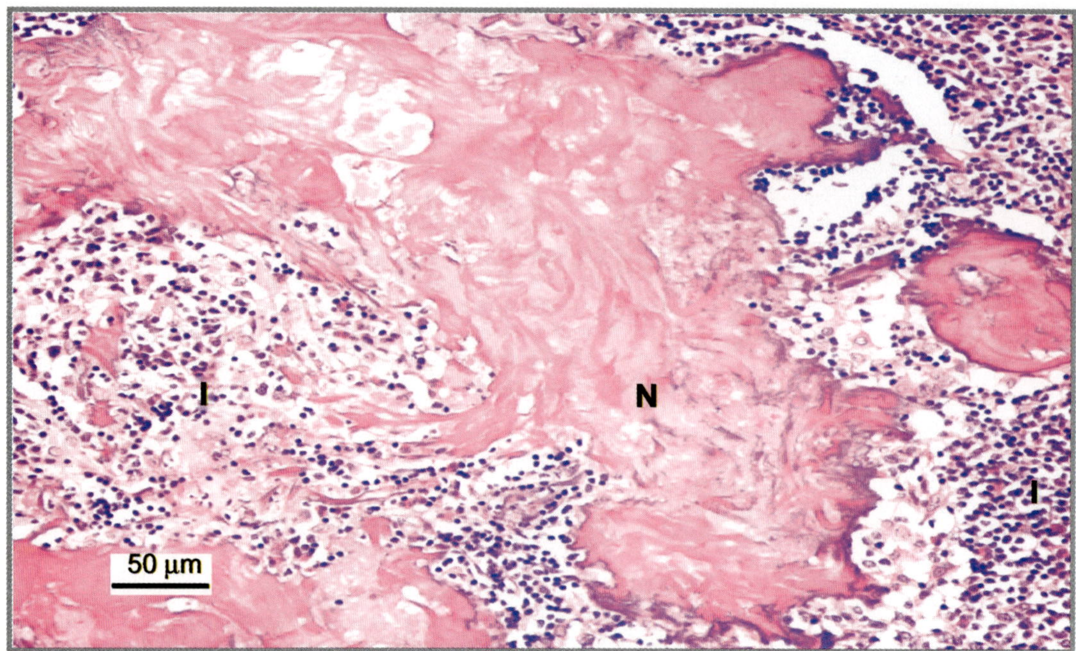

Figure 58B Knee joint cartilage implant. H & E x 20
Higher magnification of necrosis (N) of underlying bone and inflammation (I)

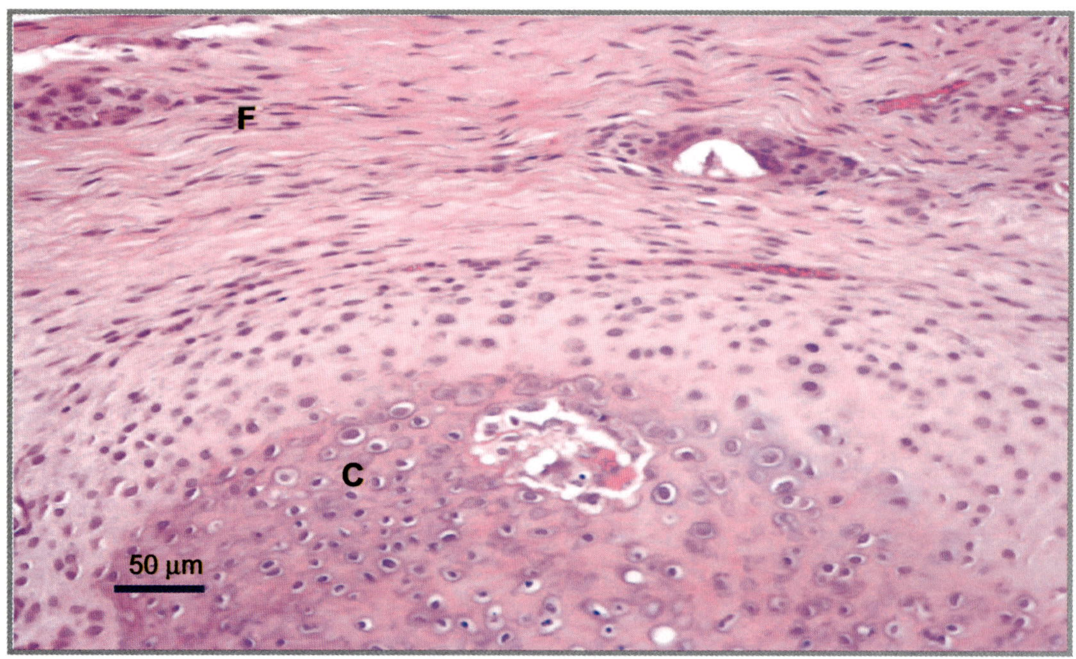

Figure 59 Knee joint cartilage implant. H & E x 20
Chondrocytes (C) and fibrosis (F)

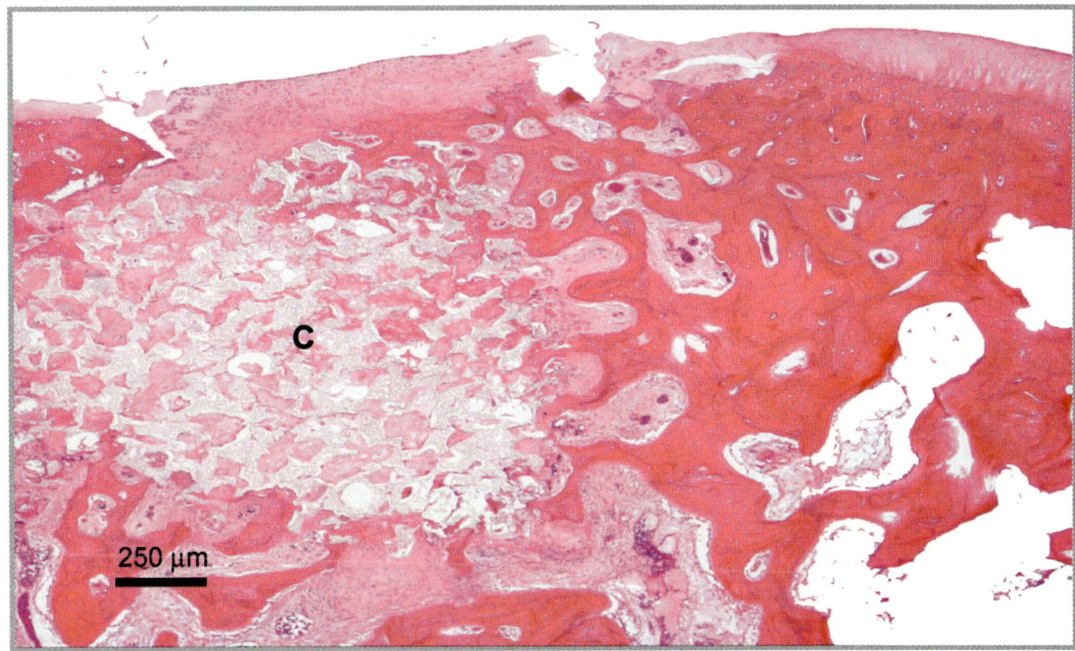

Figure 60 Tissue engineered cartilage implant. H & E x 4
Polymer scaffold with chondroblasts (C) implanted in articular surface defect made in knee joint in rabbit

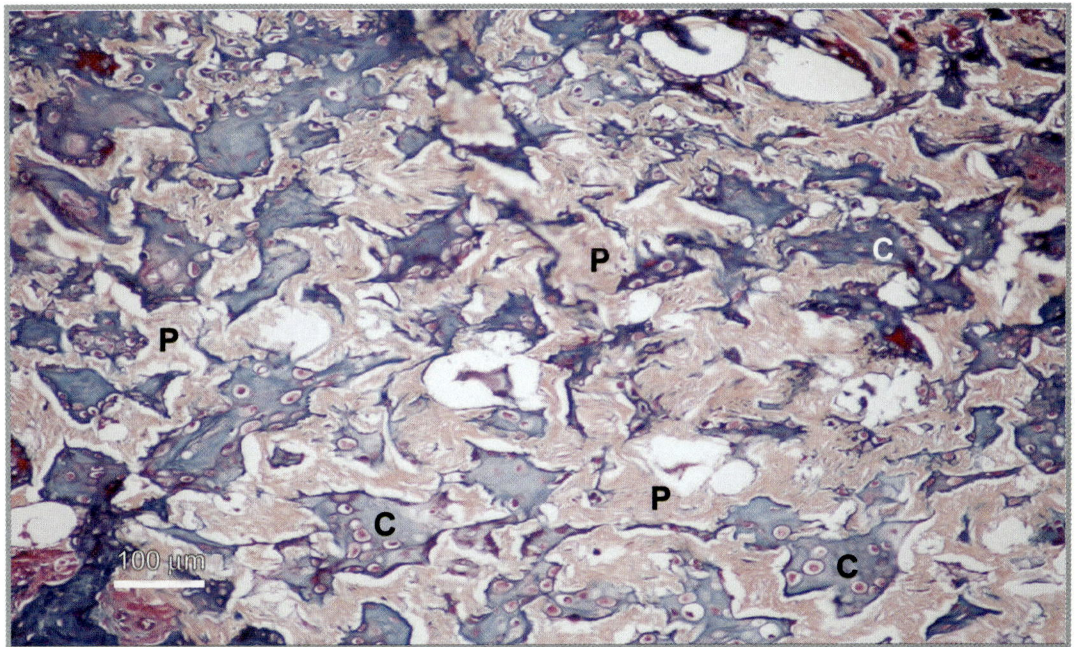

Figure 61A Tissue engineered cartilage implant. Masson's trichrome x 10
Polymer scaffold (P) with chondroblasts (C) implanted in cavity made in knee joint in rabbit

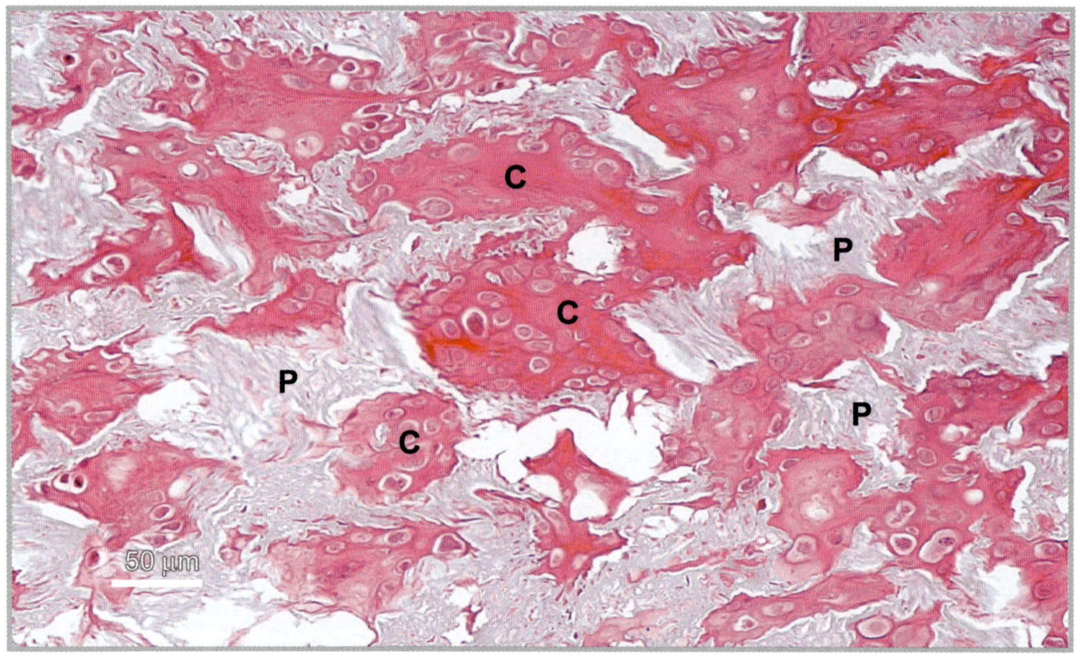

Figure 61B Tissue engineered cartilage implant. H & E x 20
Higher magnification of the polymer scaffold (P) with chondroblasts (C)

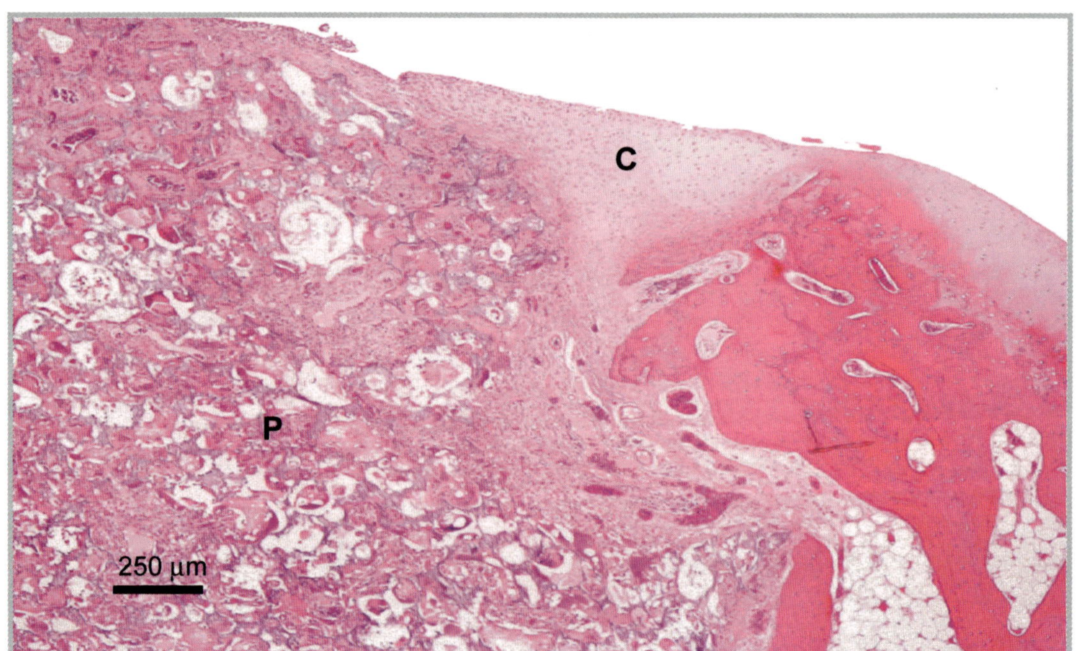

Figure 62A Tissue engineered cartilage implant. H & E x 4
As the polymer scaffold (P) degrades, inflammatory cells are seen infiltrating the material. New cartilage (C) forms above

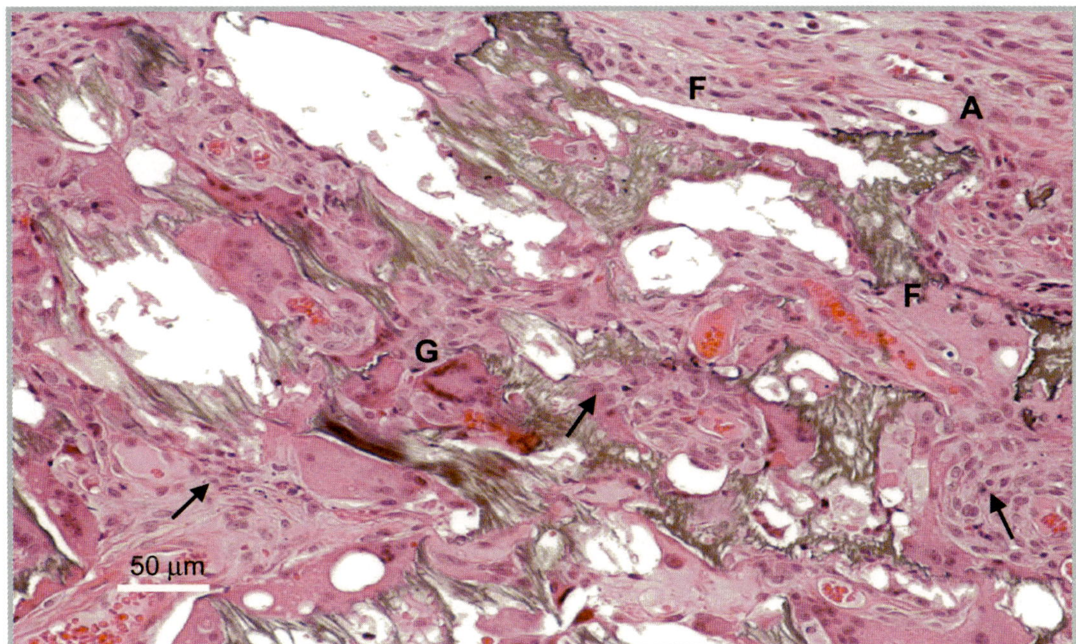

Figure 62B Tissue engineered cartilage implant. H & E x 20
As the polymer scaffold degrades, macrophages (↑) fibrocytes (F), foreign body type of giant cells (G) are seen infiltrating the material

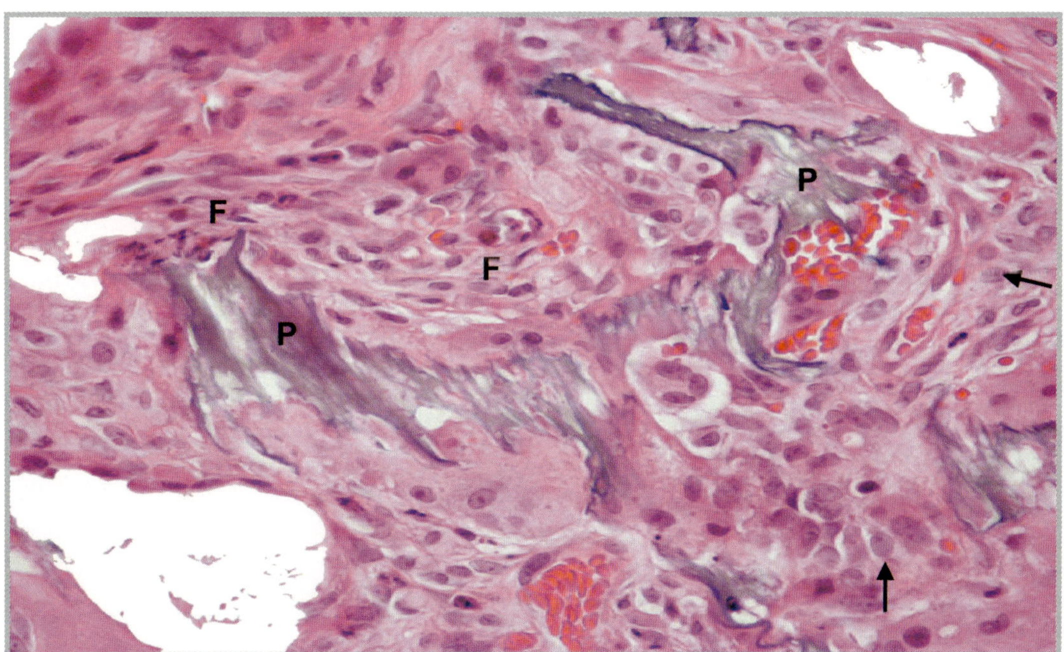

Figure 62C Tissue engineered cartilage implant. H & E x 40
Higher magnification of the degrading polymer scaffold (P) with macrophages (↑) and fibrocytes (F)

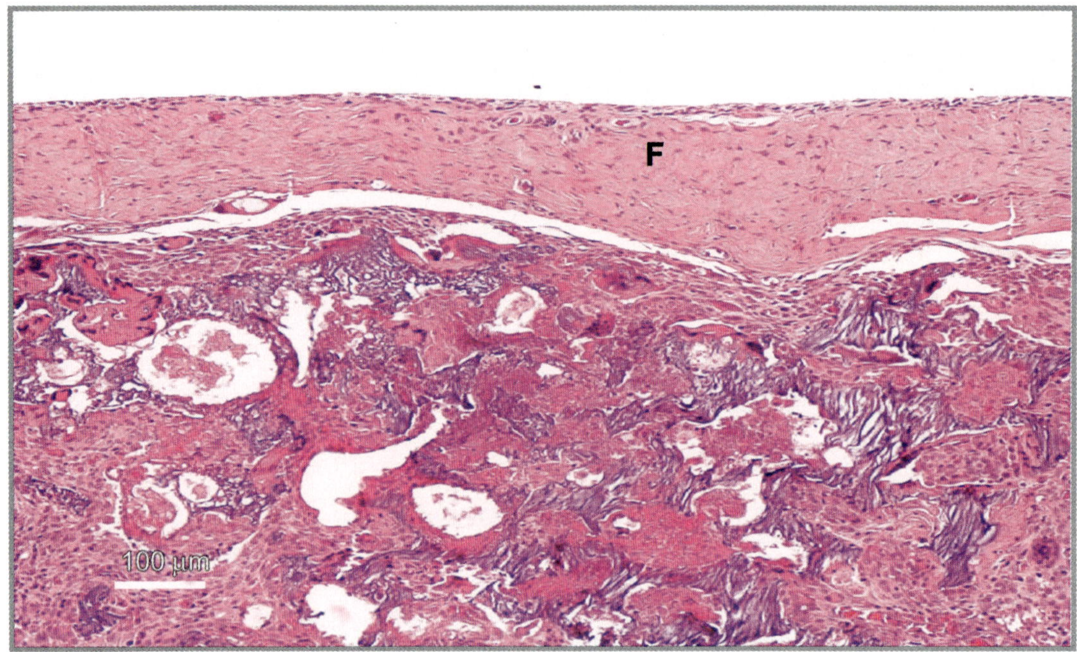

Figure 63A Tissue engineered cartilage implant. H & E x 10
Fibrous tissue (F) over polymer scaffold in articular surface defect

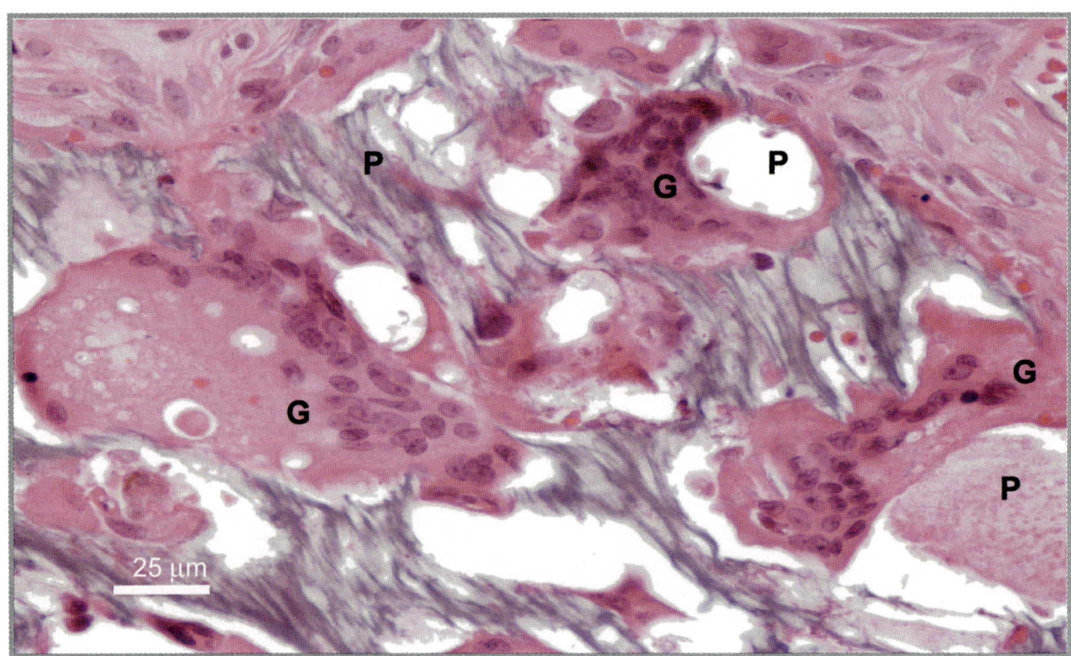

Figure 63B Tissue engineered cartilage implant. H & E x 40
Foreign body type of giant cells (G) around polymer material (P)

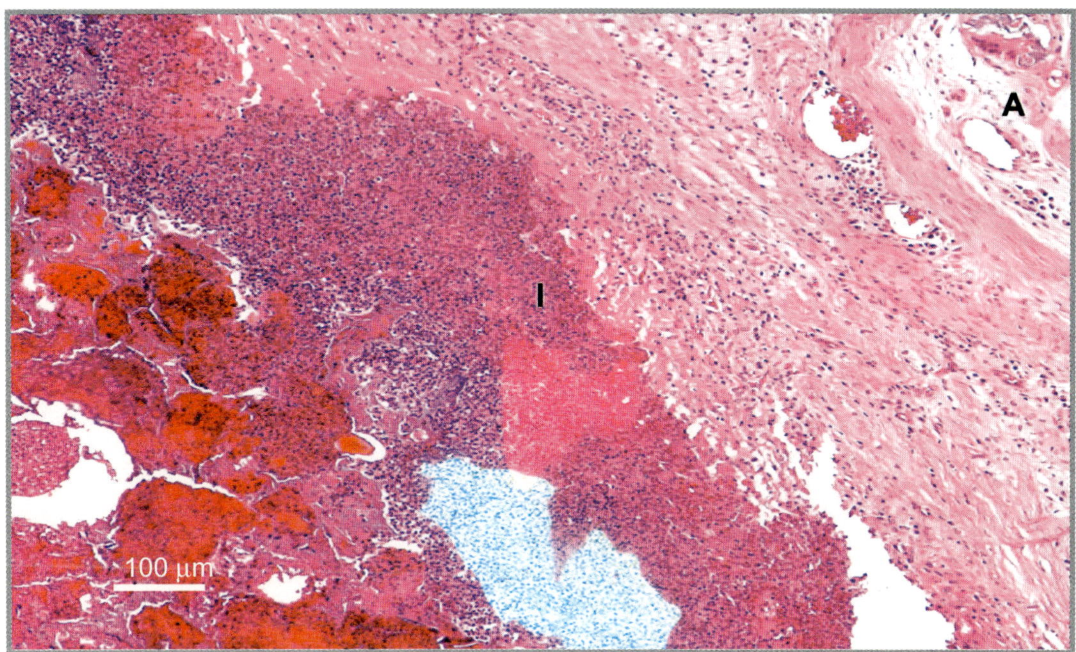

Figure 64A Tissue engineered cartilage implant. H & E x 10
Severe inflammation (I) in and around the scaffold. Angiogenesis (A) seen in periphery

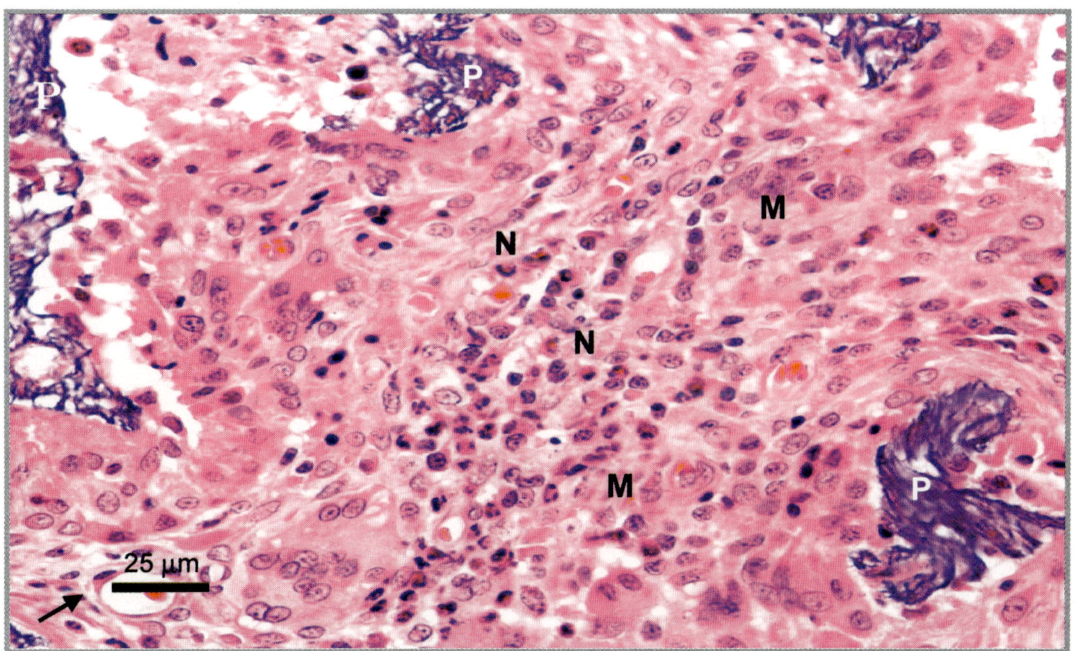

Figure 64B Tissue engineered cartilage implant. H & E x 40
Neutrophils (N) and macrophages (M) infiltrating the polymer scaffold (P)
Angiogenesis (↑) is seen in the scaffold

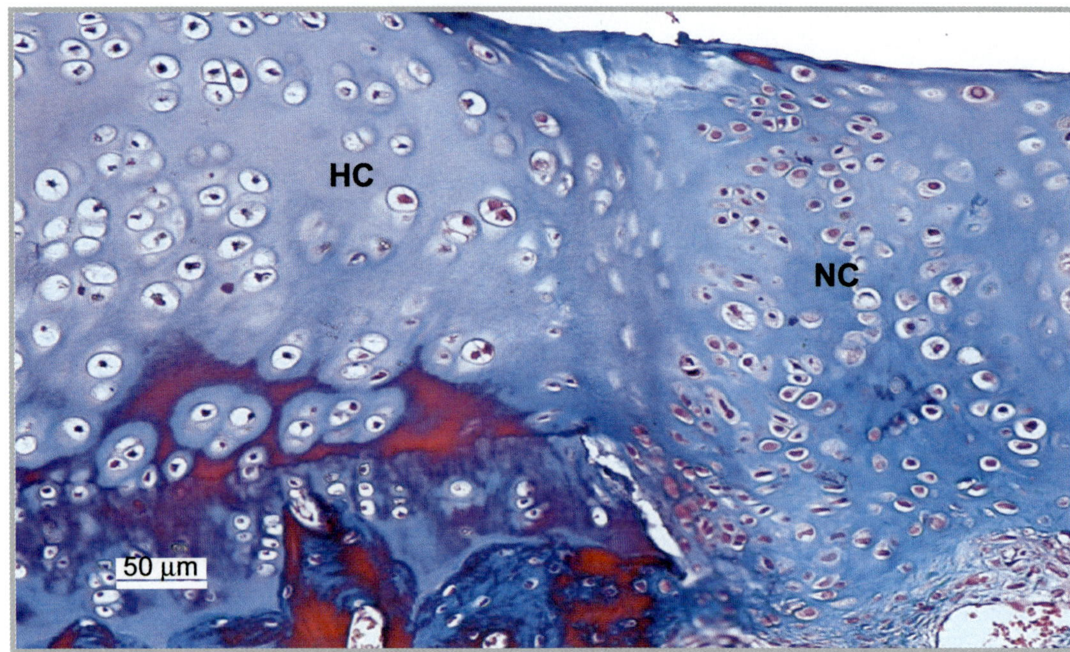

Figure 65 Tissue engineered cartilage implant. Masson's trichrome x 20
New cartilage (NC) with chondrocytes in articular surface defect. Adjoining host cartilage (HC) on left

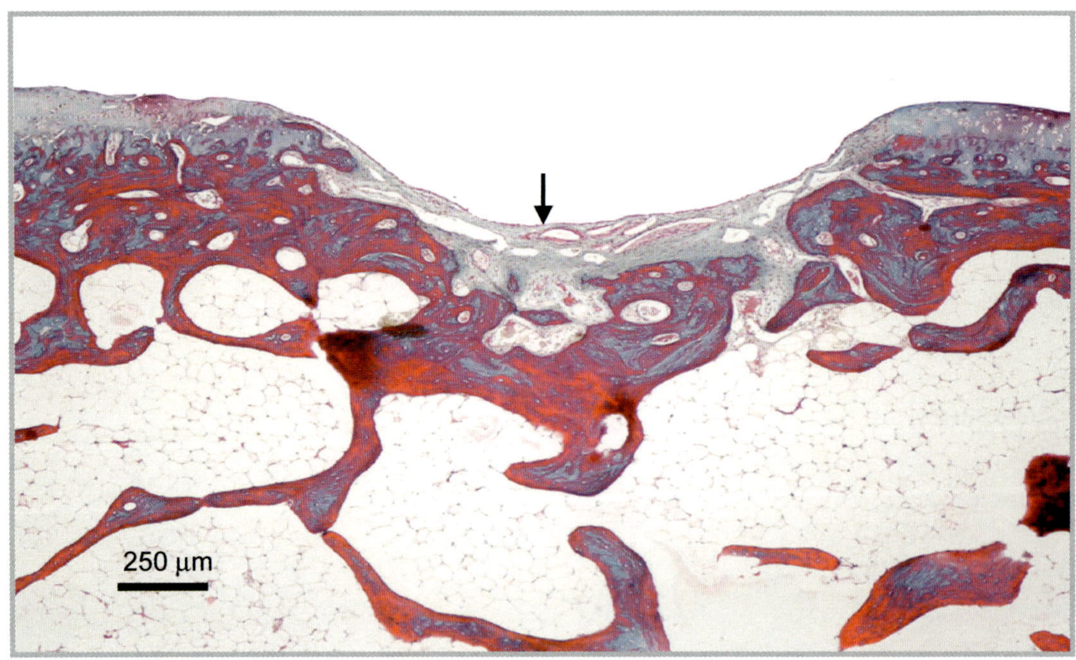

Figure 66A Tissue engineered cartilage implant. Masson's trichrome x 4
Healing in articular surface defect in joint

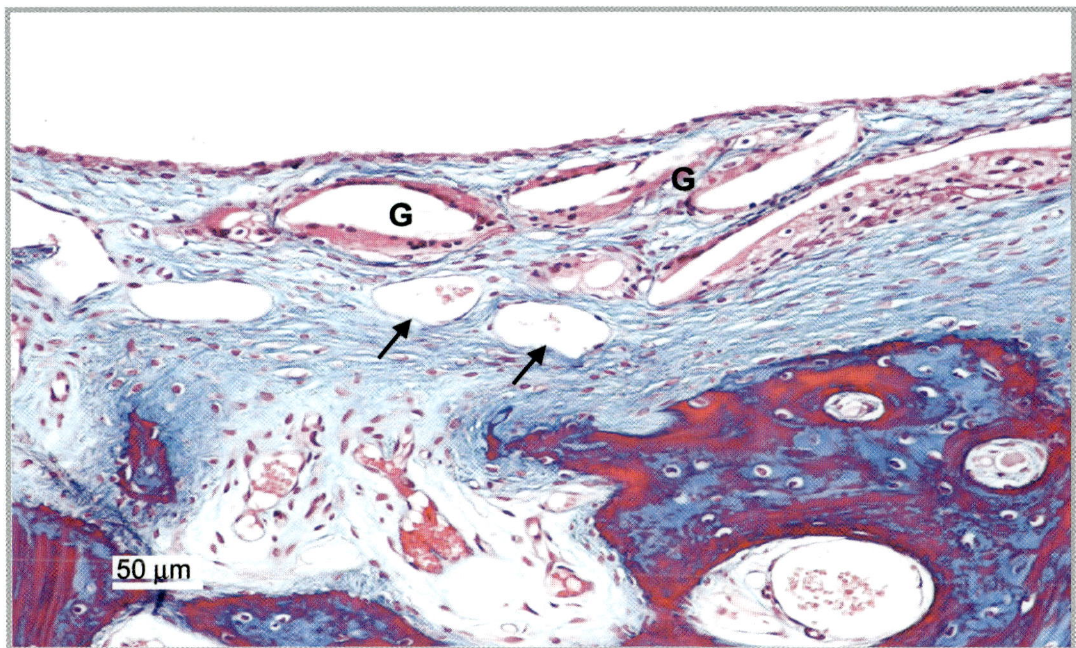

Figure 66B Tissue engineered cartilage implant. Masson's trichrome x 20
Polymer scaffold material engulfed by foreign body type of giant cells (G), angiogenesis (↑) is seen

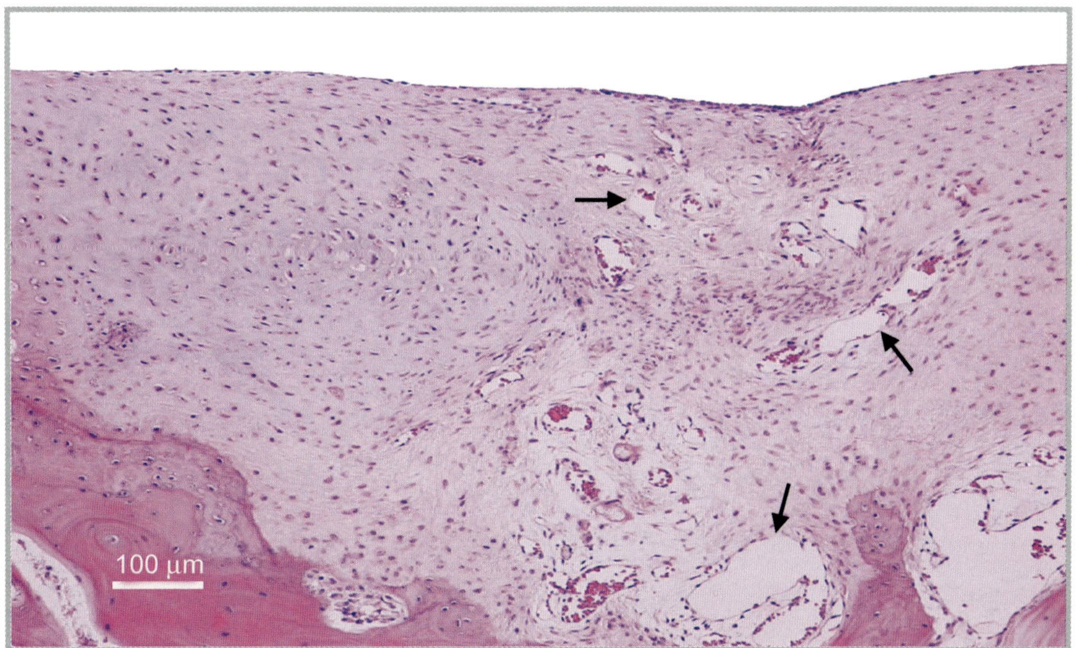

Figure 67 Tissue engineered cartilage implant. H & E x 10
Angiogenesis (↑) in healed articular surface defect

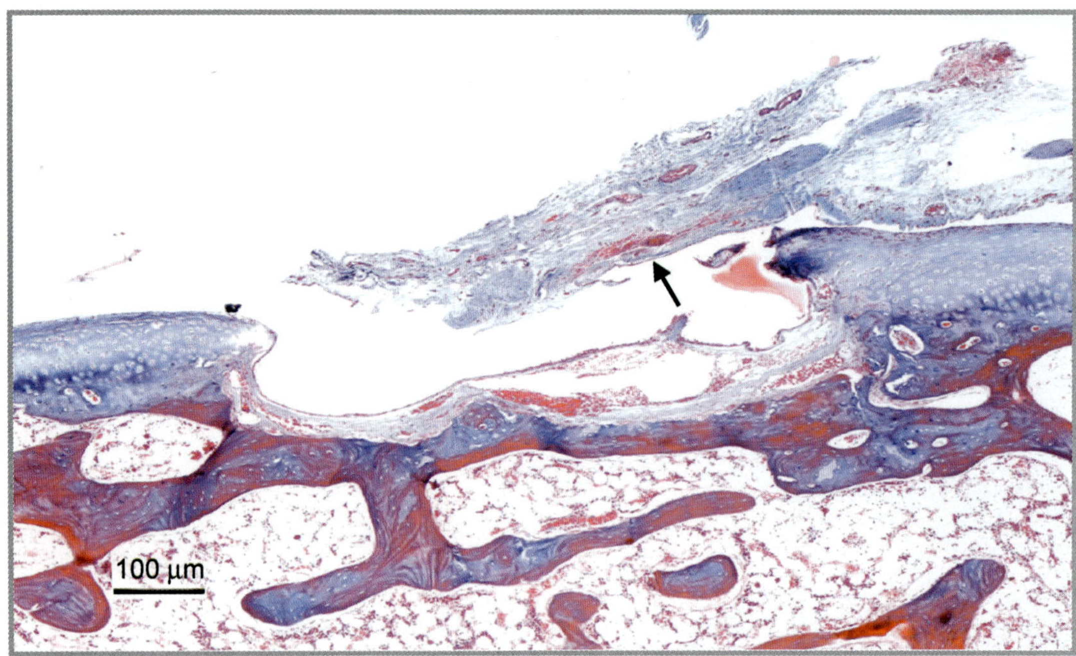

Figure 68 Tissue engineered cartilage implant. Masson's trichrome x 10
Fibrovascular tissue (↑) proliferation in articular surface defect

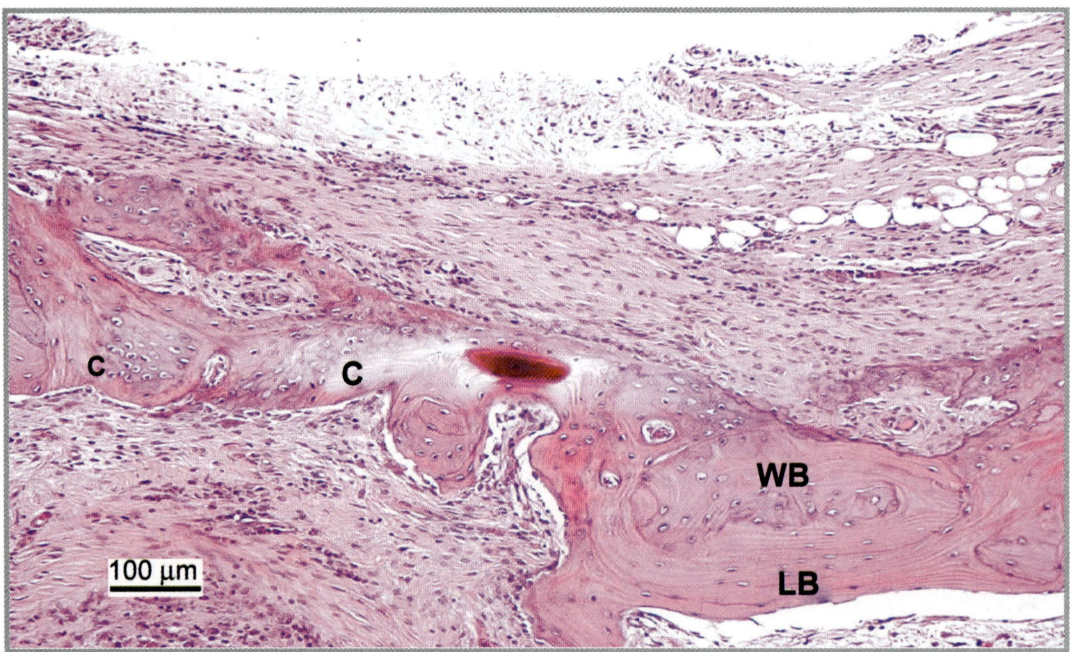

Figure 69 Tissue engineered cartilage implant. H & E x 10
New bone trabeculae at base of cavity. Areas of chondrogenesis (C) with woven bone (WB) and lamellar bone (LB)

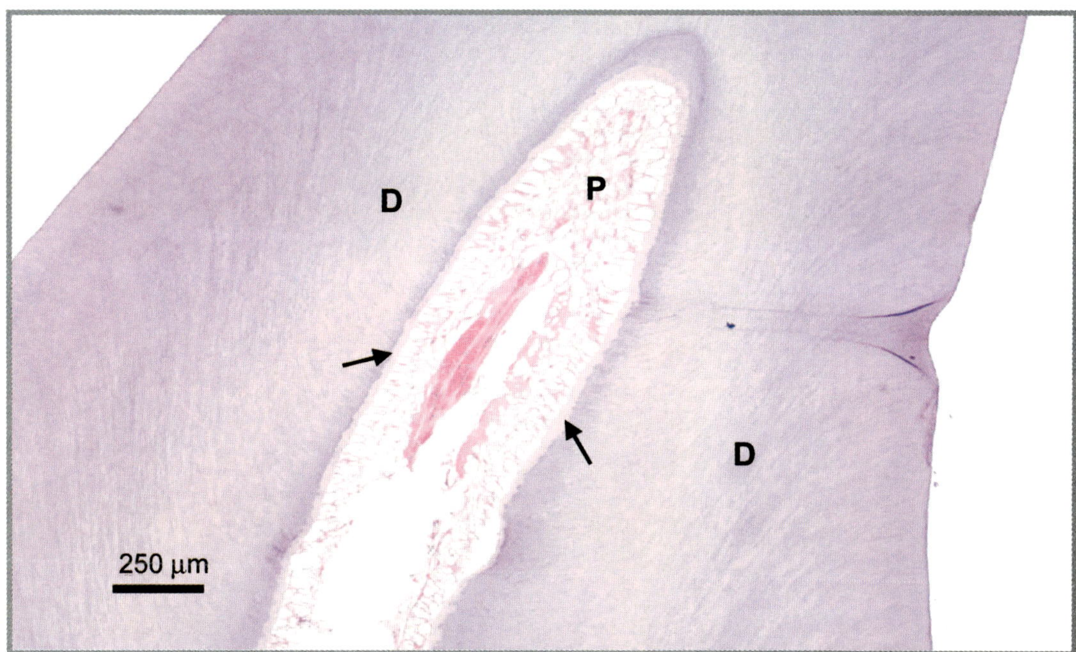

Figure 70A Normal tooth. H & E x 4
Decalcified normal tooth with dentine (D), predentine (↑) and pulp (P)

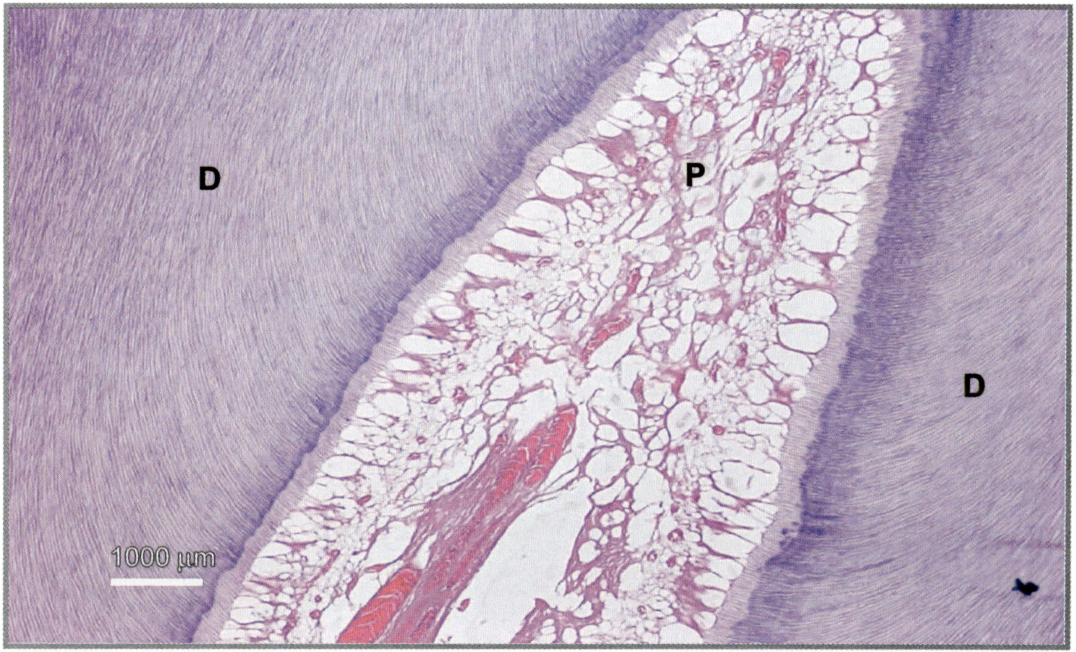

Figure 70B Normal tooth. H & E x 10
The predentine is lined by odontoblasts. The pulp (P) contains blood vessels, nerves and collagen

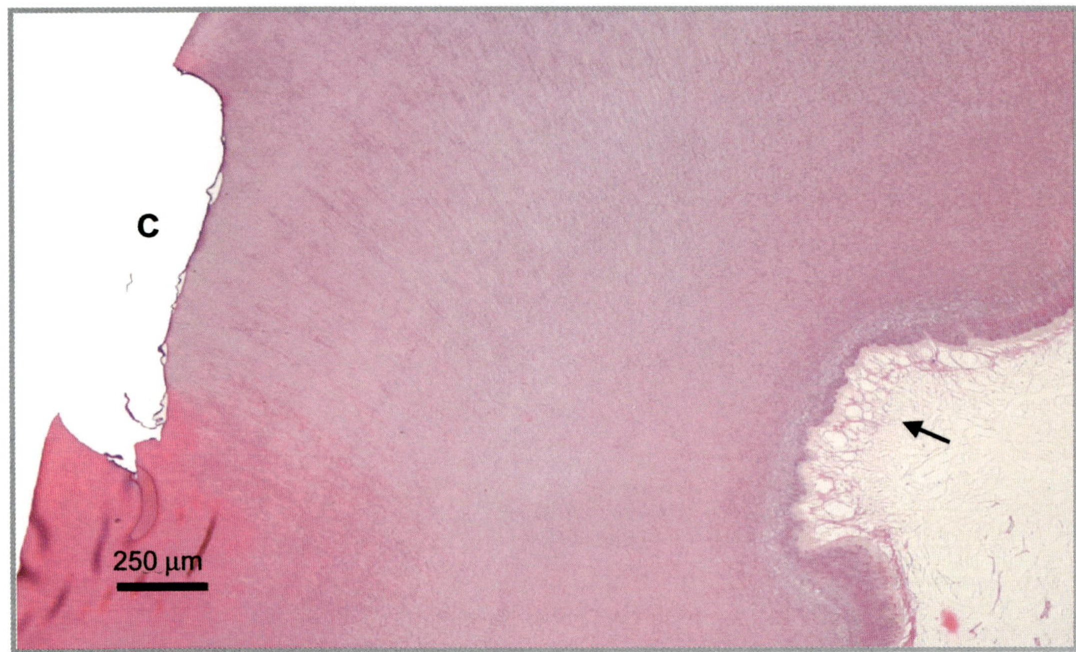

Figure 71A Dental restoratives. H & E x 4
A cavity (C) is made in the dentine and filled with dental material to be tested. The response of odontoblasts and pulp below the cavity (↑) is evaluated for biocompatibility

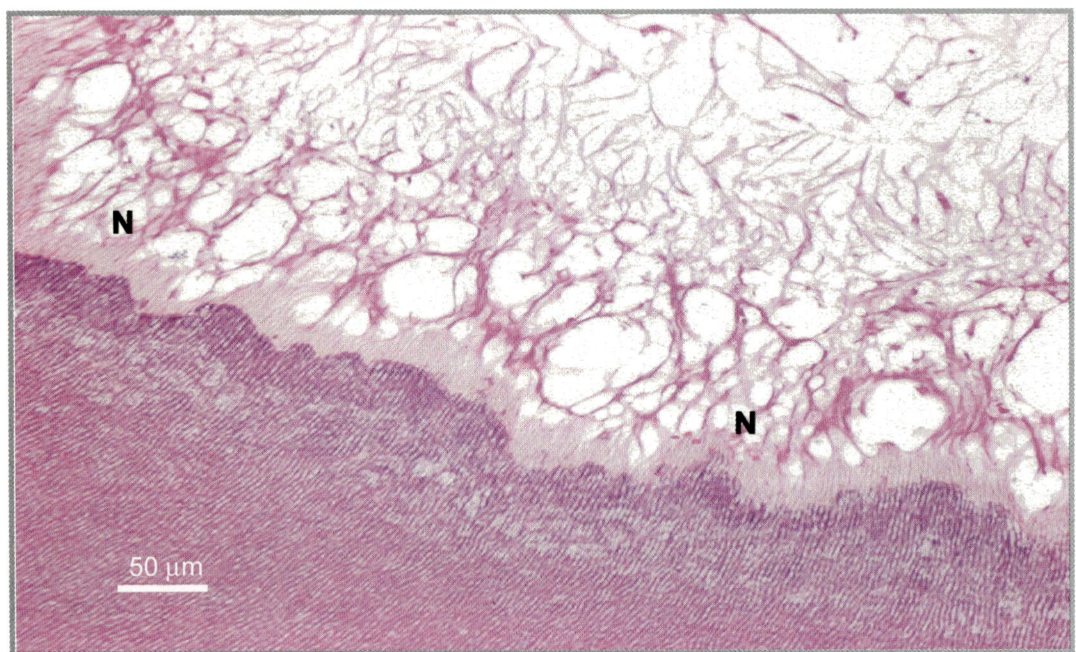

Figure 71B Dental restoratives. H & E x 20
Necrosis (N) at 7 days

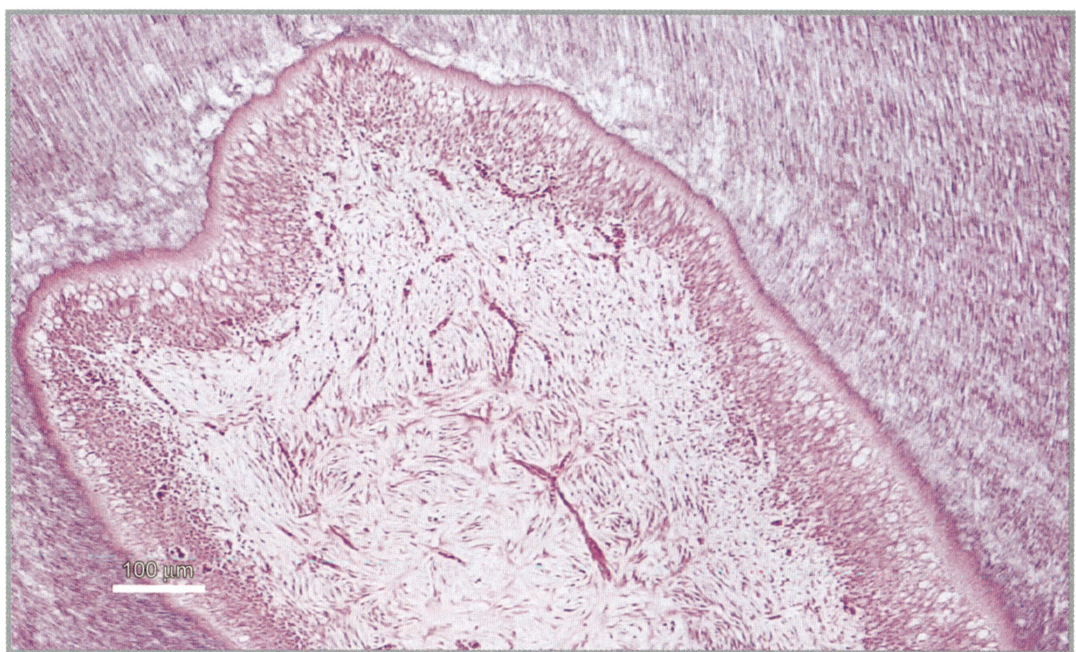

Figure 72A Dental restoratives. H & E x 10
Absence of odontoblasts at 28 days

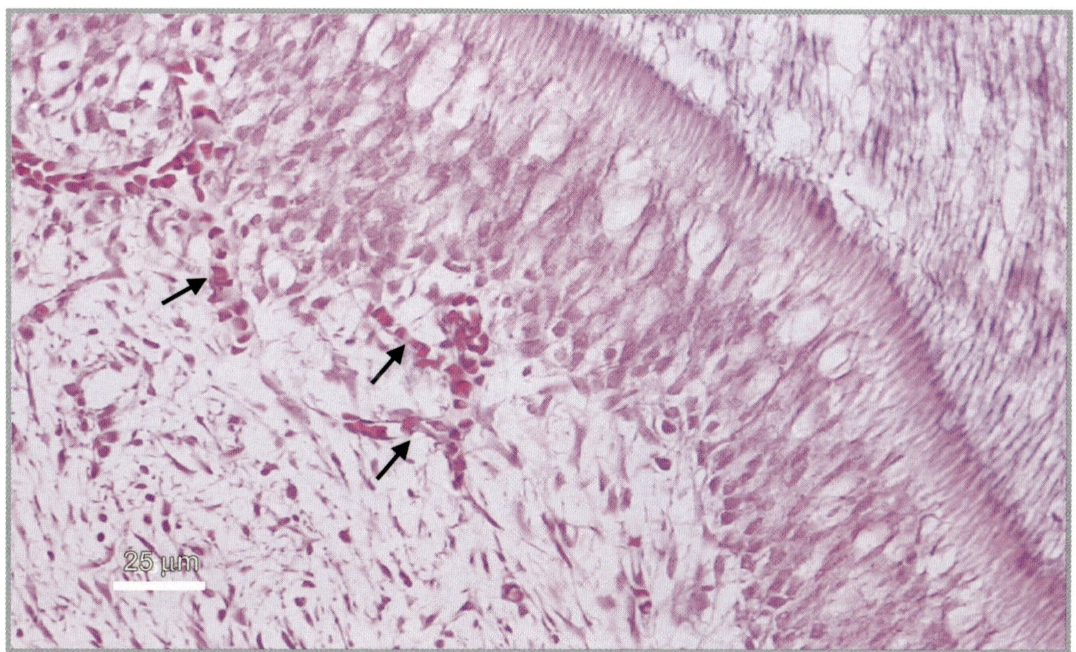

Figure 72B Dental restoratives. H & E x 40
Capillaries (↑) in the pulp

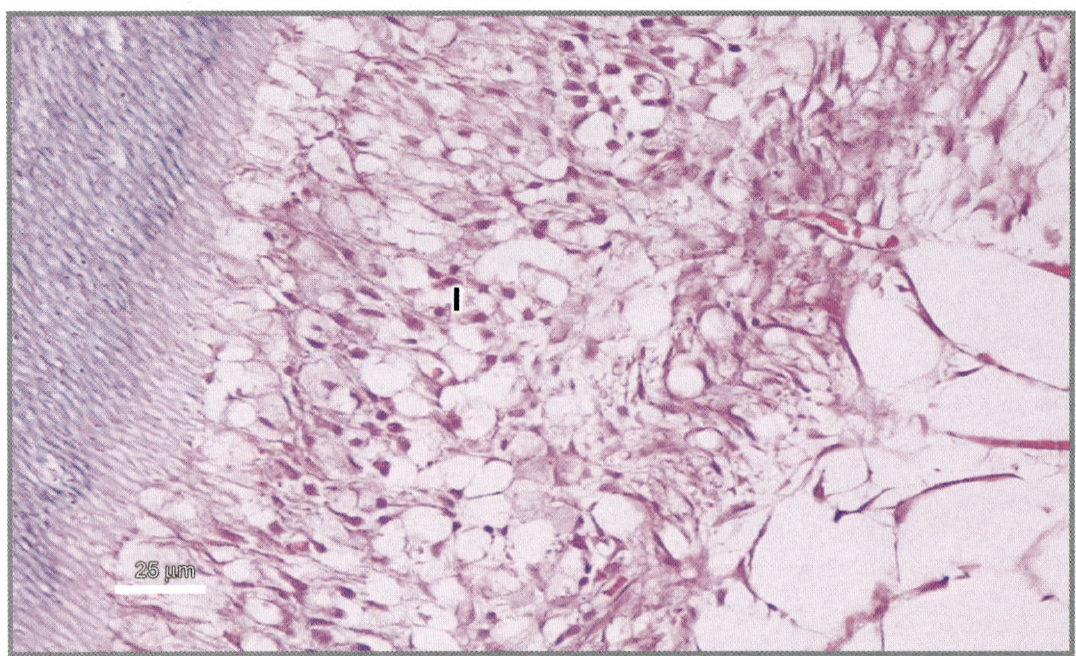

Figure 72C Dental restoratives. H & E x 40
Inflammation (I) at 28 days

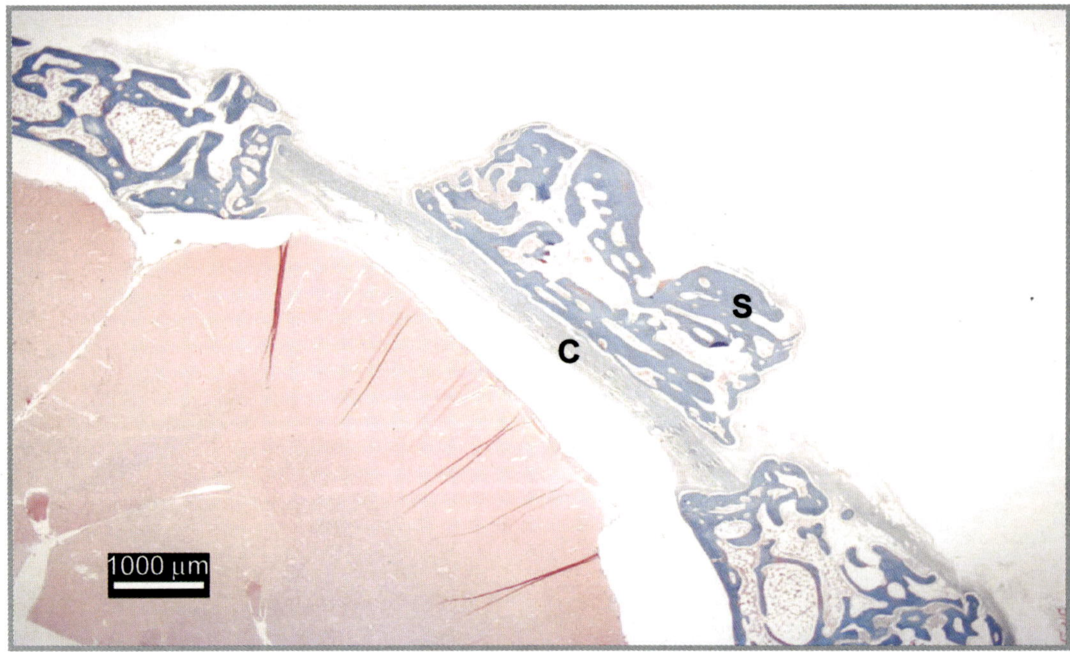

Figure 73 Dural substitute. Masson's trichrome x 1
Segment (S) of skull removed, underlying dura mater removed and replaced by a patch of decellularized collagen (C). Segment of skull replaced back. Cross-section through the brain and skull

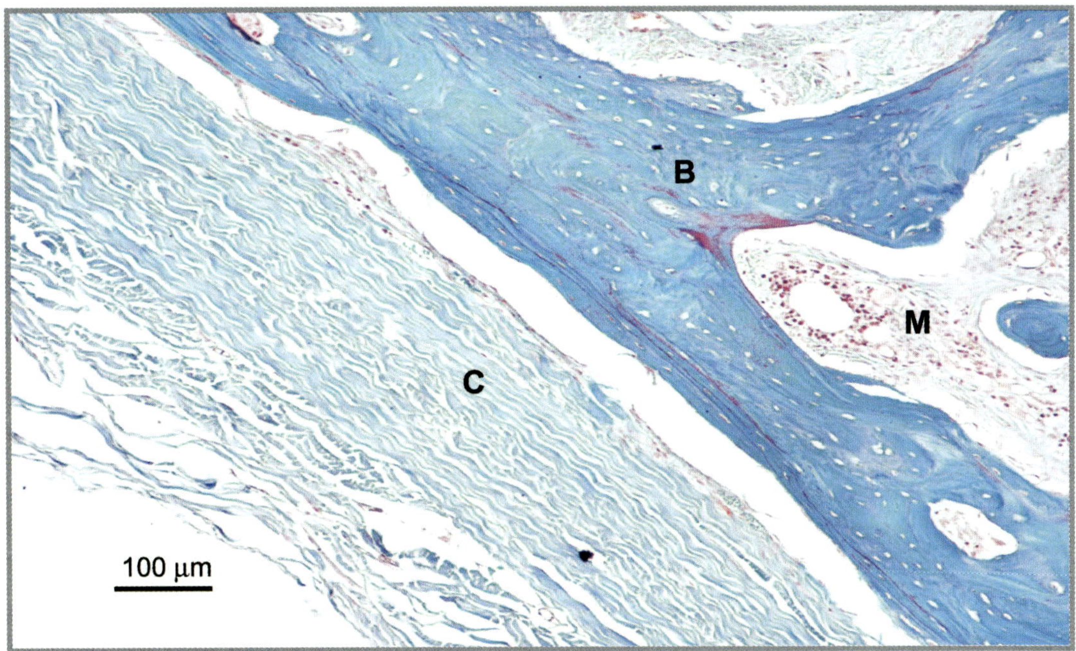

Figure 74A Dural substitute. Masson's trichrome x 10
Skull bone (B) with marrow (M) and underlying decellularized patch (C)

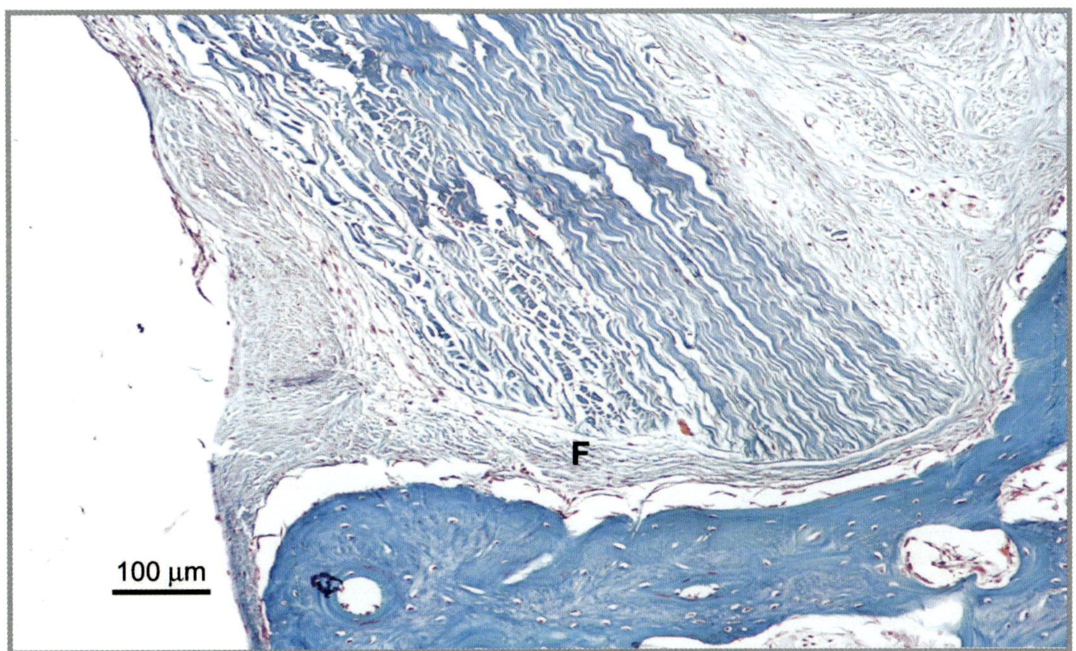

Figure 74B Dural substitute. Masson's trichrome x 10
Well-defined fibrous tissue (↑) around the patch

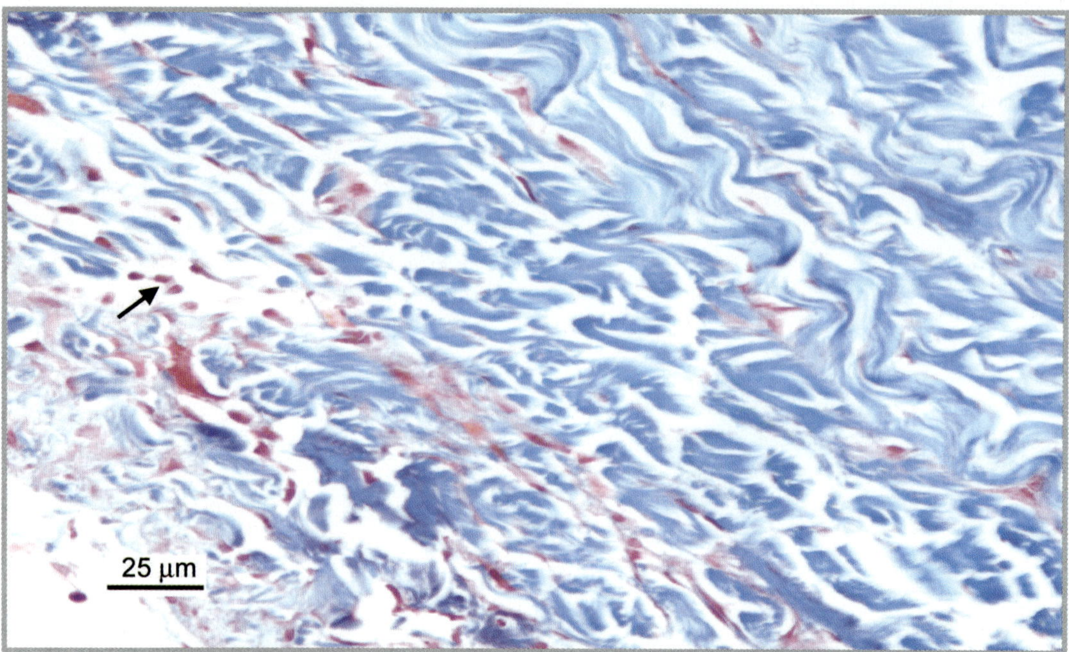

Figure 74C Dural substitute. Masson's trichrome x 40
Inflammation is absent. Occasional red blood cells are noted (↑)

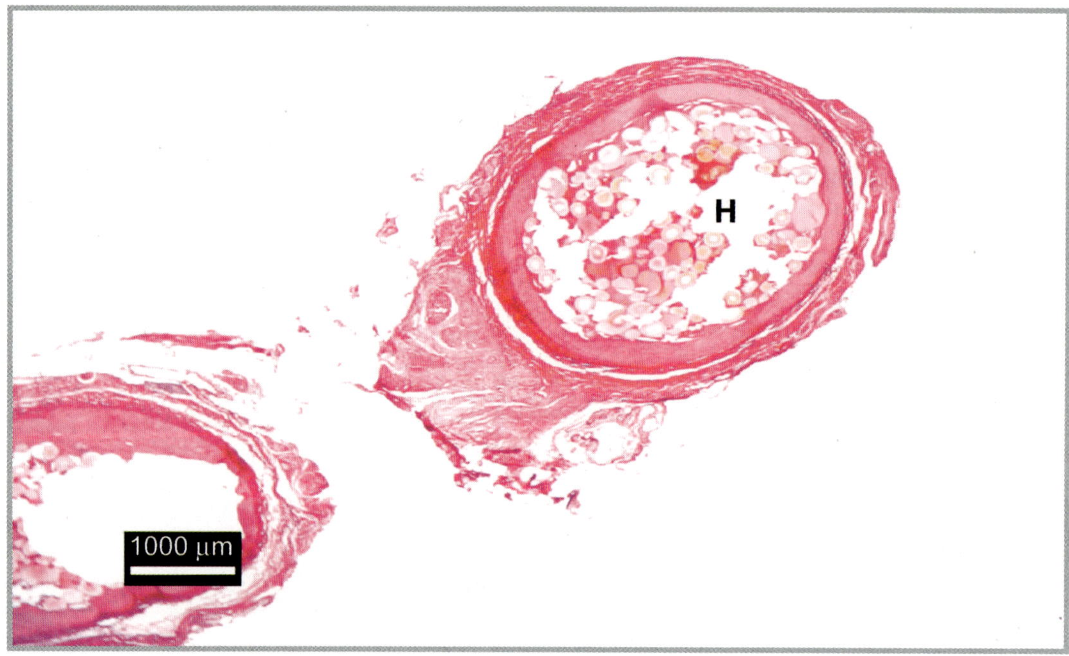

Figure 75A Embolization in blood vessels. H & E x 1
Hydrogel beads (H) injected in renal artery initiating thrombus formation

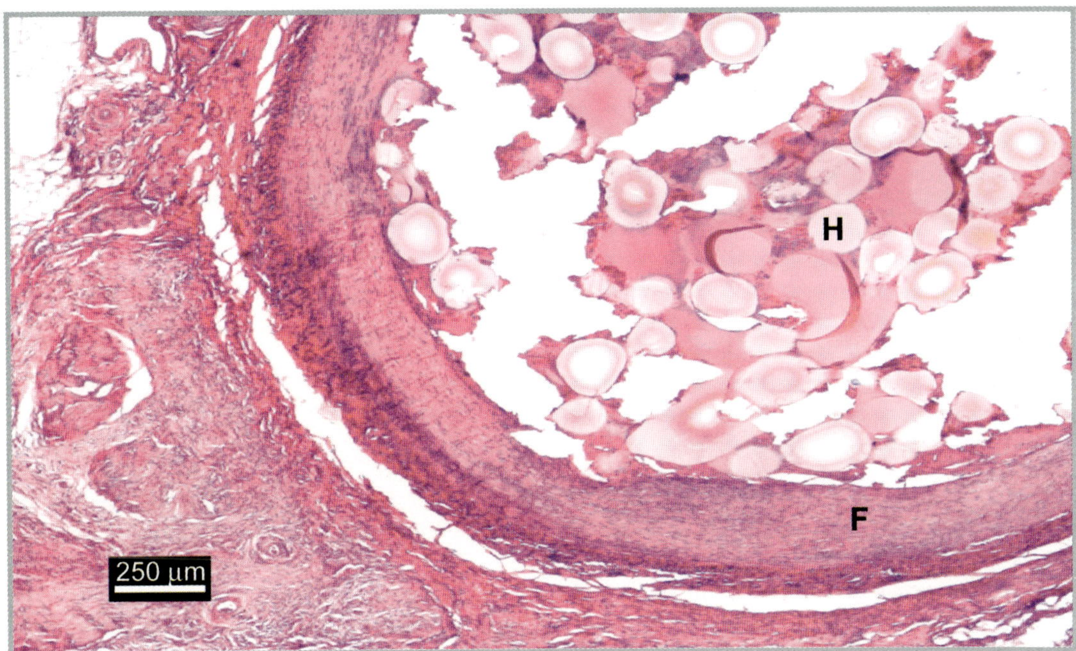

Figure 75B Embolization in blood vessels. H & E x 4
The thrombus is organized with fibrosis (F) in between and around the hydrogel beads (H)

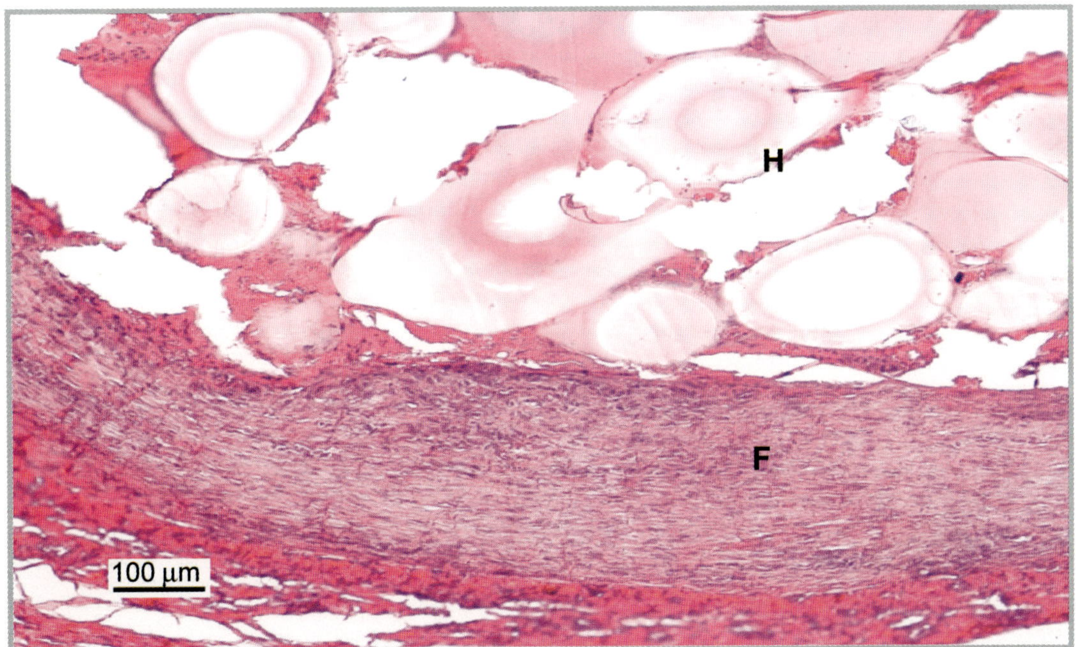

Figure 75C Embolization in blood vessels. H & E x 10
Higher magnification showing beads (H) and organized thrombosis with fibrosis (F).
Successful blockage of the blood vessel indicates the feasibility of use of this material for endovascular embolization in treatment of aneurysms

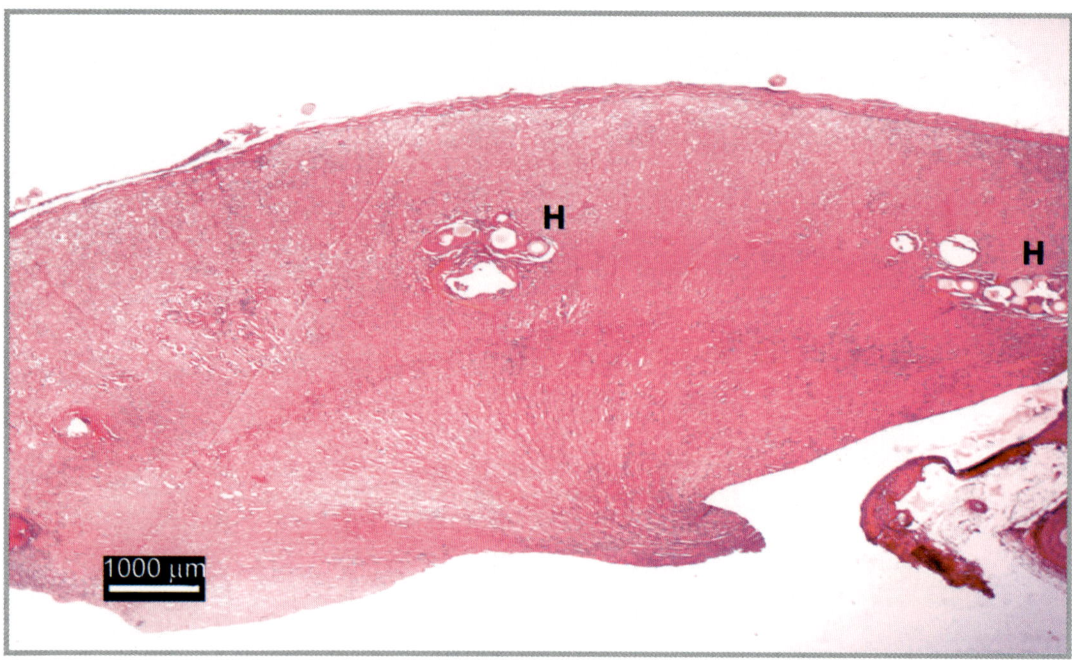

Figure 76A Embolization in blood vessels. H & E x 1
Groups of polymer beads (H) injected in renal artery, lodged in the cortical region of kidney

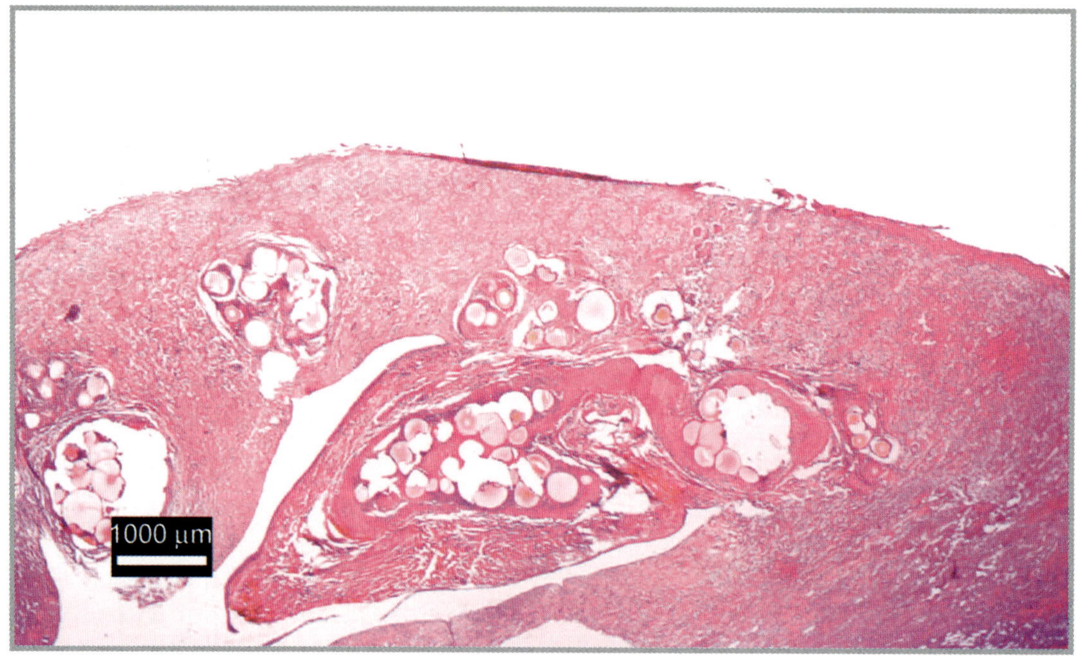

Figure 76B Embolization in blood vessels. H & E x 1
Groups of polymer beads injected in renal artery, lodged in the medullary region of kidney

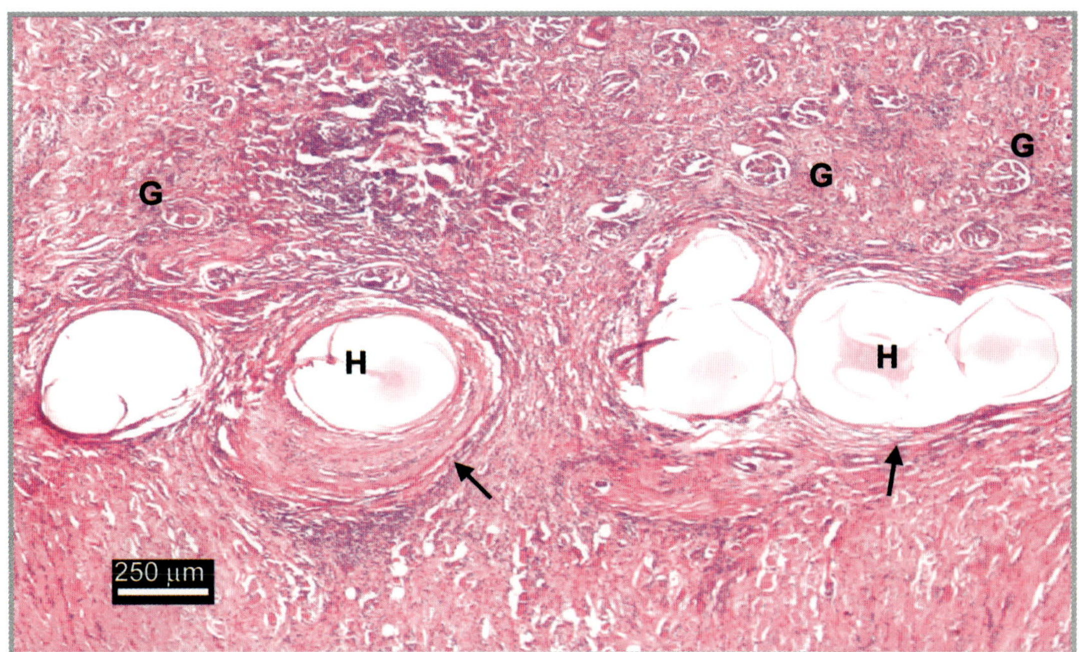

Figure 77A Embolization in blood vessels. H & E x 4
Polymer beads (H) injected in renal artery, lodged in the cortical region of kidney
Glomeruli (G) is seen

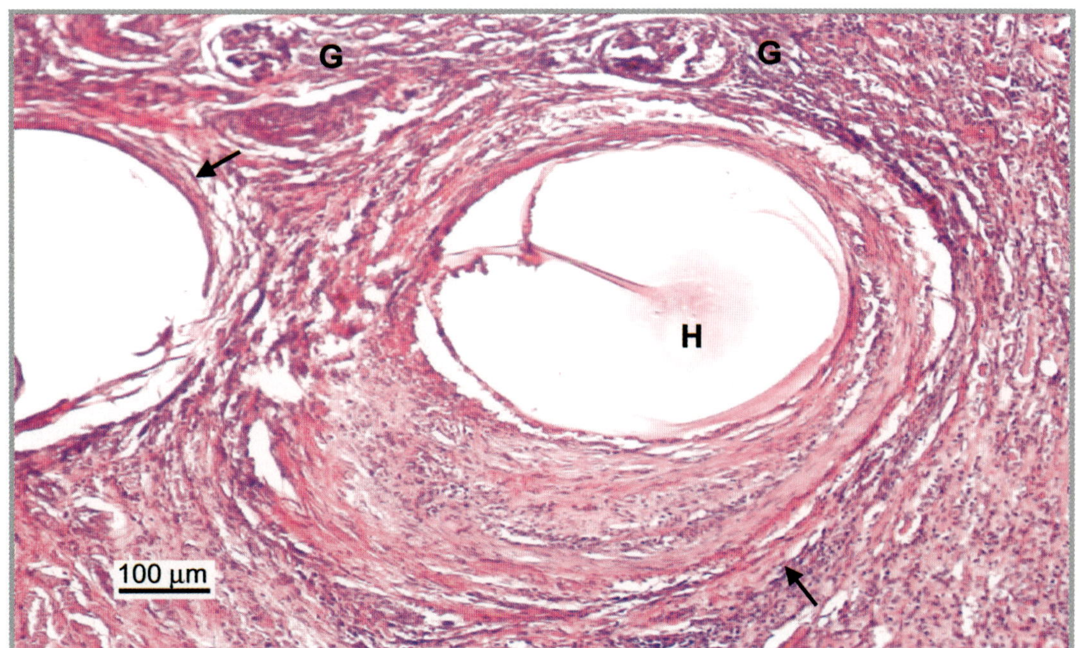

Figure 77B Embolization in blood vessels. H & E x 10
Mild inflammation and fibrosis (↑) present around the beads (H) and glomeruli (G)

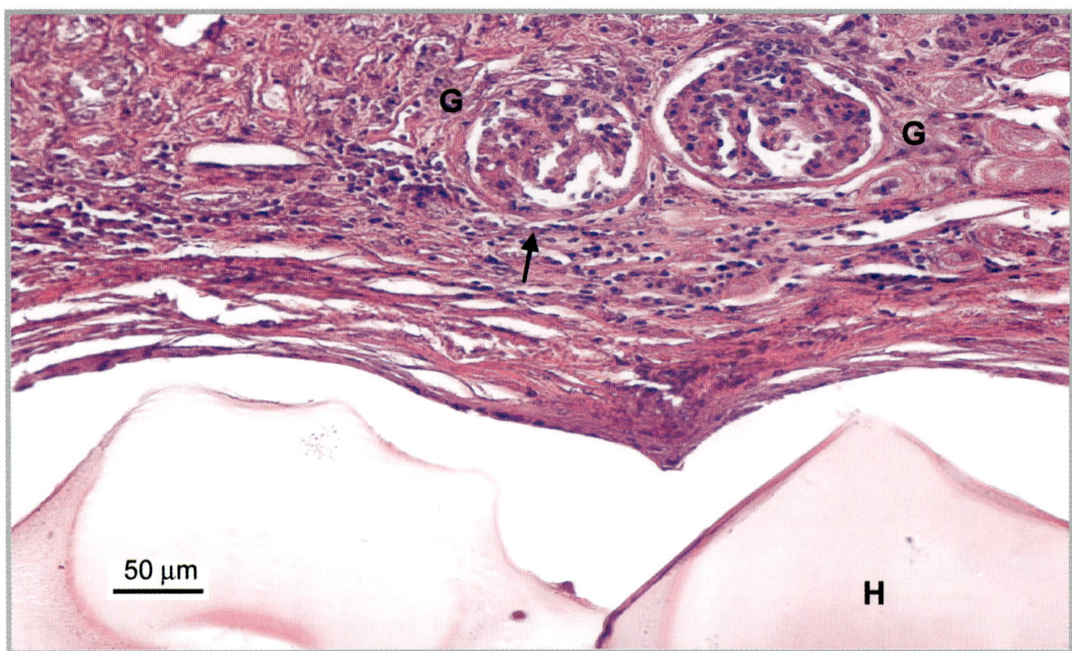

Figure 77C Embolization in blood vessels. H & E x 20
Higher magnification of mild inflammation and fibrosis (↑) present around the beads and glomeruli (G)

5

Retrieved Clinical Implants

Reports of failure of implanted devices following long term implantation in the human body have led to detailed investigation of the failed devices with adjacent tissue. Detailed study of changes of surface and bulk properties of the component material have revealed that these properties do change with long-term residence in the physiological environment. Microscopic examinations of the adjacent tissue have shown evidence of morphological and functional changes at the cellular and molecular level. Such studies have helped in developing materials with tailor made surface properties for better functioning. Material and biological changes compromise the functioning of the device with resultant failure and the need for revision surgery and replacement. Better and longer functioning devices are most needed in older patients whose health is already compromised due to geriatric changes. The study of these changes is important and will help industry in the development and manufacture of improved medical devices and will help clinicians to devise strategies to prevent adverse tissue responses leading to clinical failure.

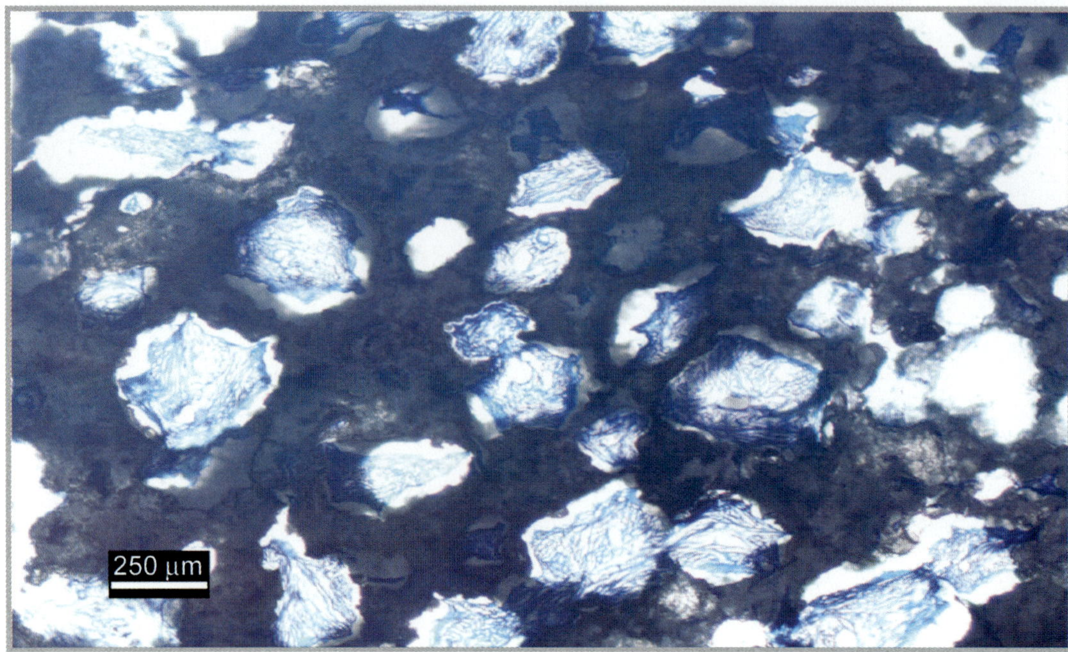

Figure 1A Porous hydroxyapatite implant in bone harvest site in iliac crest (one year), Stevenel's blue x 4
Fibrovascular tissue (blue) in the pores

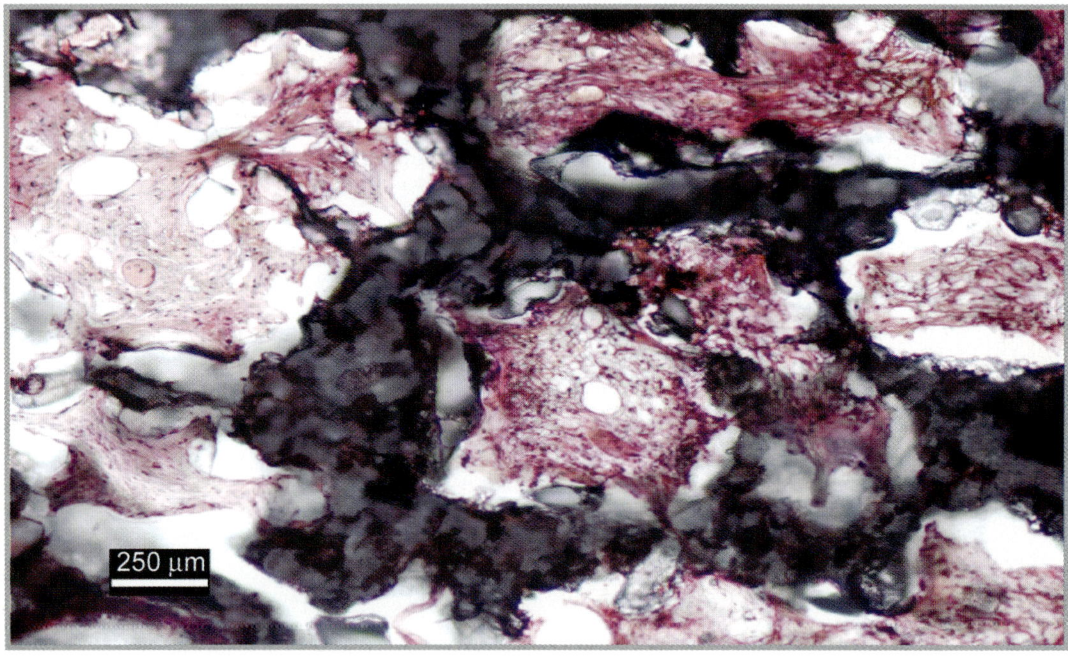

Figure 1B Porous hydroxyapatite implant in bone harvest site in iliac crest (one year). H & E x 4
Fibrovascular tissue (pink) in the pores

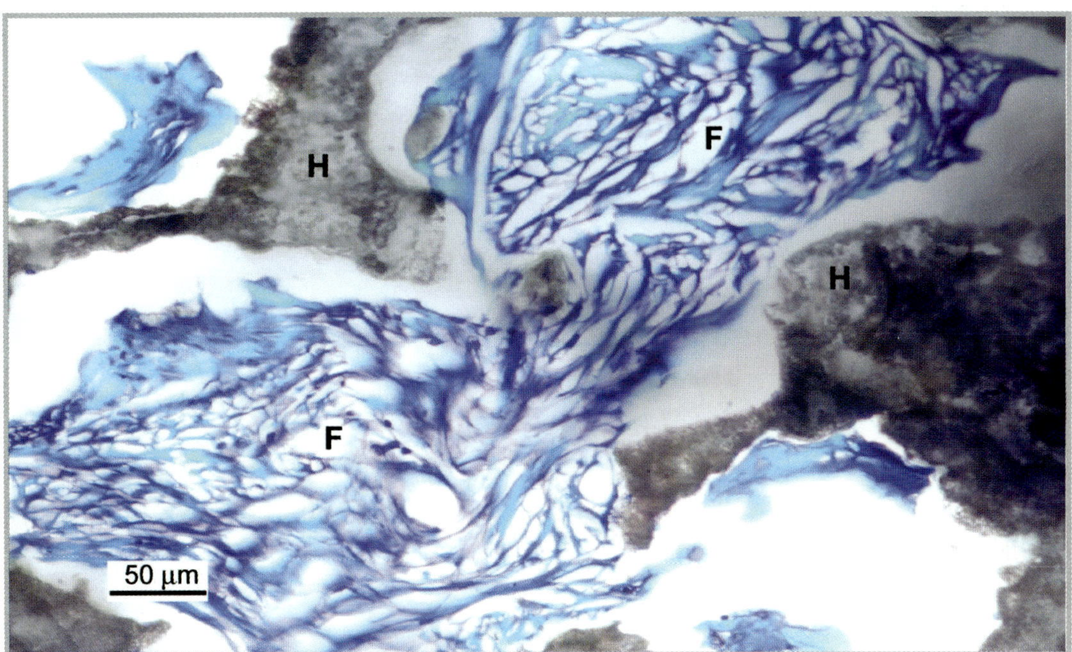

Figure 2 Fibrous tissue (F) in growth through pores in hydroxyapatite implant (H)
Stevenel's blue x 20

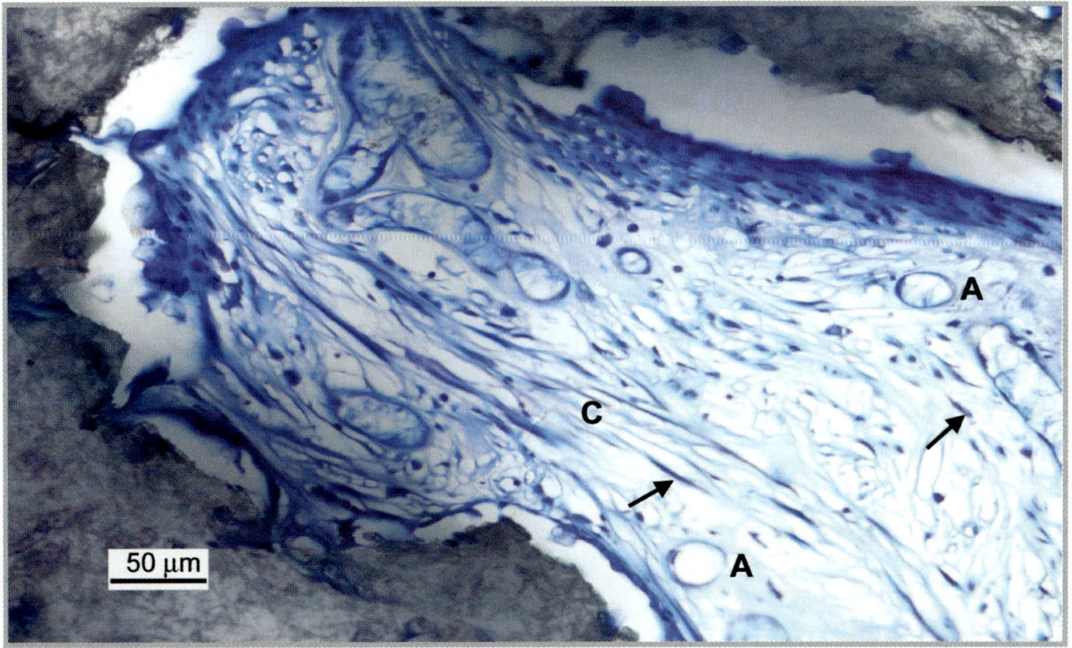

Figure 3A Fibrocytes (↑), collagen (C) and angiogenesis (A) in pore in hydroxyapatite porous implant
Stevenel's blue x 20

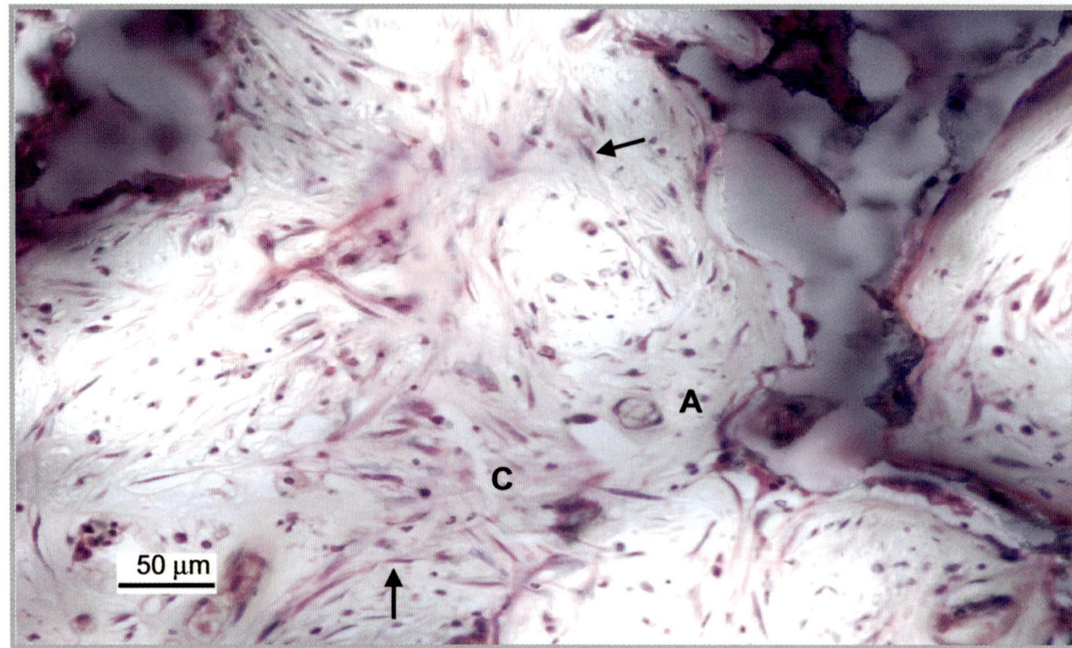

Figure 3B Fibrocytes (↑), collagen (C) and angiogenesis (A) in pore in hydroxyapatite porous implant.
H & E x 20

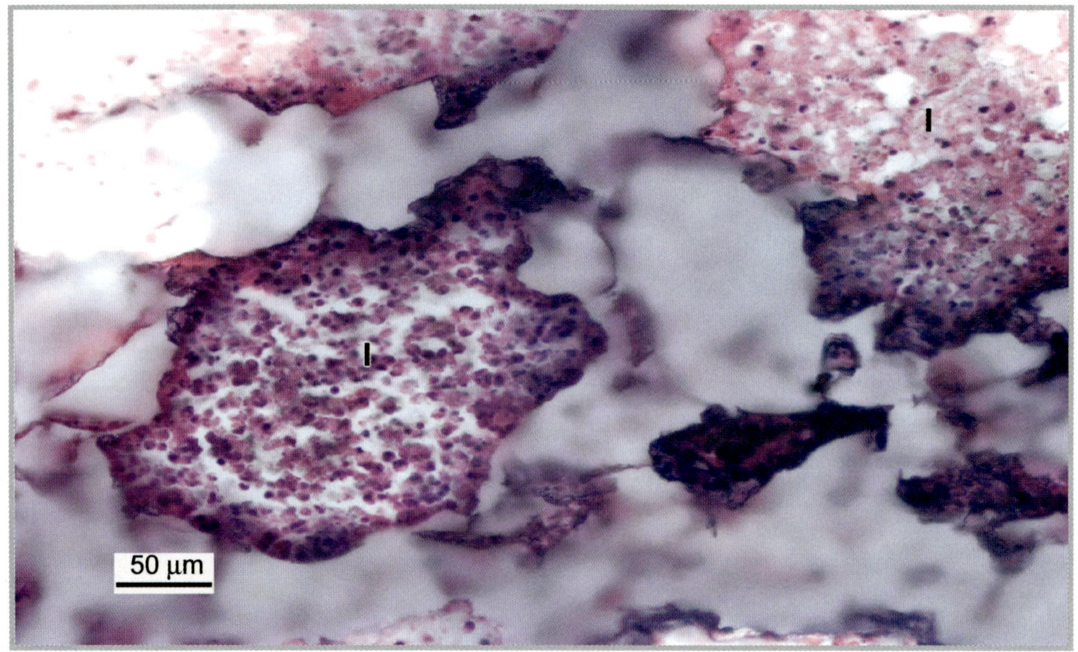

Figure 4 Inflammation (I) in pore in hydroxyapatite porous implant.
H & E x 20

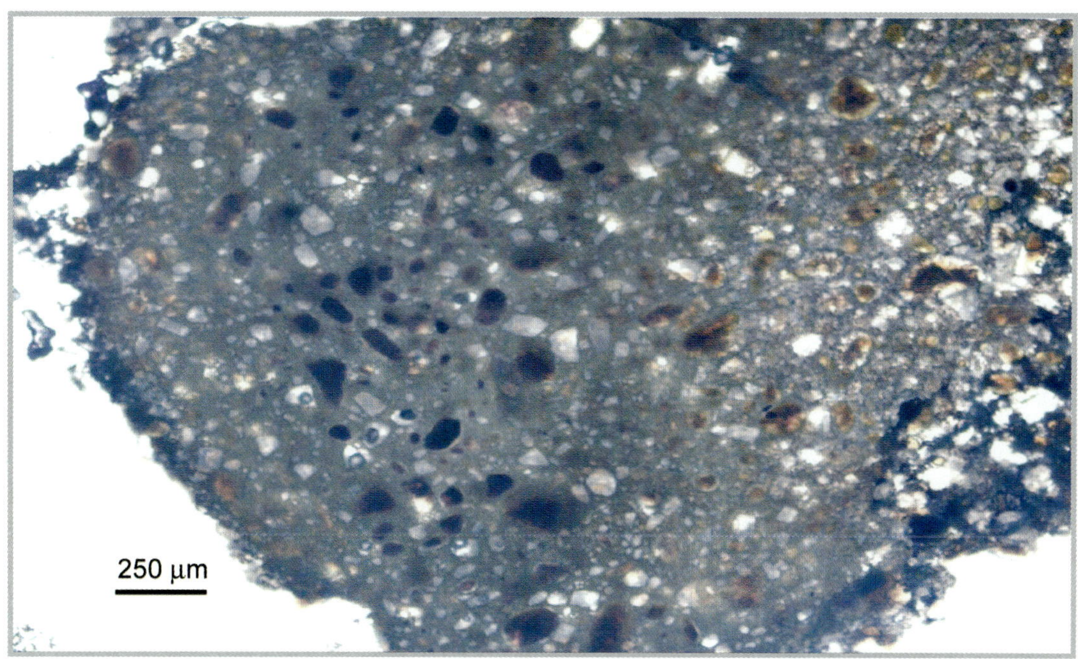

Figure 5A Absence of any tissue infiltration.
H & E x 4

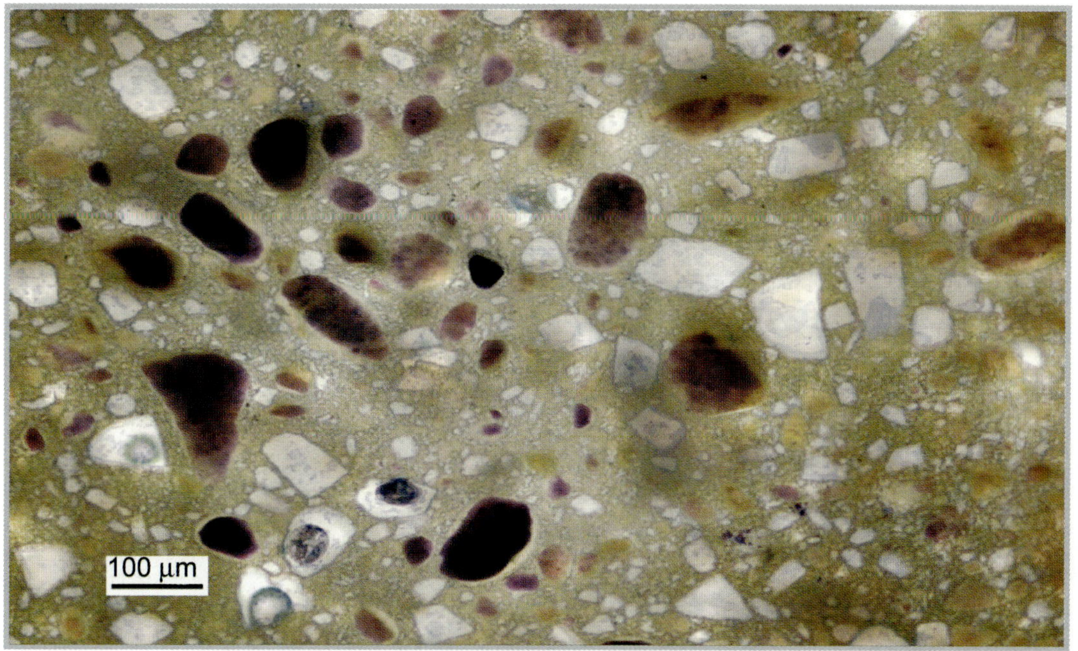

Figure 5B Absence of any tissue infiltration.
H & E x 10

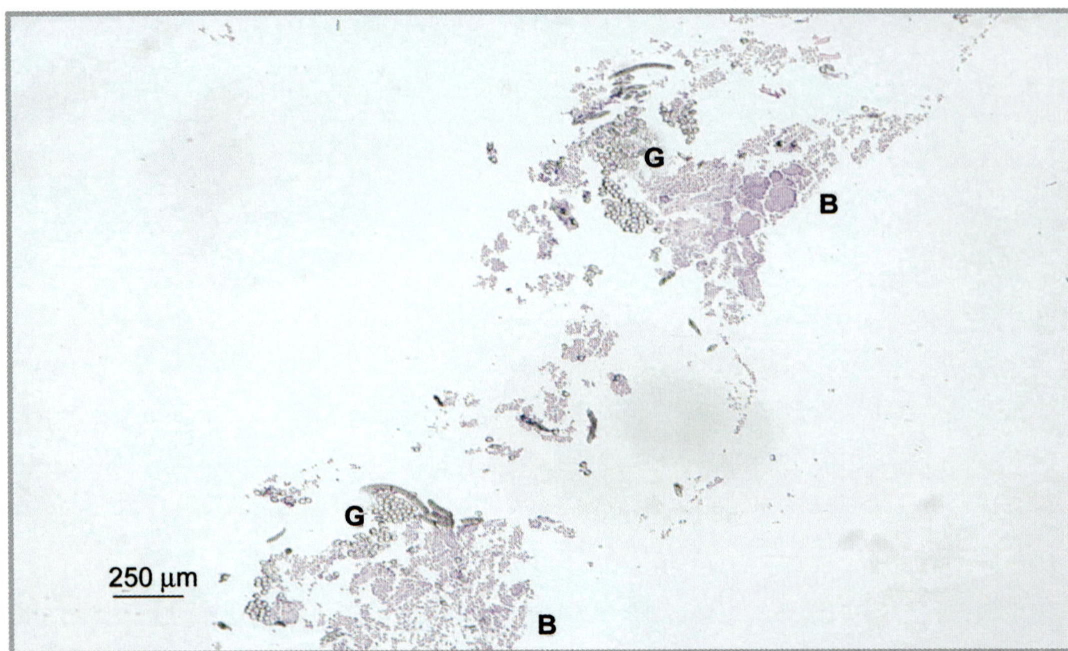

Figure 6A Cross-section of infected vascular graft (G) with bacterial colonies (B) in iliac artery, more than 1 year post implantation. H & E x 4

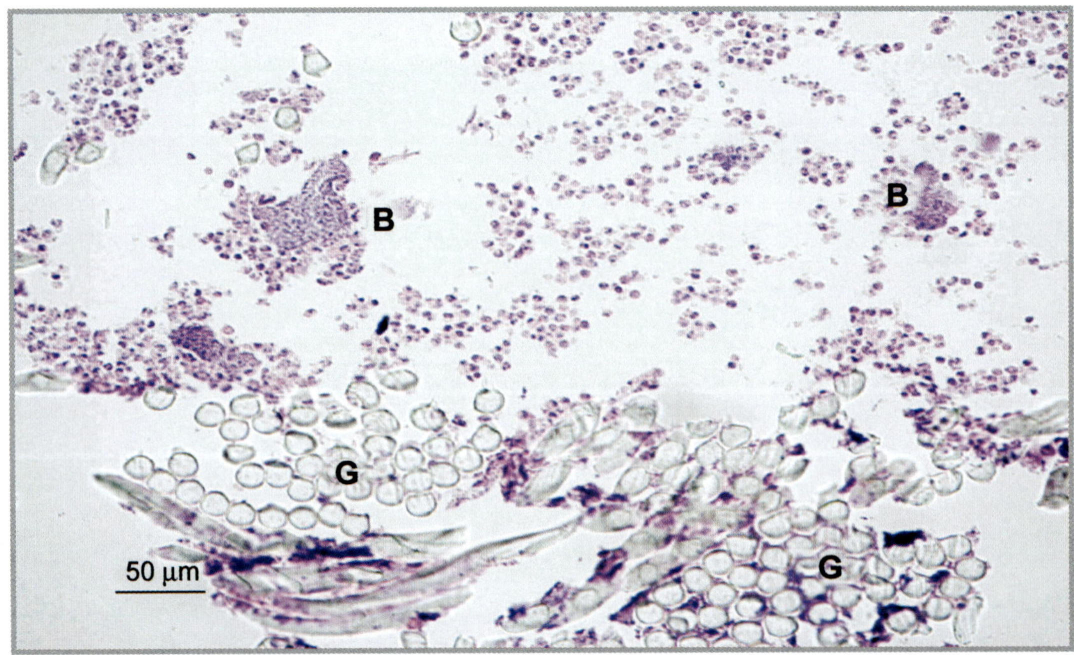

Figure 6B Higher magnification of cross-section of infected vascular graft (G) with bacterial colonies (B) between fibers of the graft. H & E x 20

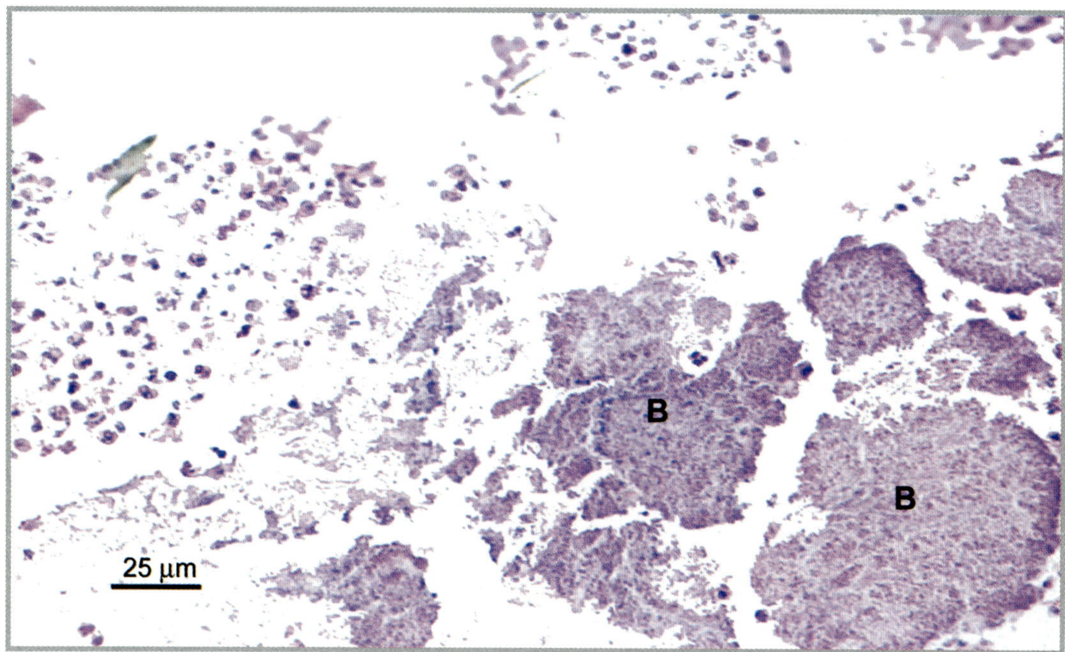

Figure 6C Bacterial colonies (B) in the graft.
H & E x 40

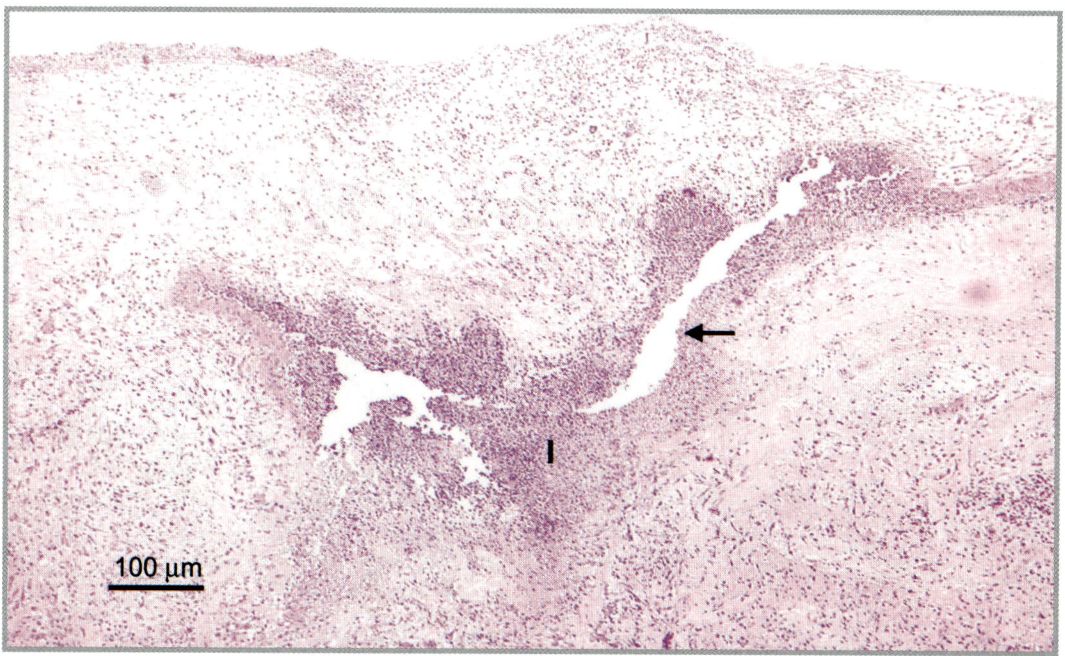

Figure 7A Inflammation (I) with macrophages at tissue interface (↑) with metal screw removed from fractured bone months after implantation. H & Ex 10

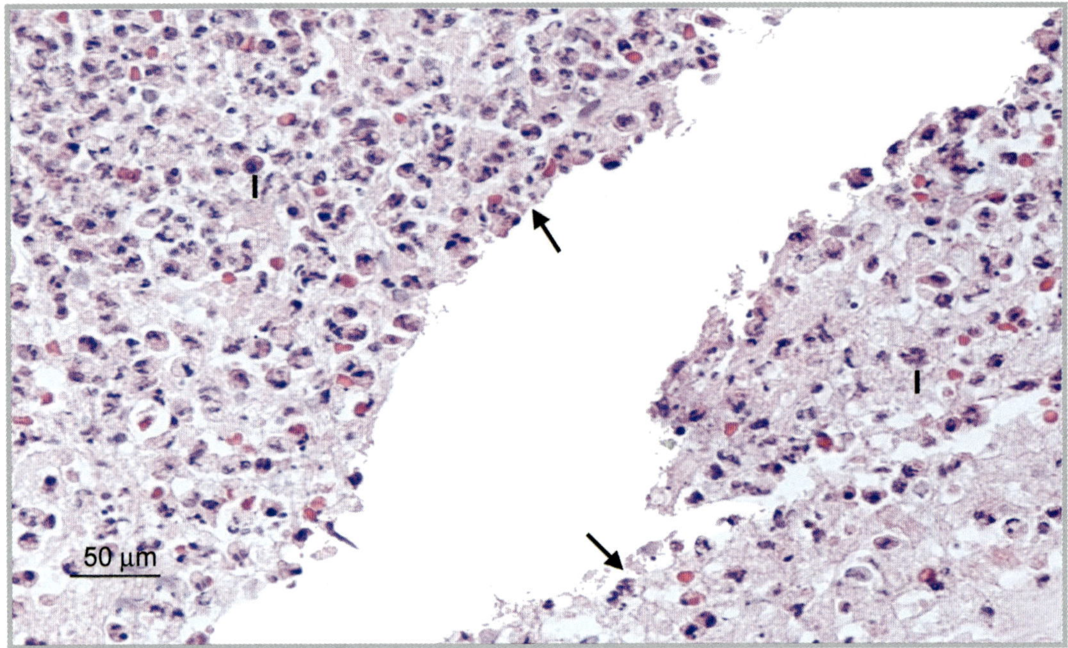

Figure 7B Severe inflammation with numerous inflammatory cells (↑) adjacent to a metal plate in bone. H & E x 20

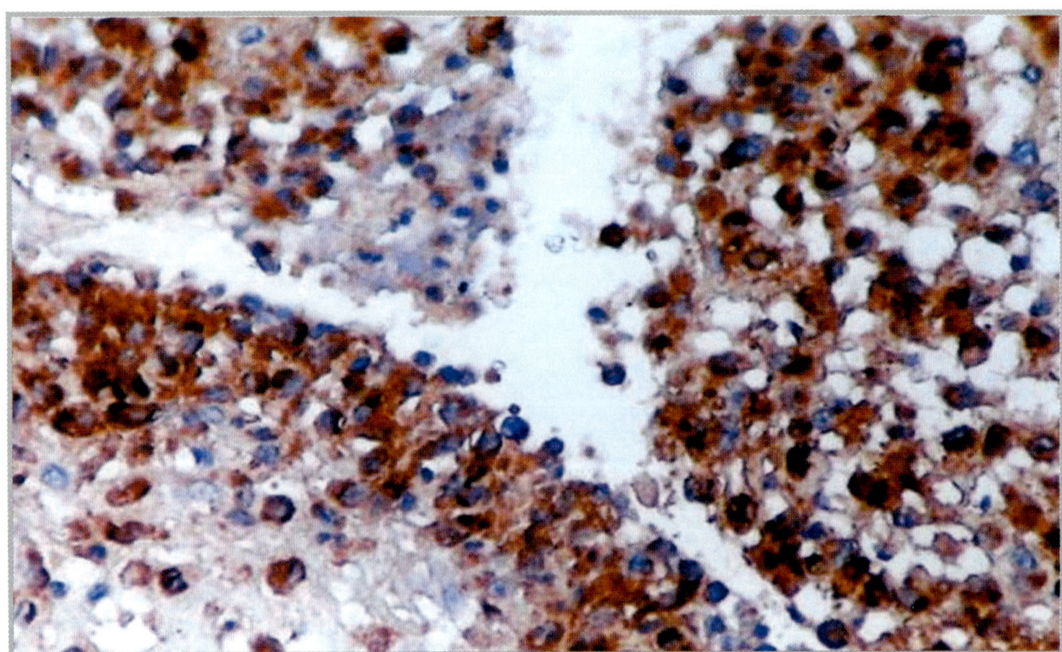

Figure 7C Macrophages stained brown with antibody, in tissue adjacent to metal plate, seven years post implantation. Immunohistochemical staining. Immunohistochemical staining x 40

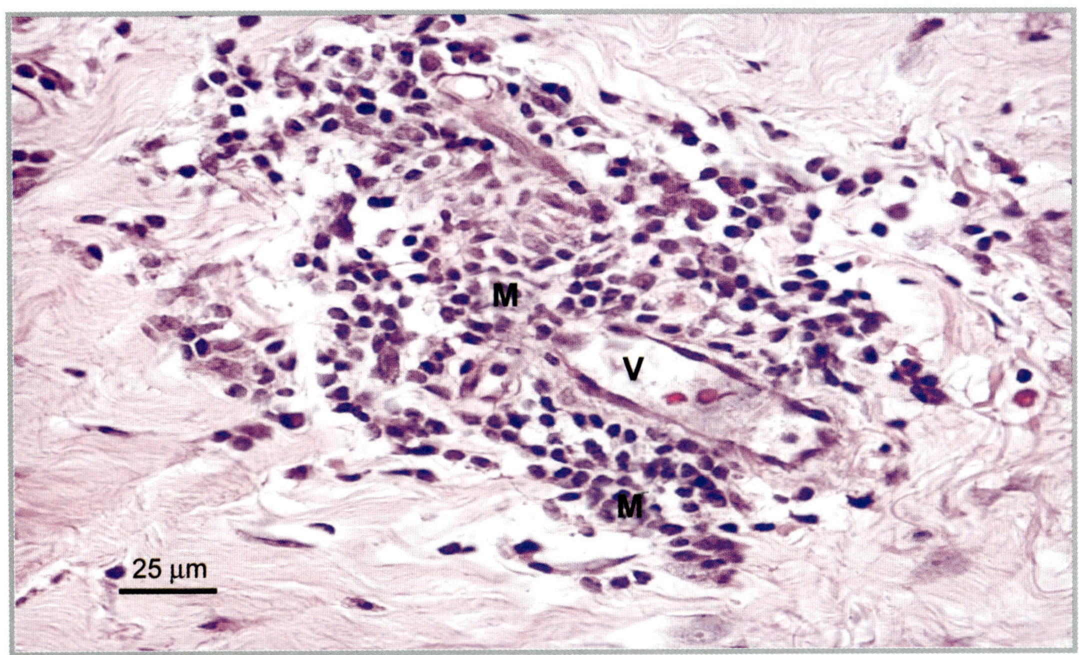

Figure 7D Perivascular inflammation in tissue adjacent to a metal plate. Macrophages (M) are seen around the blood vessel (V). H & E x 40

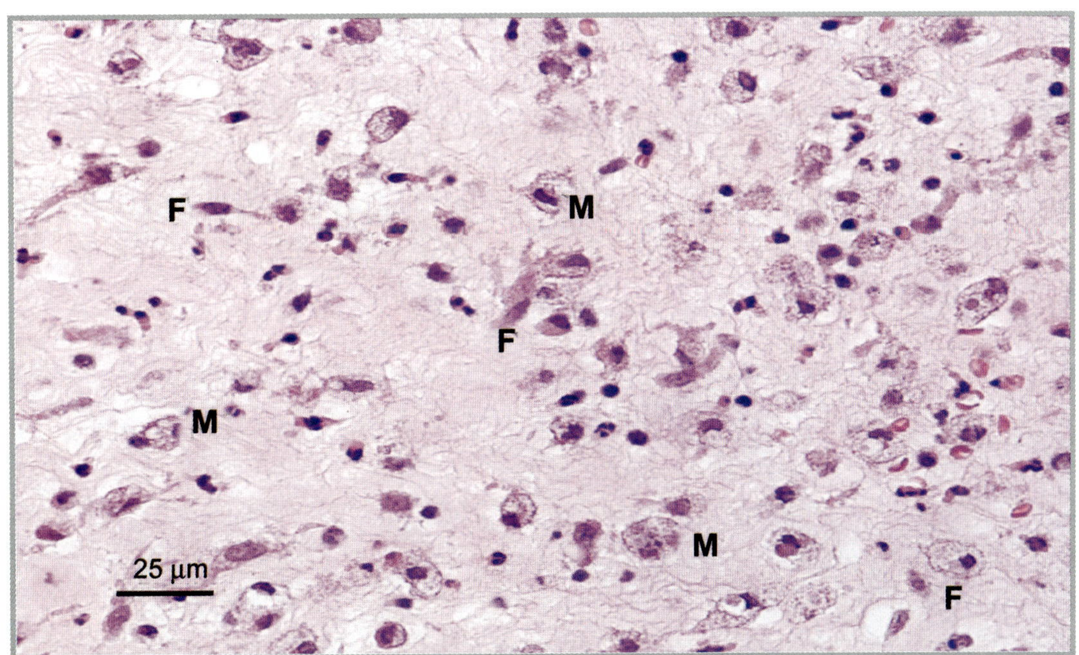

Figure 8A Foamy macrophages (M) and fibroblasts (F) in tissue adjacent to metal plate. H & E x 40

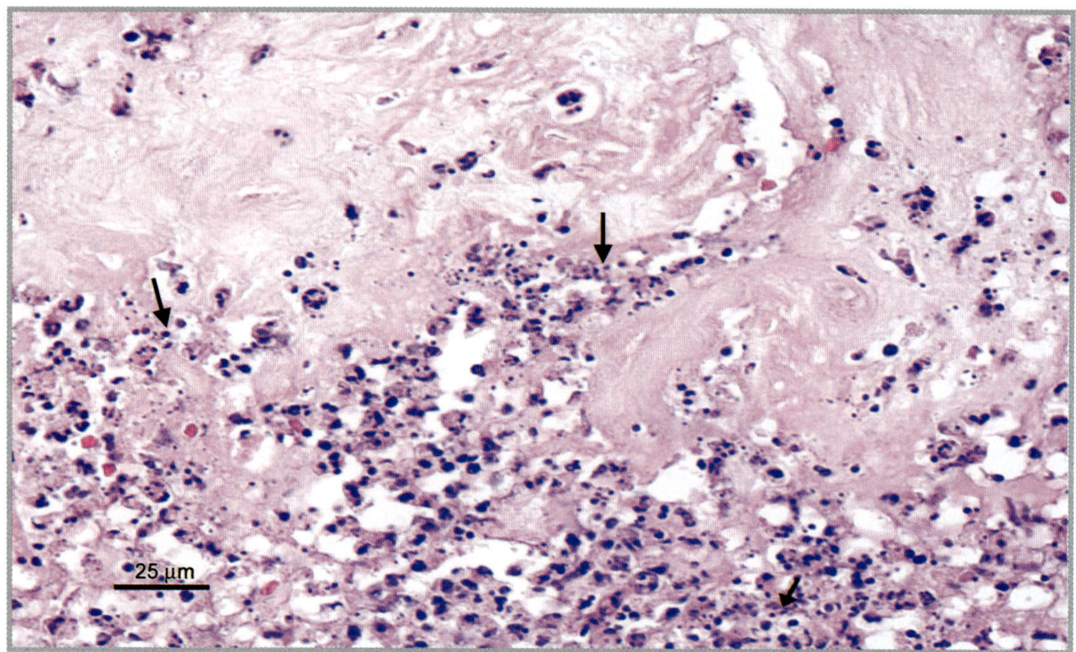

Figure 8B Cellular debri (↑) in tissue adjacent to metal plate. H & E x 40

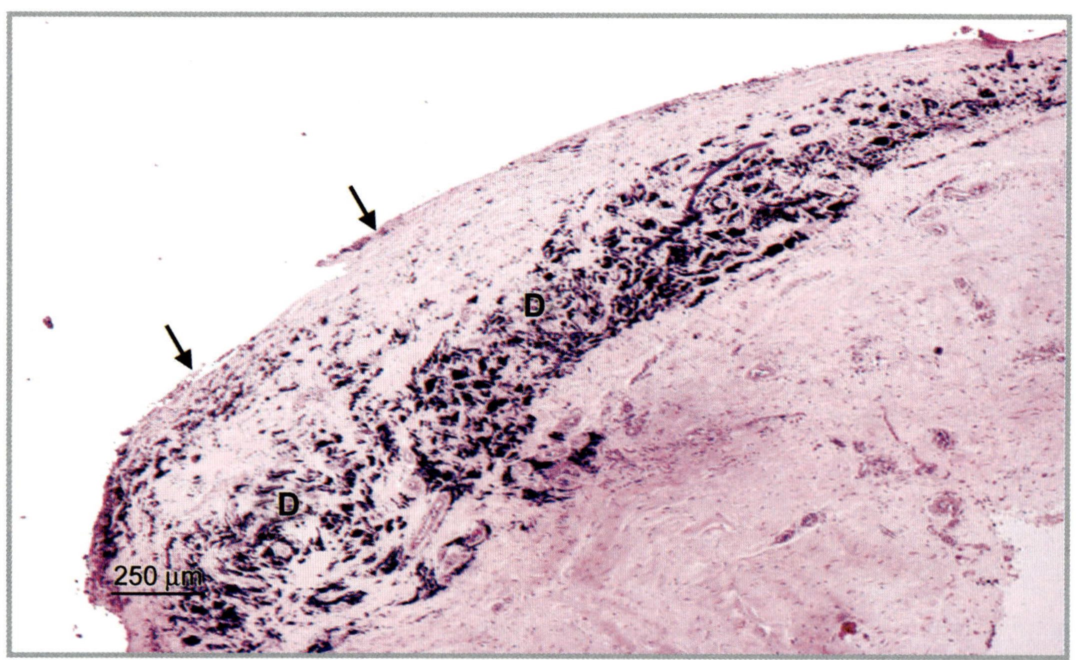

Figure 9A Dense black metal debri (D) at interface (↑) with metal plate. H & E x 4

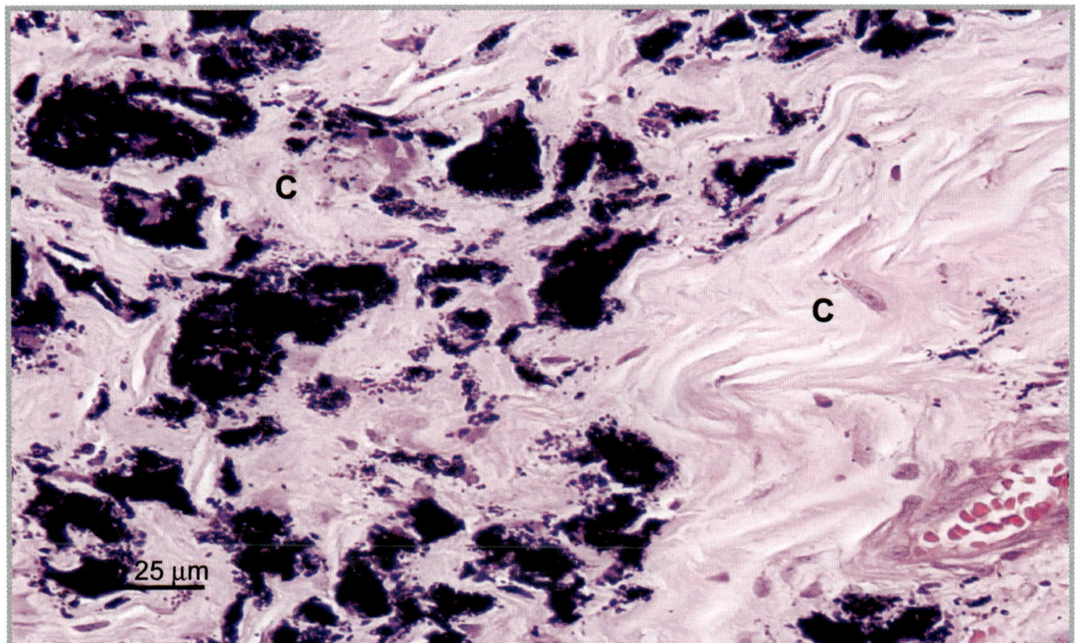

Figure 9B Dense black metal debri at interface with metal plate. Thick collagen (C) with occasional macrophages. H & E x 40

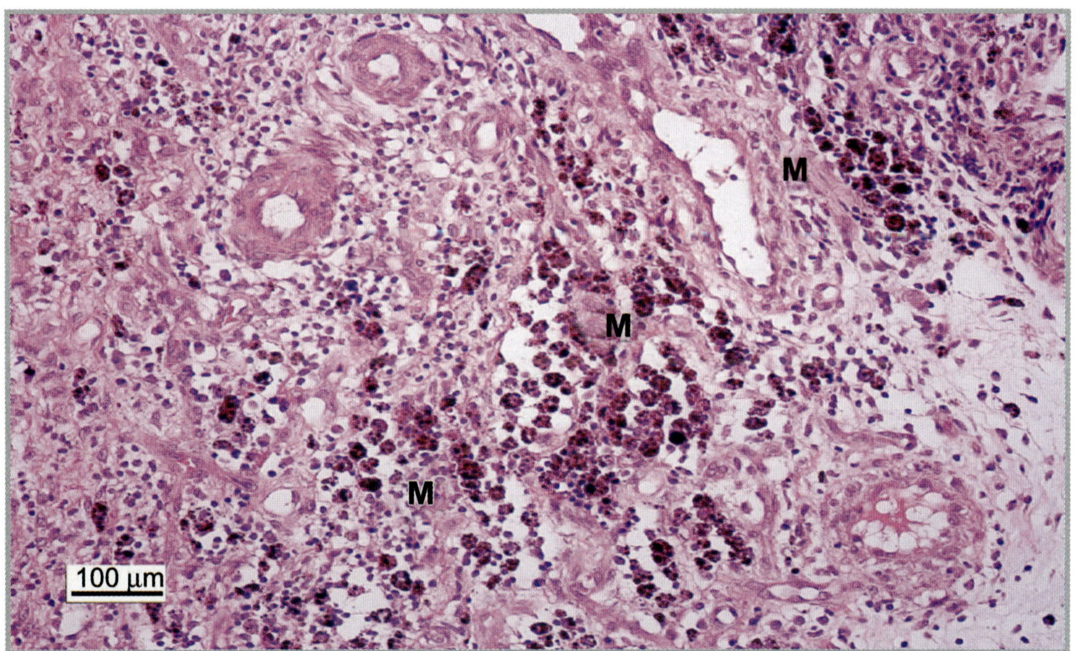

Figure 10A Golden brown hemosiderin laden macrophages (M) indicating old hemorrhage at interface with metal plate. H & E x 10

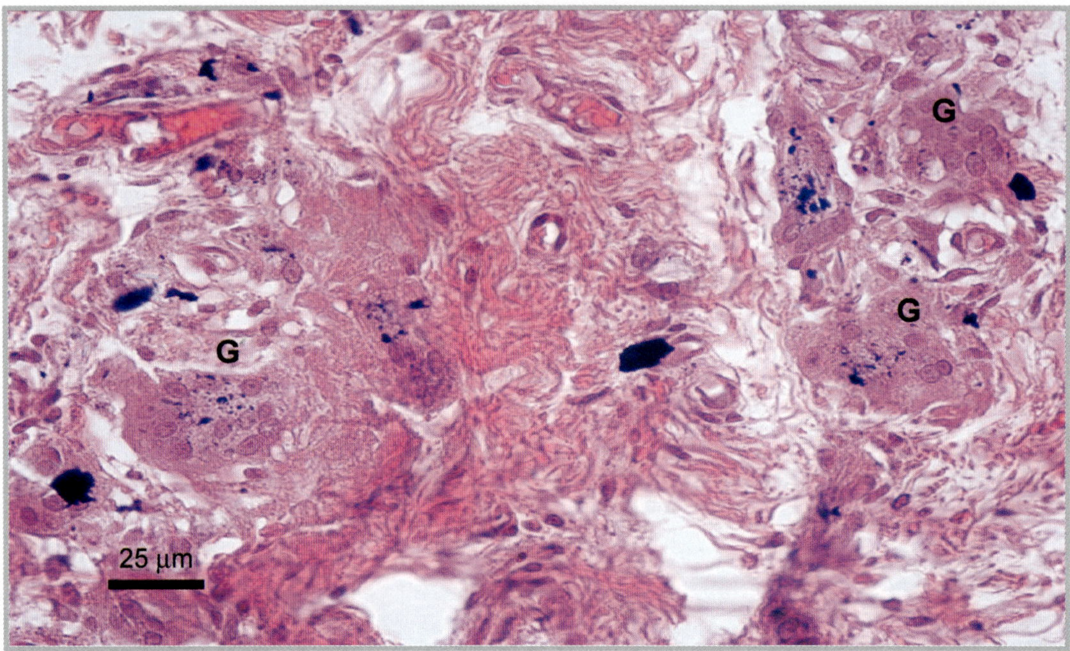

Figure 10B Black metal debri in foreign body type of giant cells (G) at interface with metal plate. H & E x 40

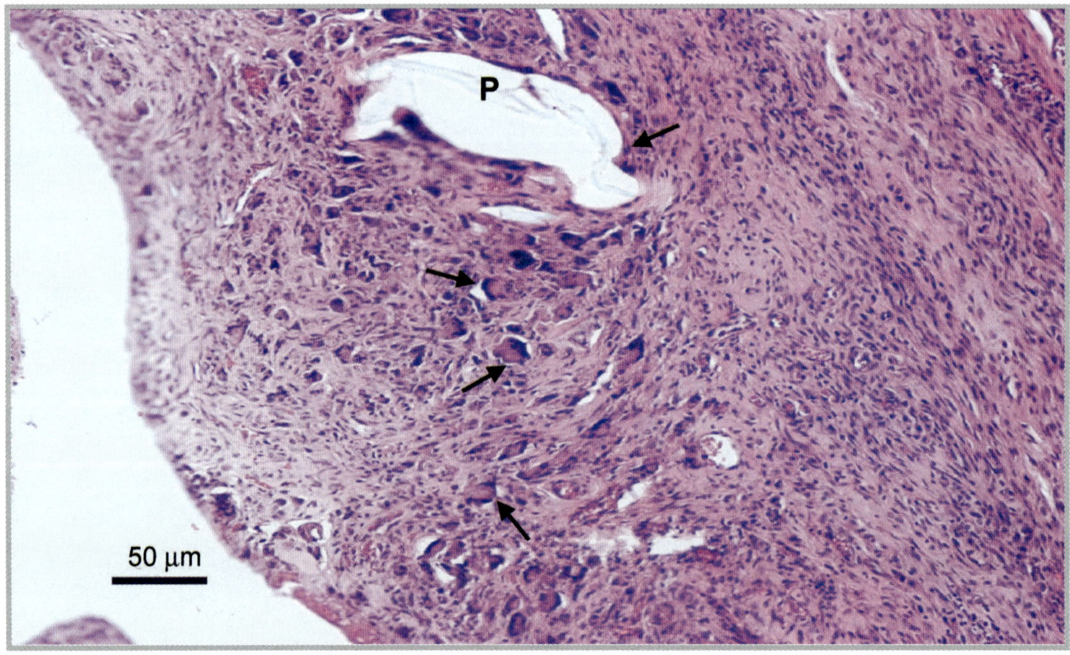

Figure 11A Severe inflammation with numerous macrophages and foreign body giant cells (FBGC) (↑) with a piece of polyethylene (P). H & E x 20

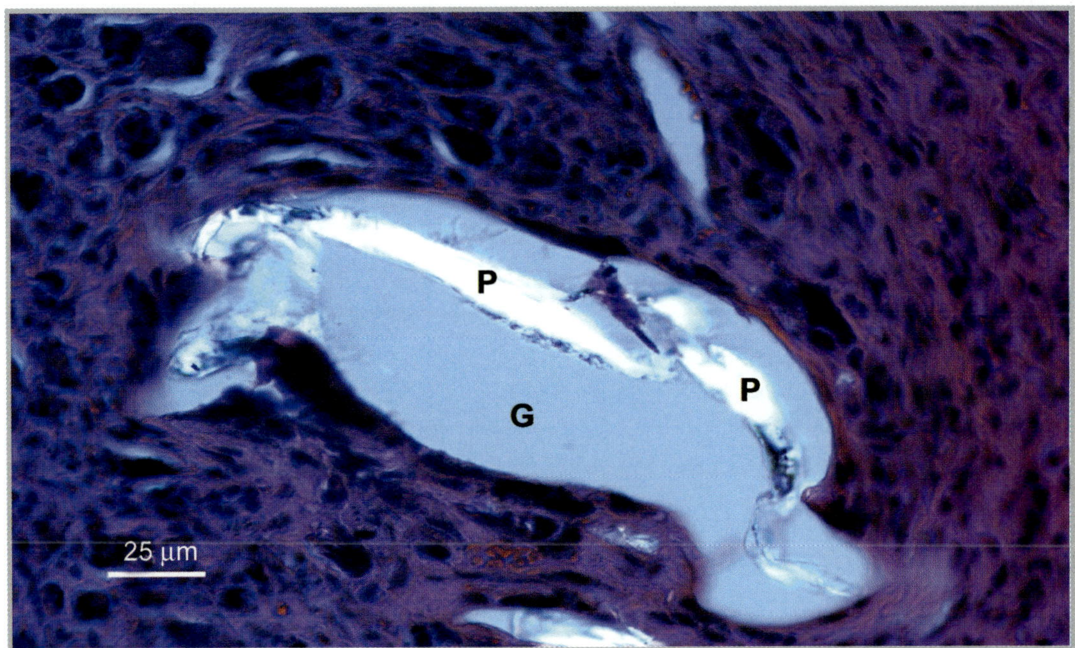

Figure 11B Large FBGC (G) with a piece of polyethylene (P). Polarized light microscopy. H & E x 40

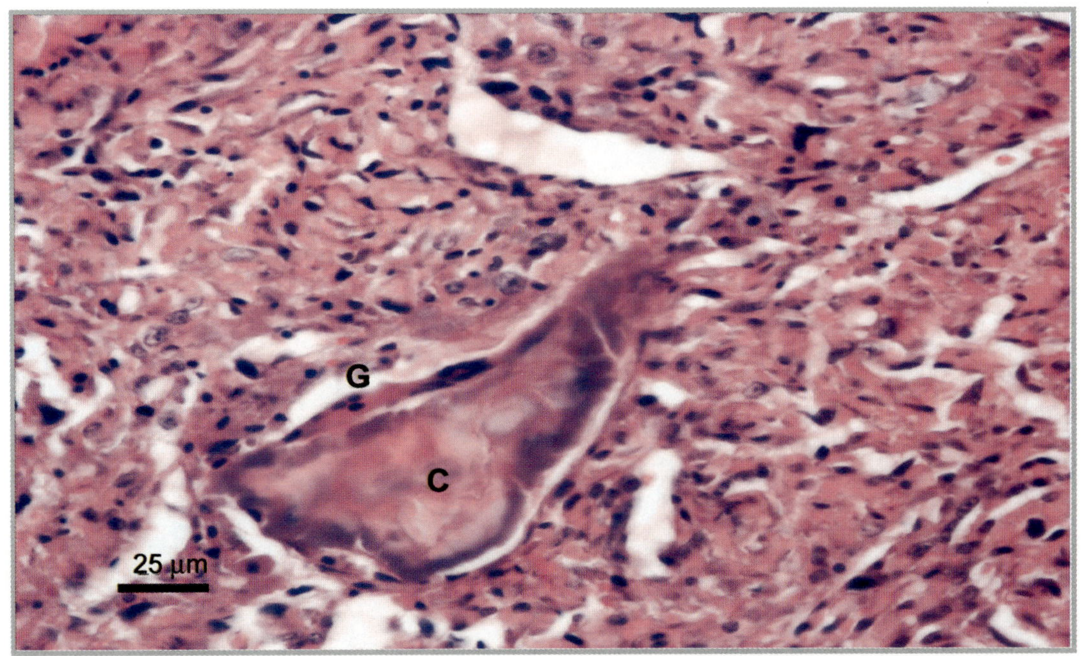

Figure 11C Cement (C) in FBGC (G). H & E x 40

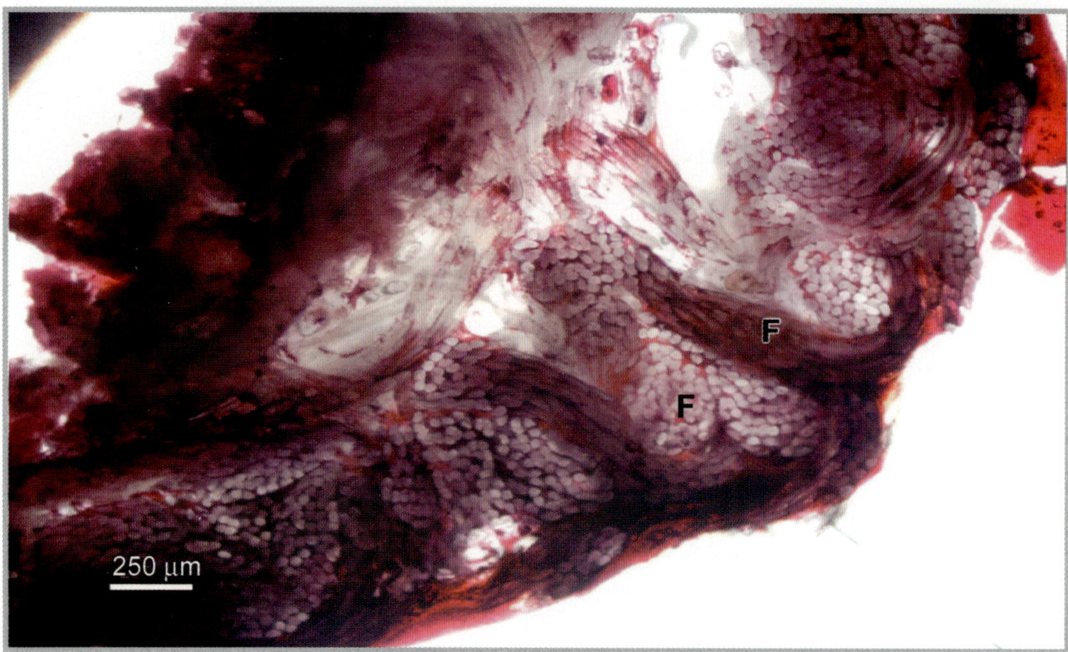

Figure 12 Sewing ring of mechanical heart valve. Pattern of fabric fibers (F). H & E x 4 Resin section

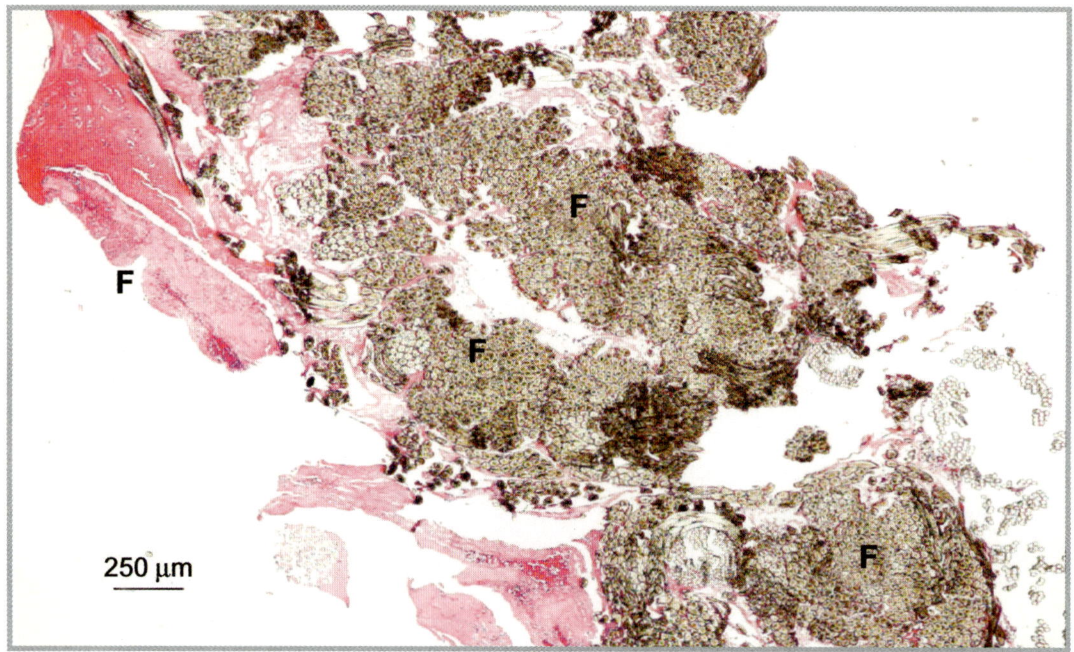

Figure 13A Sewing ring of mechanical heart valve. Fibrin thrombus at flow edge left and fibrin (F) in intercises of the sewing ring. H & E x 4 Paraffin section

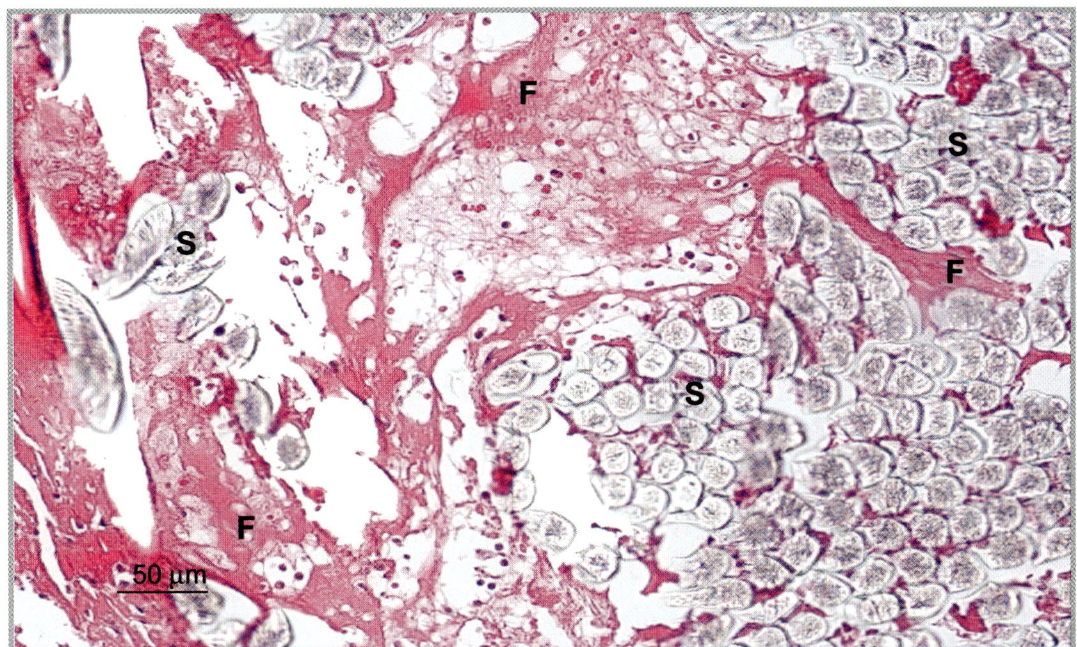

Figure 13B Sewing ring of mechanical heart valve. Fibrin (F) in intercises of the sewing ring (S). H & E x 20 Paraffin section

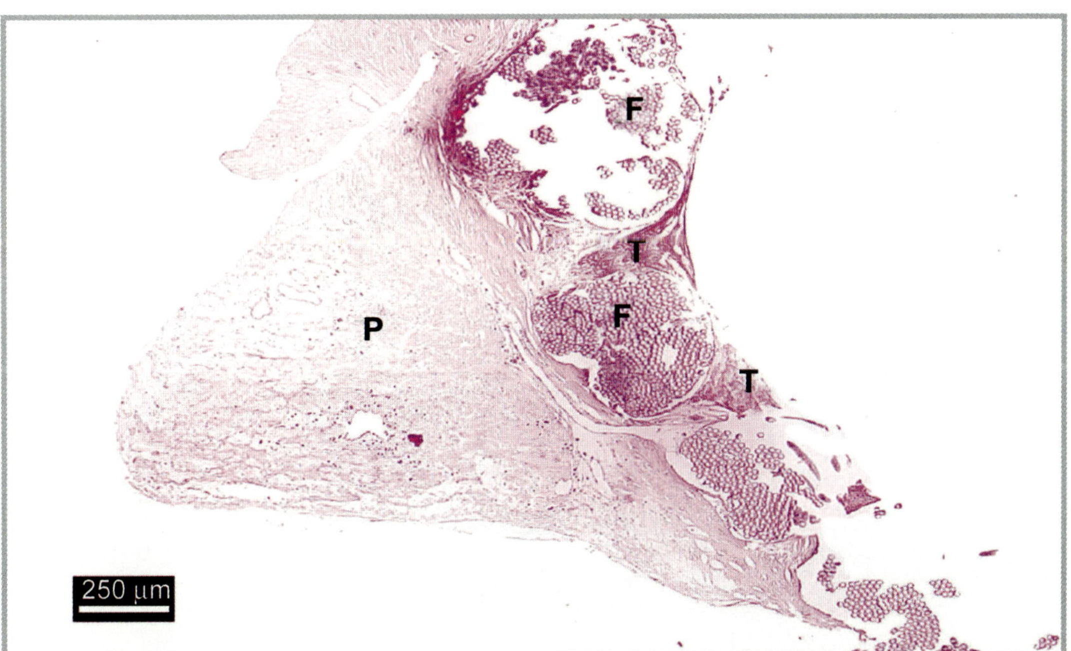

Figure 14A Tissue ingrowth (T) into pores in between bundles of fabric fibers (F) of sewing ring of mechanical heart valve. Pannus (P) formation from inner surface. H & E x 4

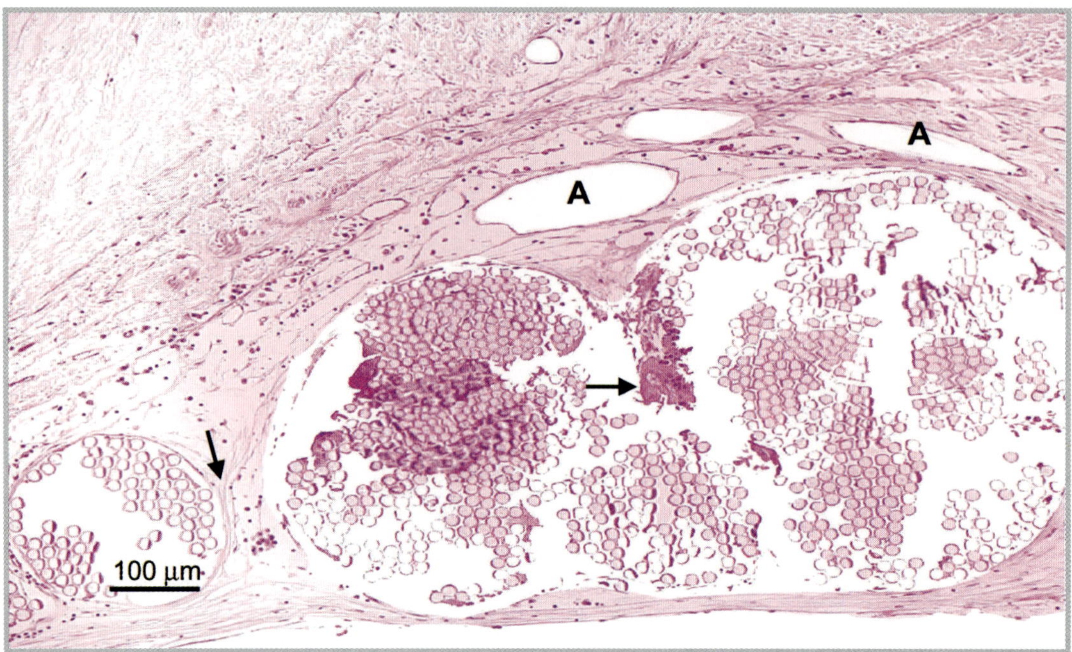

Figure 14B Mild cellular infiltration and fibrin (↑) in between individual fabric fibers. Numerous thin walled blood vessels (A) indicating angiogenesis are seen. H & E x 10

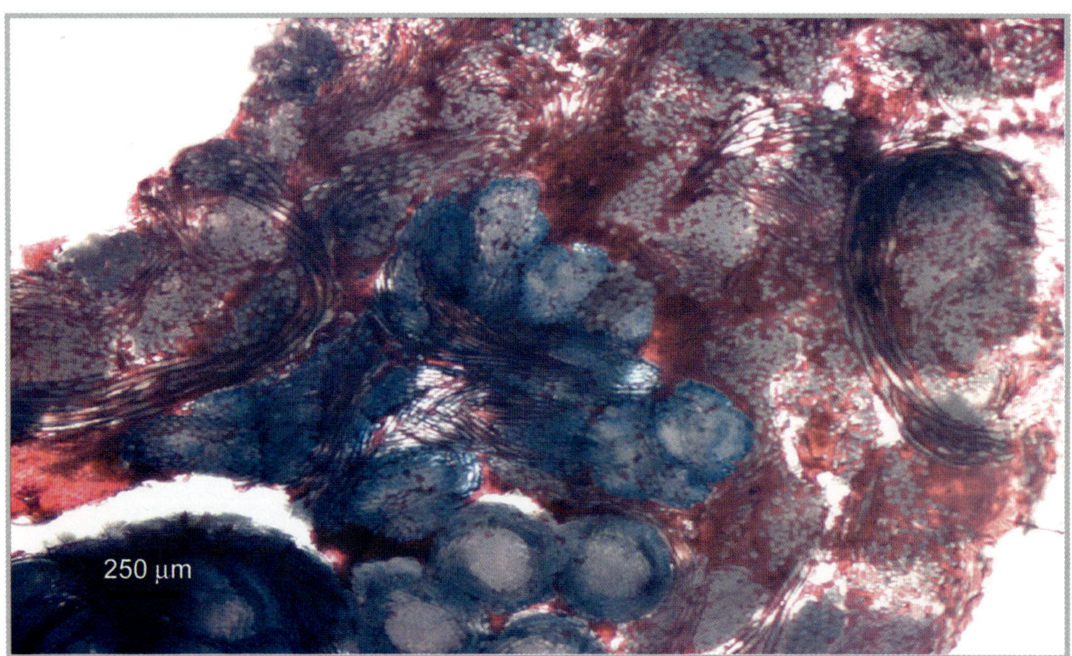

Figure 15A Sewing ring of mechanical heart valve. Different pattern of fabric fiber bundles. H & E x 4 Resin section

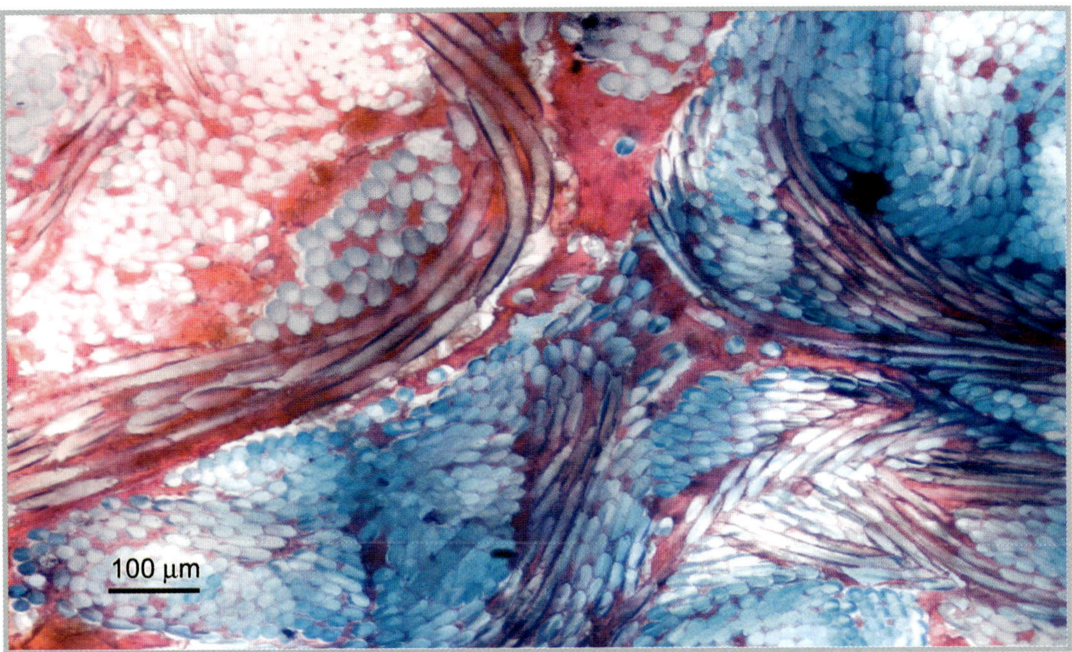

Figure 15B Different running pattern of fabric fibers. H & E x 10

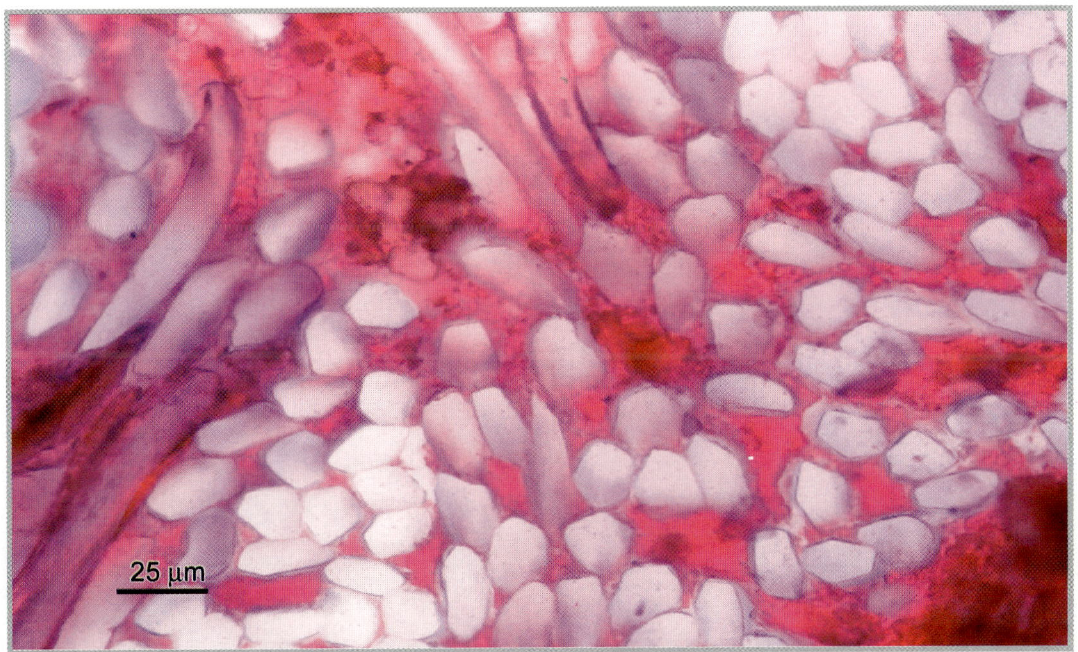

Figure 15C Higher magnification of cross-section of fabric fibers in sewing ring of mechanical heart valve. H & E x 40

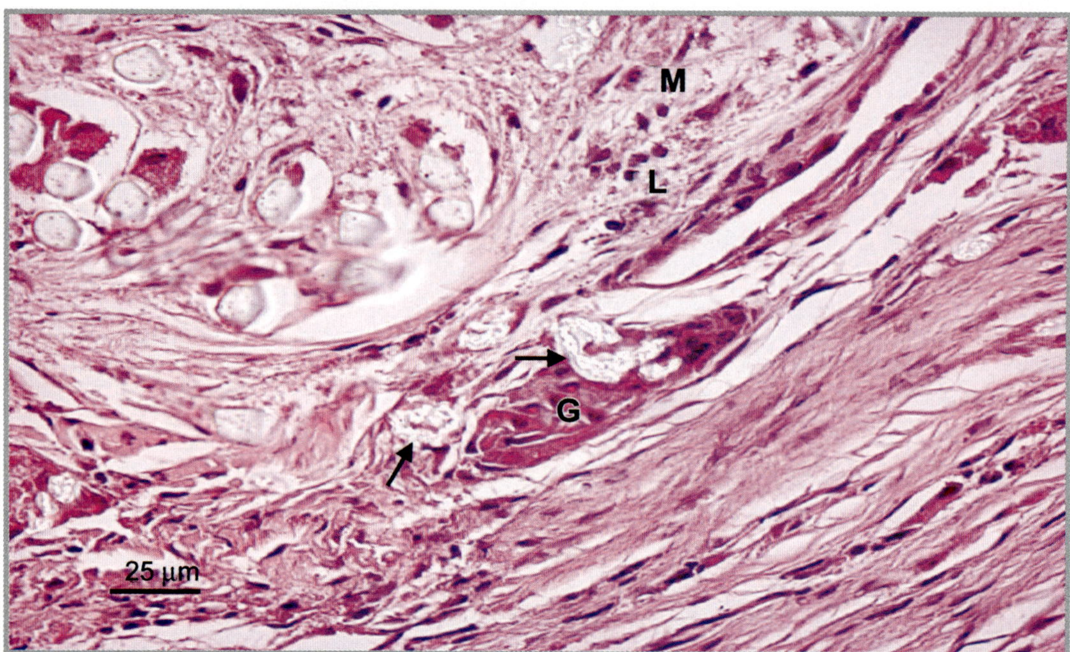

Figure 16 Foamy macrophages (M), lymphocytes (L) and foreign body type of giant cells (G) infiltrating the intercises of the sewing ring of a mechanical heart valve years after implantation. Fragments of the fabric (↑) are phagocytosed by the FBGC. H & E x 40

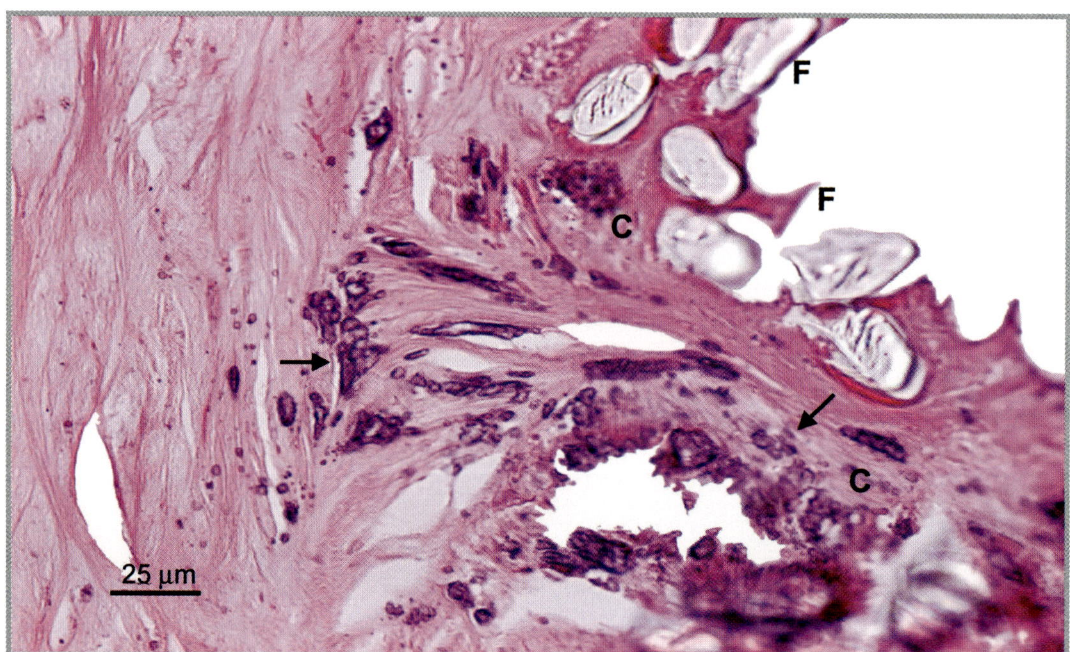

Figure 17A Spotty (↑) and moderate calcification (C) in sewing ring, in between fabric fibers (F) years after implantation. H & E x 40

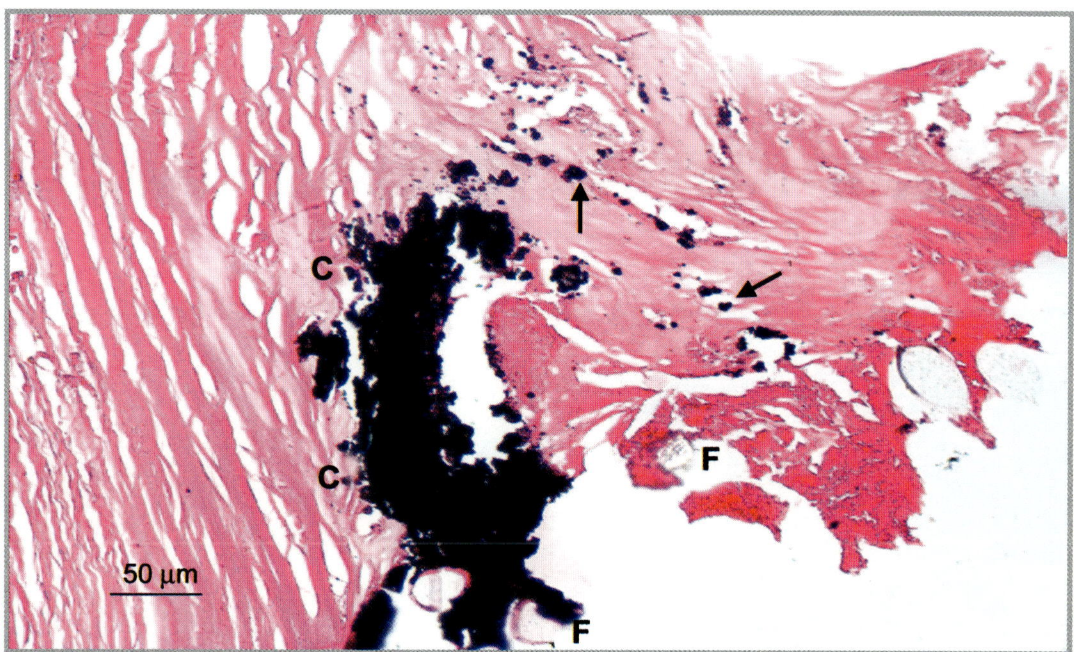

Figure 17B Calcified areas (C) and spotty calcification (↑) specifically stained with Von Kossa, in tissue in between fragments of fabric (F). Von Kossa x 20

6

Artifacts

Sometimes, when the section is seen under the microscope, we may see objects which should not be there in the section. These are called artifacts. The viewer should be aware of such artifacts during observation and not view them as part of the tissue response.

Some of these artifacts are accidentally introduced during the implantation procedure and elicit a tissue response adjacent to the implant. In such cases, it is not proper to evaluate the response to the implant material itself. Some artifacts can also occur due to improper processing, cutting and staining of the sections.

This chapter has few images of such artifacts.

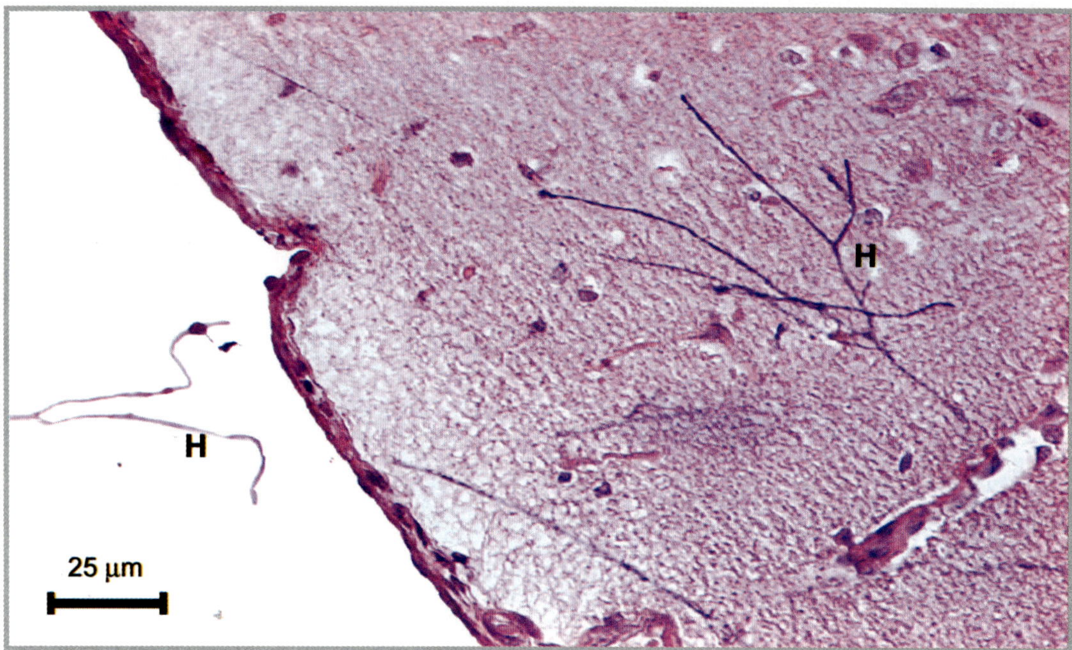

Figure 1 Fungal hyphae (H) on a section. The staining solution is contaminated with fungus. H & E x 40

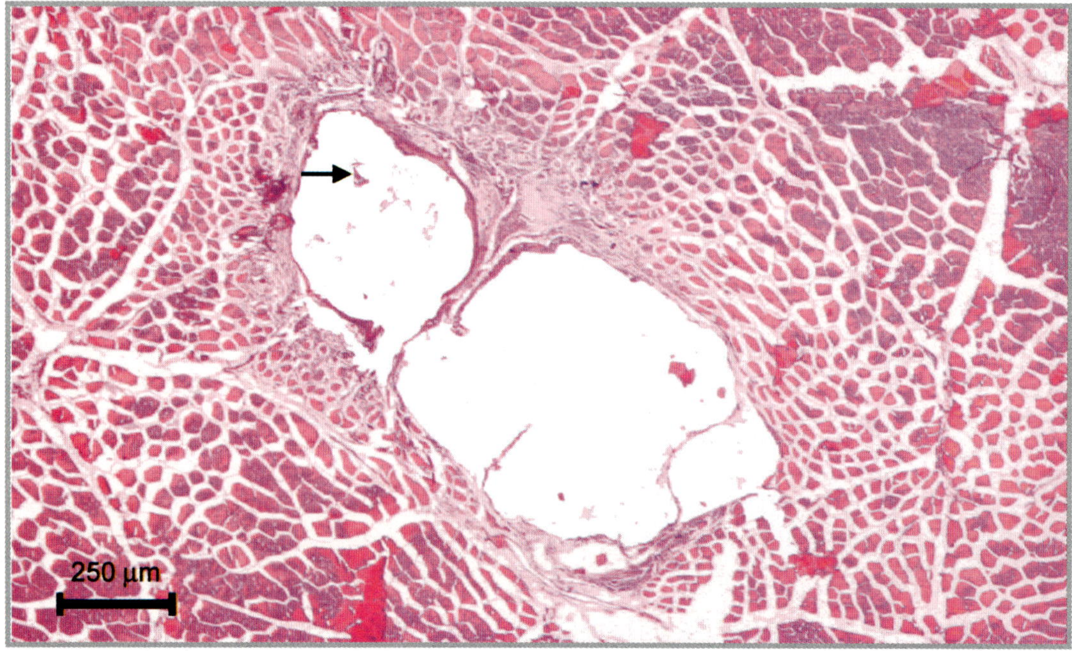

Figure 2A Fragments of hair (↑) introduced during implantation cause an inflammatory response adjacent to implant site. This section should not be evaluated for biocompatibility. H & E x 4

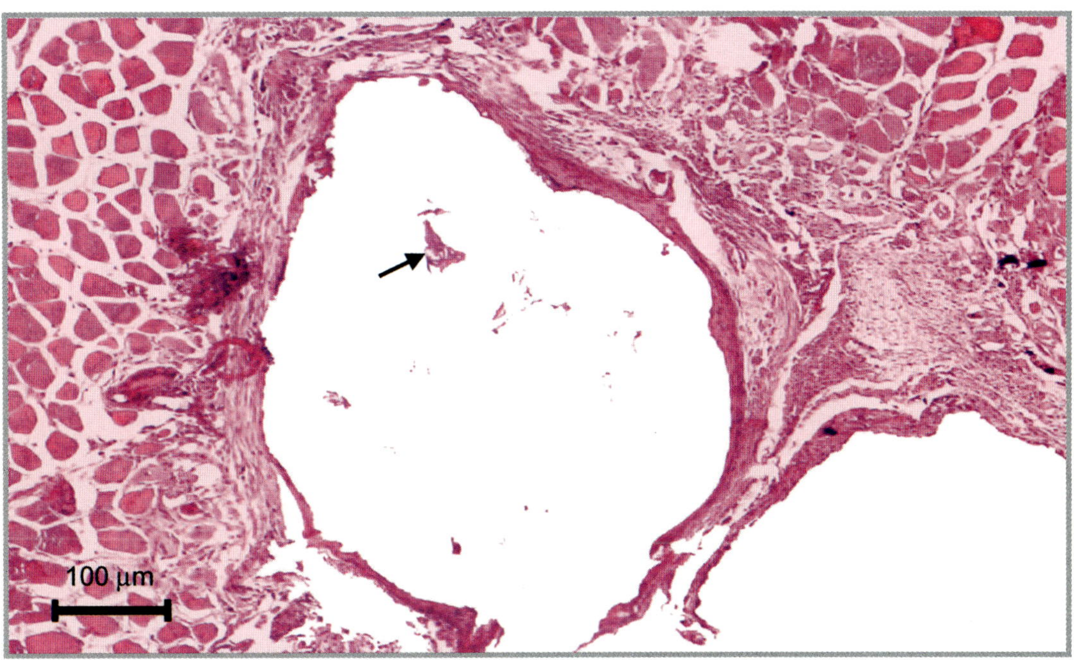

Figure 2B Higher magnification of fragment of hair (↑).
H & E x 10

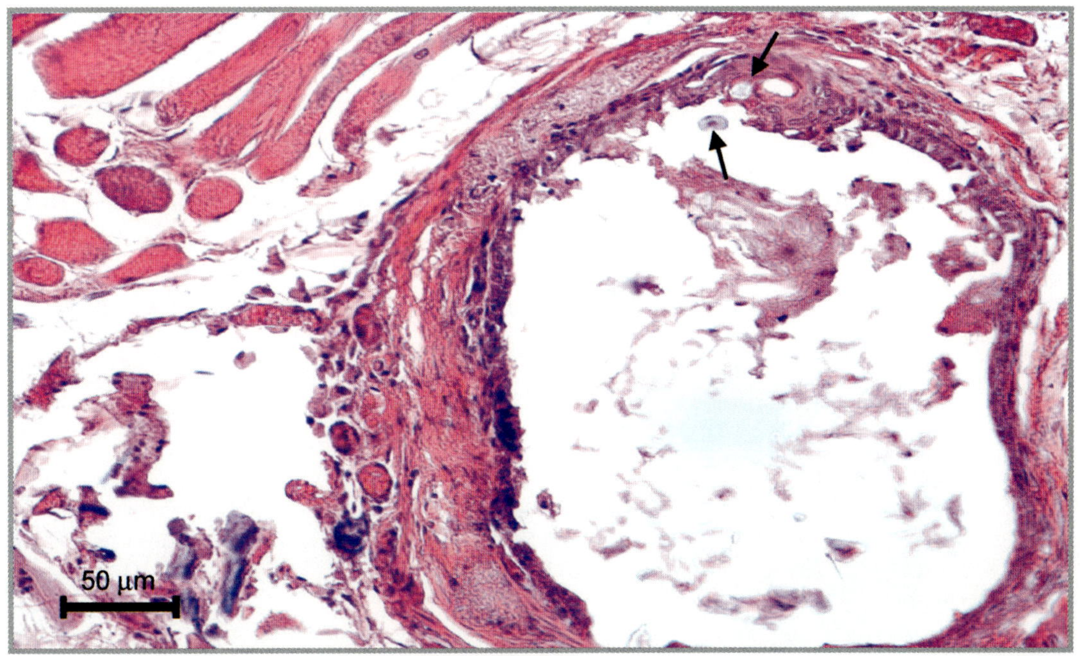

Figure 2C Fragments of hair (↑) introduced during implantation.
H & E x 20

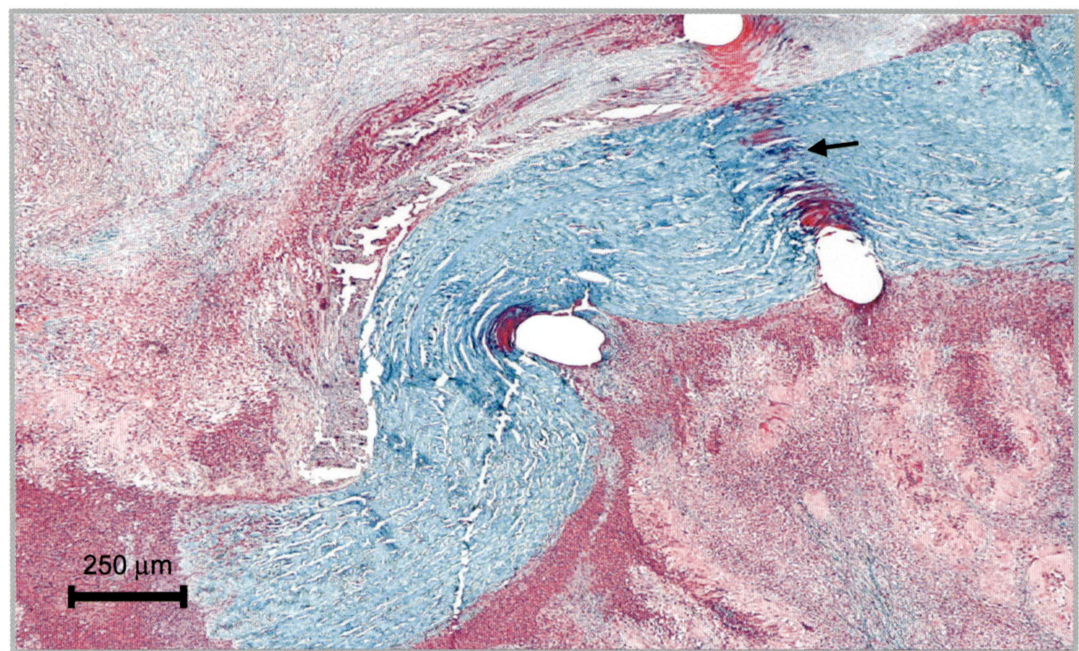

Figure 3 Damaged knife causes nicks (↑) in section.
H & E x 4

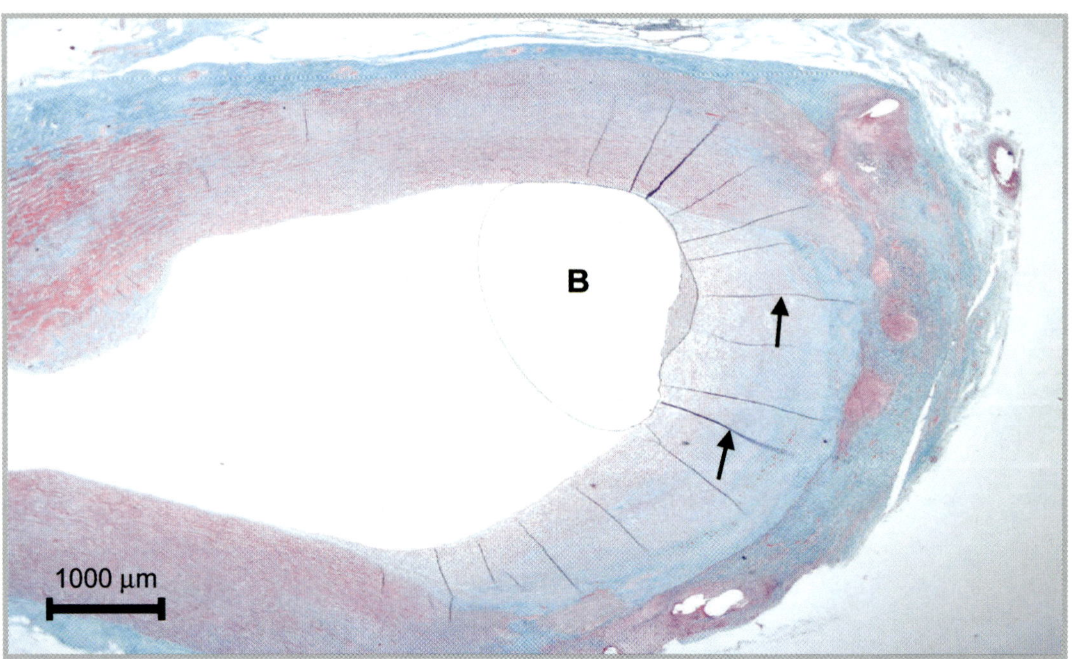

Figure 4 Air bubble (B) introduced during coverslipping of paraffin section. Folds (↑) in section due to improper expansion of section on water bath. H & E x 1

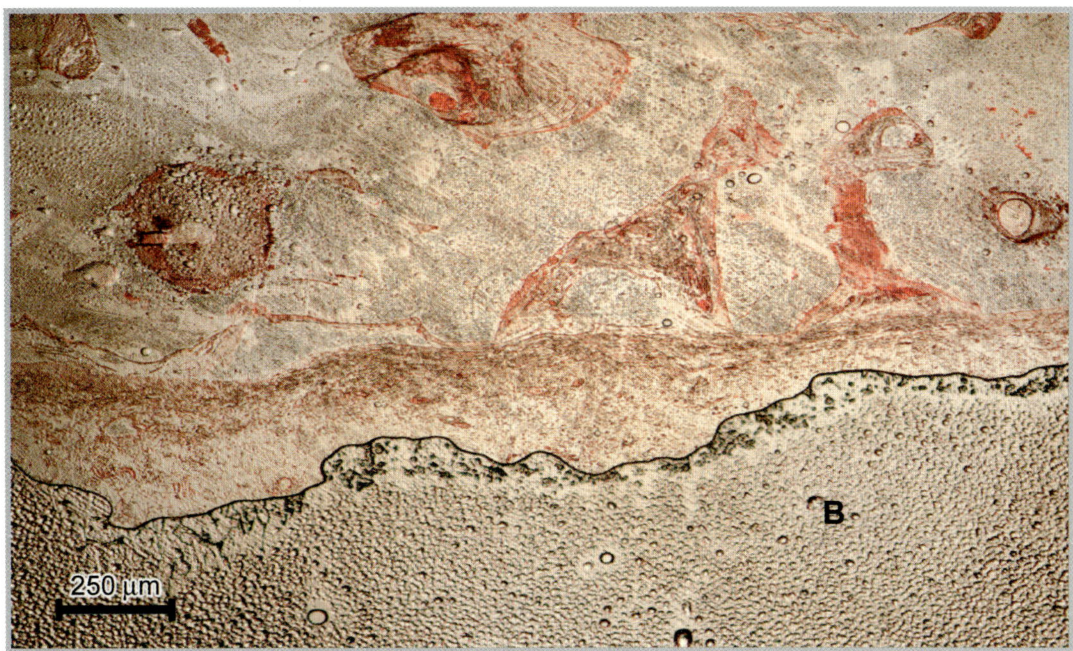

Figure 5 Section not properly rehydrated during staining (brownish color) and multiple air bubbles (B) due to improper coverslipping. H & E x 4

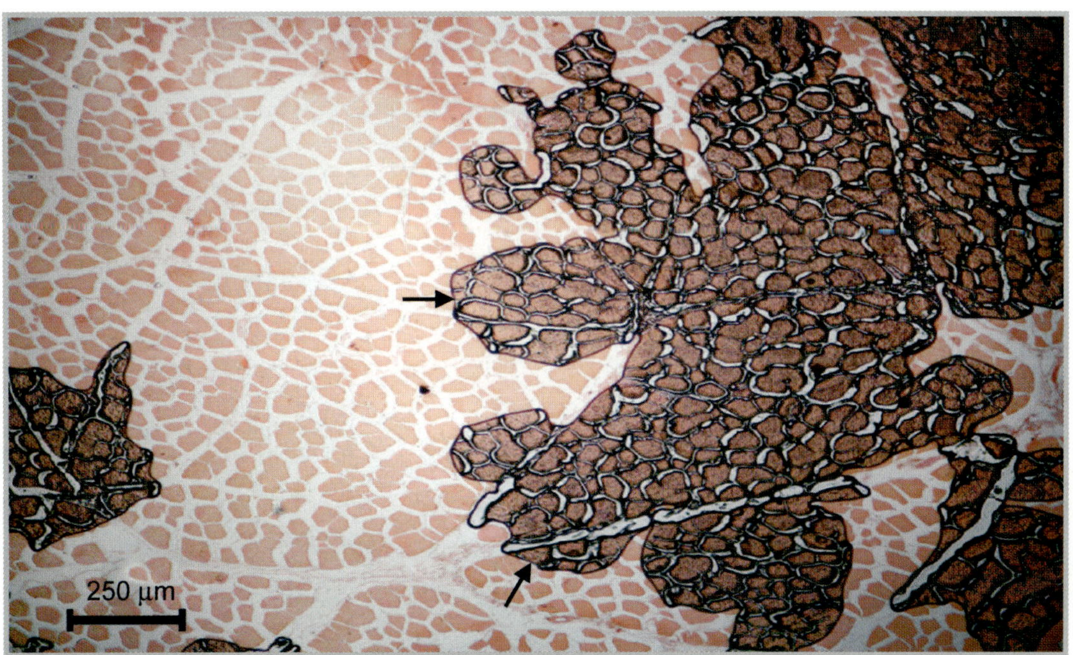

Figure 6 Mountant between coverslip and section has dried (↑).
H & E x 4

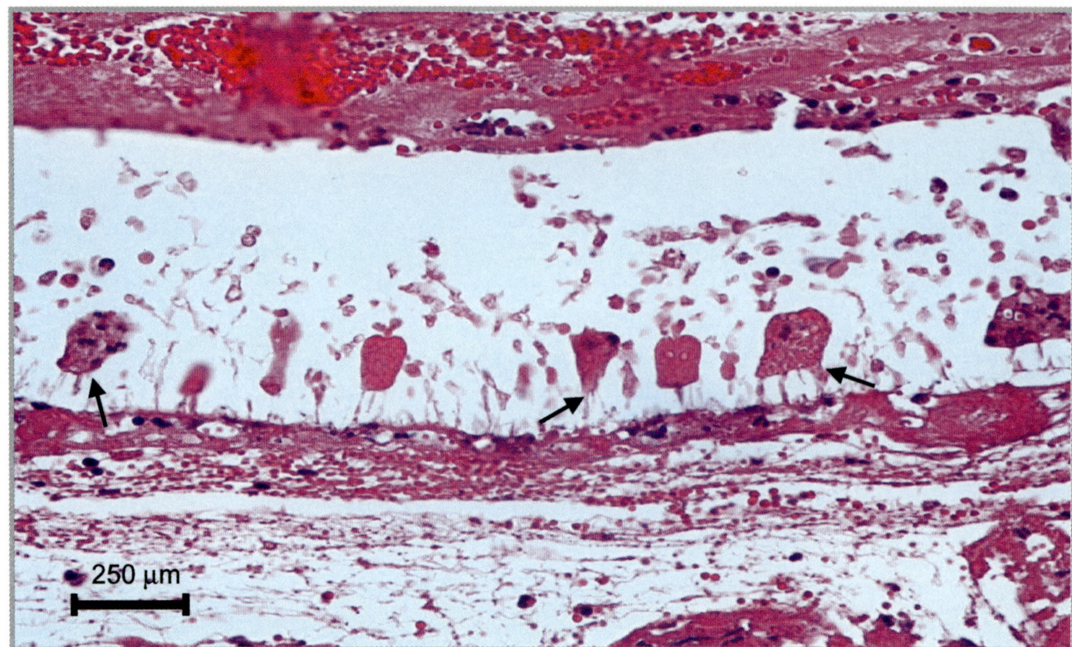

Figure 7 Melting of polymer (↑) due to high temperature during processing. The characteristics of the polymer implant with respect to alcohol, xylene and temperature to be ascertained before processing to prevent loss of implant. H & E x 4

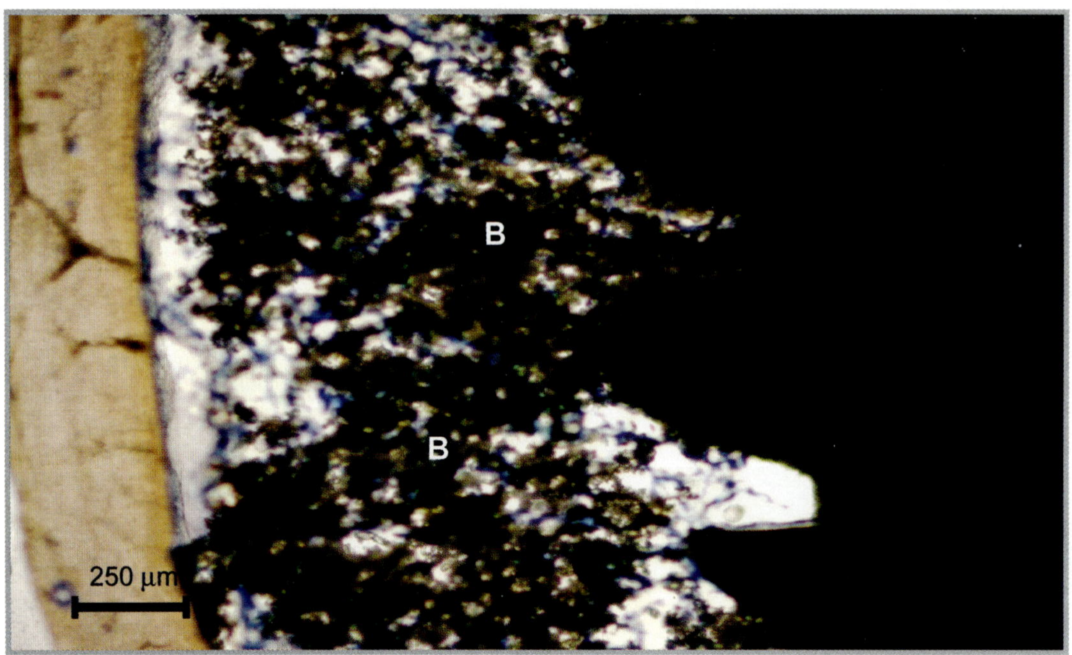

Figure 8 Air bubbles (B) introduced during embedding of tissue in resin. H & E x 4

BIBLIOGRAPHY

1. Williams DF (Ed). Techniques of biocompatibility testing. Volume 1 (CRC Series in Biocompatibility. Edited by Williams, David F). CRC Press lnc, 1986.
2. Williams DF (Ed). Techniques of biocompatibility testing. Volume 2 (CRC Series in Biocompatibility. Edited by Williams, David F). CRC Press lnc., 1986.
3. Yuehuei H An, Kylie L Martin (Eds). Handbook of histology methods for bone and cartilage. Humana Press, 2003.
4. Bancroft JD, Gamble M (Eds). Theory and practice of histological techniques. Churchill Livingstone, 2002.

INDEX